Developing Professi
Health and Sc

G000161136

Addressing the changing world of professionalism, this text combines theory, research and practice, using real case studies, to investigate the process of becoming professional. Mapping the journey from allied or associate practitioner positions through qualifying and into advanced practitioner status, it is a valuable companion for health and social care, social work and allied health students from the beginning of their studies.

Developing Professional Practice in Health and Social Care is an accessible text, including case studies, reflective exercises and activities, chapter aims and summaries and further reading boxes throughout. It covers:

- the context for professional practice, including historical perspectives, policy and discussion of relevant competencies and frameworks
- the concept of professionalism, exploring what it means to be a professional
- values and ethics underpinning professional practice
- professional identity development, including formation and changes in identity
- professional practice in complex environments, paying particular attention to working in organisations
- becoming a critical and globally aware practitioner
- the role of evidence and knowledge in professional practice
- working with supervision.

Maintaining a strong focus on the ethical dimensions of professional practice, this text emphasises how health and social care practitioners can contribute to social justice and challenge social exclusion.

Adam Barnard is Senior Lecturer in Health and Social Care in the Department of Social Work and Health at Nottingham Trent University. He has worked in higher education for over twenty years and runs the Professional Doctorate in Social Practice. He has taught across a range of undergraduate and postgraduate programmes and courses and teaches on the BA (H) Health and Social Care degree. His research interests are varied and include research into visual methodologies; enabling environments; the self in professional practice; pedagogies of reflection; and critical theory about professional practice. His publications include *The Value Base of Social Work and Social Care* (with Horner and Wild, 2008), which has been internationally translated, and the edited volume *Key Themes in Health and Social Care* (2012). He has conducted contract and evaluative research with local authority partners.

Developing Professional Practice in Health and Social Care

Edited by Adam Barnard

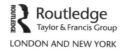

Routledge
Taylor & Francis Group

LONDON AND NEW YORK

First published 2017
by Routledge
2 Park Square, Milton Park, Abingdon, Oxon OX14 4RN

and by Routledge
711 Third Avenue, New York, NY 10017

Routledge is an imprint of the Taylor & Francis Group, an informa business

British Library Cataloguing in Publication Data
A catalogue record for this book is available from the British Library

Library of Congress Cataloging in Publication Data
Names: Barnard, Adam, editor.
Title: Developing professional practice in health and social care / edited by Adam Barnard.
Description: Abingdon, Oxon; New York, NY: Routledge, 2017. | Includes bibliographical references and index.
Identifiers: LCCN 2016030845| ISBN 9781138806719 (hardback) | ISBN 9781138806726 (pbk) | ISBN 9781315751535 (ebook)
Subjects: LCSH: Allied health personnel. | Social workers. | Medical care. | Social service--Practice.
Classification: LCC R697.A4 D485 2017 | DDC 610.73/7069--dc23
LC record available at https://lccn.loc.gov/2016030845

ISBN: 978-1-138-80671-9 (hbk)
ISBN: 978-1-138-80672-6 (pbk)
ISBN: 978-1-315-75153-5 (ebk)

Typeset in Joanna
by Saxon Graphics Ltd, Derby

Printed and bound by CPI Group (UK) Ltd, Croydon, CR0 4YY

Dedication

Thanks to all the creative and reflective practitioners, staff and students that I've had the privilege to work with on my journey in health and social care. It's been an adventure.

To my dead Dad and living Mum. I summon the weight of ancestors to let the fairies be free.

Many thanks to the supportive team at Routledge and the professionalism of Rachel Norridge for making this book possible.

Finally, thanks to my long-suffering partner for being herself at all times; the two troublesome monkeys Ngaio and Edie; and a big shout out to anyone else who knows me.

Contents

List of figures

List of tables

Notes on contributors

Adam Barnard is a Senior Lecturer in Health and Social Care in the Department of Social Work and Health at Nottingham Trent University. He has worked in higher education for over twenty years and runs the Professional Doctorate in Social Practice. He has taught across a range of undergraduate and postgraduate programmes and courses and teaches on the BA (H) Health and Social Care degree. Dr Barnard's research interests are varied and include research into visual methodologies; enabling environments; the self in professional practice; pedagogies of reflection; and critical theory about professional practice. His publications include *The Value Base of Social Work and Social Care* (with Horner and Wild, 2008), which has been internationally translated; and the edited volume *Key Themes in Health and Social Care* (2012). He has conducted contract and evaluative research with local authority partners.

Jane Challinor is Principal Lecturer and Subject Lead in Health and Social Care at Nottingham Trent University. She has worked in higher education since 2006, teaching both undergraduates and postgraduates, and is a Senior Fellow of the Higher Education Academy. Formerly a senior NHS manager and management consultant, Jane has also been Programme Leader of a BAC Accredited Diploma in Person Centred Counselling and has over ten years' experience working as a UKCP-registered counsellor and clinical supervisor in primary care.

Kevin Flint was the Joint Programme Leader for the Professional Doctorate programme incorporating the Doctor of Education, Doctor of Legal Practice and Doctor of Social Practice awards at Nottingham Trent University. He taught methodology and philosophy on the Professional Research Practice Course that is organised for PhD students from a number of schools within the university. He was also Cluster Leader for the group of researchers working with issues of social change, justice and equality.

Ricky Gee is Senior Lecturer based in the Division of Sociology at Nottingham Trent University. He currently teaches on a range of programmes at undergraduate and postgraduate level. These include the BA Sociology, Sociology and Politics, Psychology and Sociology, Youth Students and the Postgraduate Diploma in Careers Guidance. Richard is also Chair of the School of Social Sciences Student Forum. This position enables the student voice to engage with the School's Learning and Teaching Committee so as to influence policy decisions made to enhance the student experience at NTU. He has been sponsored by Nottingham Trent University to undertake a professional doctorate to explore pedagogic practice to enhance the teaching and exploration of 'career' from multiple perspectives.

Catherine Goodall is a KTP Associate – a Design and Implementation Analyst, on a 30-month Knowledge Transfer Partnership project between Nottingham Trent University and Nottinghamshire County Council. She is the lead on the project, which will employ a range of methods to research and assess the current provisions within the Children, Families and Cultural Services Department, to improve and transform service delivery. As the KTP Associate, Catherine is responsible for both completing the project and project management. Functioning as an intermediary between the organisations, the role involves ensuring that the goals of the project are achieved, and that knowledge is continually transferred between herself and both organisations.

Nick Hartop has worked in the higher education sector as a Senior Lecturer for eight years, leading courses and modules in the fields of Offender Management, Youth Justice, Drug and Alcohol Work and Criminology. He has previously spent over a decade working in youth justice practice as a Drug and Alcohol Specialist and Senior Practitioner leading on 'Priority and Prolific' offender management strategies. Nick has research interests around multi-agency working, inter-professional education, drug and alcohol work and social practice.

Simon Howard teaches on a wide range of qualifying and continuous professional development (CPD) post-qualifying social work courses at Nottingham Trent University. Simon is a child (and adult) care social worker by background and was a postgraduate CPD child care candidate in 2000, gaining a full post-qualifying award. He is a Health Care Professions Council (HCPC)-registered social worker and Fellow of the Higher Education Academy (HEA). Simon's current professional interests are: leadership and management within social work practice; competence and practice – direct work; emotional abuse, neglect and domestic violence; and emotional intelligence and social work.

Linda Kemp works as a Research Assistant at Nottingham Trent University and is a PhD candidate at the University of Sheffield. Publications include *Immunological* (2014) and *Blueprint* (2015) and an album, *speaking towards* (2015, enjoy your homes press).

Vicky Palmer currently teaches on youth justice on the BA (Hons) Youth Studies and MA Advanced Social Work Practice at Nottingham Trent. In addition, she will shortly be taking over the role of Course Leader for the BA (Hons) Youth Justice course. Vicky has successfully completed the Professional Doctorate in Social Practice. She is presently in the process of editing parts of her professional doctorate theses for journal publication. Her research interests are children in conflict with the law, mental disorder, autism and learning difficulties and their connection to youth offending, the proliferation of managerialism in youth justice practice and the re-introduction of diversion techniques for young offenders.

Hannah Sawtell is a freelance illustrator who lives in Nottingham with her husband, two children, some fish and a cat called Pippa.

Chris Towers' main teaching specialism is social policy and he is the Module Leader on a Year One course at Nottingham Trent University. He has a background of research and expertise in this subject, having taught social policy for a number of years both at Nottingham Trent University and elsewhere. His PhD related both to social policy and elderly care, which is a particular interest of his. In addition, Dr Towers teaches on a range of other subjects and makes a number of contributions to the BA (Hons) Health and Social Care degree. His work also involves administration, research and writing for journals – including areas such as pedagogical issues as well as social policy. Dr Towers also prepares teaching resources, in particular audio-visual materials, and he has involved students in their preparation.

Siân Trafford works one-to-one with students in the School of Social Sciences at Nottingham Trent University. Siân provides discipline-specific sessions on academic writing for a range of courses within the School of Social Sciences to improve composition skills.

Mick Wilkinson is a former Senior Lecturer in Social Work at Nottingham Trent University.

Andy Wolfe has worked in the FE and HE sectors. He has been appointed Dean of the new Diocesan Younger Leadership College for the Church of England across Nottinghamshire. He was formerly Vice Principal at Nottingham Emmanuel School, a 1000-pupil Church of England secondary school in central Nottingham.

Preface

Writing a book is like an elephant's pregnancy, a long gestation with the delivery of a thing of beauty. Orwell advises in *Gangrel* (1946), 'writing a book is a horrible, exhausting struggle, like a long bout with some painful illness. One would never undertake such a thing if one were not driven on by some demon whom one can neither resist nor understand'. He goes on to say there are different degrees to writing: sheer egoism, aesthetic enthusiasm, historical impulse and political purpose. This work is a blend of each degree. It is for reflective readers to make up their own minds.

Acknowledgements

Table 1.1 is provided by Stan Lester and is available at: http://devmts.org.uk/profnal.pdf

Figure 1.1 is from Finlay, L. (2008) Reflecting on 'Reflective Practice', Practice-Based Professional Learning Centre, Open University Press, available at www.open.ac.uk/pbpl

The figures in Chapter 2 were commissioned from Hannah Sawtell. She has been identified by the *Guardian* as one of the 'creatives' to watch out for. She can be contacted at: www.hannahsawtell.co.uk

A version of Andy Wolfe's chapter (Chapter 13) has appeared in Wolfe, A. (2016) *Journeys of Faith: Personal Stories and Faith Development in Church Schools*. Cambridge: Grove Education, although the copyright rests with the author.

Introduction

Health and social care is a growing and necessary area. When one needs health and social care services there is nothing more important or nothing more needed in one's life. We can all expect health and social care to gain importance in our lives as the time we live in becomes less certain and more complex. There is a need for a critical and essential friend and this is the book that provides the critical capacity to develop and reflect upon practice in health and social care. This book is an indispensable guide and essential resource for professionals working with people. The guiding principle that runs throughout the book is the focus on professions' contributions to social justice and challenging social exclusion.

This book makes a significant contribution to professional practice in the social professions. It will allow and facilitate philosophical and conceptual reflection on the issues facing professional practitioners, so the book can act as a pedagogically informed training resource and contribute to changing, improving and creating excellent practice.

This text is designed to be a critical resource for those in health and social care. It will be a companion for those who have qualified, or are about to qualify, as health and social care professionals. It is for developing professional practice both personally and professionally.

Making use of tried, tested and accessible course materials in health and social care, staff expertise has created this volume to contribute to the challenges faced by professionals in changing and uncertain times and environments. As times become more uncertain, the integrity of professionals working in social and supportive professions becomes more vital. The promotion of a values-based perspective through promoting social justice as a core principle for health and social care professionals is a key objective of the book.

The development of professional practice concerns an increasing awareness and ability to address issues of social justice, challenging structural inequalities across all social divisions, and the realisation of human and citizenship rights. There are key issues that the health and social care practitioner faces and needs to develop the professional practice to effectively deal with in promoting social justice, talking about inequalities and realising rights.

Social justice operates as a regulatory heuristic for professions, professionalisation and professionality. The values-based perspective on practice and the contribution that can be made by professionals to promoting social justice is the focus for each chapter and is returned to at the end of each chapter. The philosophical focus, pedagogical features and contribution to professional practice make this a distinct text for professional practitioners.

To make this the trusted companion for developing professional practice, each chapter has clear aims and outcomes to provide a coherent and cohesive approach to each substantive discussion. Reflective exercises consolidate learning and understanding, making this an essential resource for professionals.

The book will cover a spectrum of 'becoming a professional' to address the changing world of professionalism within helping professions: health and social care and social work. Although an ambitious remit, this makes the contribution of the book unique. This book combines theory, research and practice, using real case studies to investigate the form, function and nature of becoming professional; that is (a) the process of becoming professional and (b) the person becoming a professional.

The value of the book is in the contemporary mapping of the field of professionalism which provides a companion to learning how to become professional with specific skills development embedded in the discussion. The book will address the lack of literature on associate professionals (a growing area of the health and social care service market) and higher end or 'advanced' practitioners. Its focus is on the neglected area of the experience or journey of becoming a professional, starting from pre-qualification entry right through to advanced practitioner.

The pedagogical features make this a clear, accessible and engaging book to meet the needs of a range of professionals. The principal focus is for qualifying professional programmes in social work and health and social care. The skills development component is another key feature, with reflective exercises and learning needs assessment activities to contribute to the ongoing development of professionals.

The further contribution this text makes is in the focus on themes within health and social care as understood in its broadest sense. Each chapter will have a summary of the contribution the chapter makes to social work, health and social care, and the promotion of social justice.

Structure and themes of the book

1. The current context and climate of professionals (Adam Barnard)

This chapter sets the scene for professionals and defines the core themes that will be discussed in the other chapters. The question 'What does being a professional encompass and what does it exclude?' will be the core focus to provide the contours, parameters, shape, form, function and purpose to professions. The different views of professions, historically and from different disciplines, draw on seminal and contemporary literature to define professionals, professionalism and professionality. Becoming a professional is a necessary discussion for all those involved in health and social care, particularly in uncertain times. The competency and capability frameworks for becoming a professional are also discussed. The contested nature of professionalism, the contextual tensions between instrumental approaches and an ethos of professionality are also discussed within the context of the possibilities, demands and increase in interprofessional working.

2. Philosophy for professionals (Adam Barnard and Hannah Sawtell)

This chapter examines philosophical traditions of thought and the contribution they make to contemporary professional practice. The traditions of critical theory, phenomenology, pragmatism, postmodernism and feminism will be considered to provide an orientation to professional practice. The provision of philosophy for professionals is a neglected source of rich learning and the philosophical orientation is a necessary element to high-quality professional practice. Opening the door to allow the crossing of the threshold for professionals is facilitated by an engagement and exploration of philosophical systems, thoughts, thinkers and ideas. The potential a philosophical engagement holds is high and strong, but this an area for development that will be pursued in forthcoming editions.

3. Values and ethics for professionals (Adam Barnard)

The ethics of professionalism is a terrain of contradictions and tensions. This discussion will provide a navigational chart through value-based perspectives and the ethics of professionalism. Taking a historical approach, shifts in values and ethics are mapped to arrive at a horizon of possibilities for ethical practice. Illustrative examples facilitate engagement with ethical debates around practice and deeper exploration of the ethics of professionalism.

4. Professional identity (Nick Hartop, Adam Barnard and Mick Wilkinson)

This chapter reviews the contributions of understandings of identity and the way in which personal and professional identities contribute to professional practice. The concept of professional identity in social work education is a relatively neglected topic. The difficulty in formation, maintenance and review of a stable identity in problematic circumstances is enhanced by reflective exercises.

5. Working in organisational systems (Simon Howard)

Taking an ecological approach, this chapter explores the contingent and contextual nature of professions working in organisations. It explores the 'shadow side' of organisations, and points up the difficulties of new public management challenges and managerialist approaches to practice. The chapter discusses reflective pluralism as an alternative to 'brittle' managerial approaches and identifies effective supervision in the importance of reflective practice. Learning organisations are identified as the basis for a reflective organisation that is protective of wellbeing for the organisation and workforce and promotes a social learning culture, 'communities of practice', a cultural ecology and appreciative inquiry. It presents case studies to illustrate the challenges to the promotion of social justice in fluid and changing circumstances. It critiques leadership and management in complex organisations.

6. Critical practice (Linda Kemp)

Linda takes a critical lens to some commonplace areas of health care, touching on practices relating to mental health care and examining the mediation of language. This activity unfolds in the context of neo-liberalism and the way that individual problems mask societal issues. The advocacy of mental health service user groups calls for the need for an UnRecovery star. The act of measurement and performance targets mitigates against the challenges raised by people experiencing mental health difficulties. This is often taken further evidence of their non-compliance rather than the societal problems giving rise to mental health difficulties and against holistic wellbeing. The horizon of possibilities presented by opening 'closed discourses' is a step forward in health and social care and mental health. The contextual understanding of dissociation and its social-ness is necessary for a dynamic notion of becoming 'healthy' rather than an intrumentalised measurement of recovery.

7. Globalised practice (Adam Barnard)
This chapter examines the challenges presented to professionals in a globalised world. The neo-liberal orthodoxy of McProfessionals is deconstructed to provide a more ethical, critical and holistic professional motivated by promoting social justice.

8. Reflections on conditionality (Chris Towers)
This chapter examines the issues surrounding conditionality and how far or in what way conditionality can deliver modification in behaviour and action of people in receipt of welfare. It also addresses the tensions experienced by practitioners and emerging practitioners wrestling with the purpose of welfare and health and social care service delivery. The pedagogical provision of role play is a key technique in facilitating emerging professionals' reflective understanding.

9. Professional supervision (Jane Challinor)
Exploring purposes and different models of supervision, this chapter reviews the essentials of what supervision can offer and how to manage the supervisory process, both as a supervisor and a supervisee.

10. Reflective writing for professional practice (Siân Trafford)
This chapter addresses the core and necessary skills for professionals to be able to communicate clearly in a written form and to keep accurate and up-to-date records of their professional work.

11. Contemplating 'career' across disciplines (Ricky Gee)
This chapter addresses the challenges and opportunities for professionals as they develop through and across their careers. It conceptualises the skills necessary to develop the 'troublesome' concept of career.

12. Personal development planning as reflection (Catherine Goodall)
This reflection on personal development planning provides a form of structured reflection for the early career stages of a developing professional. Using skills-based competencies the reflective journey is part of an emerging professionalism.

13. Journeys of faith (Andy Wolfe)
This narrative and story-based focus provides personal stories from faith schools as an interesting examination of 'becoming' stories of self. The 'journeying' of personal and professional practice is part of this spiritual encounter.

14. A personal learning journey (Vicky Palmer)

This chapter is a personal narrative account of the 'journey' of an early career professional as they develop the knowledge, understandings, skills and attributes of what it means to be a professional.

15. 'Tain from the mirror (Kevin Flint, Vicky Palmer and Adam Barnard)

Deconstructing reflective practice and engaging with Bronfenbrenner, this chapter discusses the absence of human beings and the need for a concept of human beings to unify the knowledge, thinking, skills and competencies of this book.

16. Conclusion (Adam Barnard)

This chapter concludes the professional journey and provides a manifesto for professional development. The call to advanced and expert professionalism is considered as part of continuing professional development.

Core themes that will be discussed

The professional and becoming professional journey is:

Allied or associate, unqualified professional	End of qualifying programme	Entry into profession	Senior professional	Advanced practitioner
Becoming professional	Becoming a professionally qualified professional			

For each of the stages the following are to be considered by 'becoming professionals': knowledge and intellectual abilities; personal qualities, skills and attributes; governance and organisation; engagement, influence and impact.

This book makes a contribution to the professional journeying that people in helping professions undertake. The book has made reference to the Benchmarking Statements, Professional Capabilities Framework, Professional Regulatory Bodies' Codes of Practice including guidance from professional bodies such as Social Work Action Network (SWAN), British Association of Social Workers (BASW), International Federation of Social Workers (IFSW), Health and Care Professionals Council.

The key features of the book are a range of pedagogical features to enhance readers' understanding of the key features of professions; historical and philosophical theory to add to the thought that informs professionalism; reflective exercises and learning needs assessment activities. The clear, open and accessible style of writing with engaging activities encourages engagement with clear signposting throughout the book on opening chapters and in chapter summaries.

The book is written with key heuristic principles. The first is a 'surface skim' of ideas, theory and concepts before a 'deep dive' into the material. The style, register and voice of the contributors vary to provide a holistic way of reflecting from various vantage points.

As the book progresses and key knowledge, understanding and skills are developed, voices from the field are invited to add to the discussion and debate. Emerging as a professional, professional career 'journeys' and effective writing for professionals are considered.

The book as a whole is a critical friend and companion that will accompany you on your journey in developing as a professional. The first phase of the book is characterised by thinking about themes in professional practice; the second part of the book is a reflection on skills. Each contributes to the theory and practice nexus of the linkages between thinking and doing. Each chapter has a high value and use for the 'emerging' and 'becoming' professional, and are important contributions to the professional journey.

Chapter 1
The current context and climate of professionals

Definitions and history

Adam Barnard

Chapter outline

This chapter will introduce:

- the current context
- definitions of key terms
- understanding professions
- being and becoming
- practice
- reflection
- social justice.

This chapter will set the scene for professionals. Mapping and defining what being a professional encompasses and what it excludes will provide the contours, parameters, shape, form, function and purpose to professions. The different views of professions historically and from different disciplines will define professionals.

Becoming a professional is a timely and necessary discussion for all those involved in health, social care and social professions, particularly in uncertain times and in an age of austerity with savage public sector cuts to services. The competency and capability frameworks for becoming a professional will also be discussed. The contested nature of professionalism and the contextual tensions between rational instrumental approaches and an ethos of professionality will be considered, along with the possibilities, demands and increase in interprofessional working.

Context

The contextual discussion of professional practice is always set in a complex context of profound structural changes taking place in the ecological, political, economic, technological and social context of government and public services. Practice, and the ethics and values that underpin it, depends heavily on the ideologies of governments, social and economic situations and public opinion (Seden et al. 2011). Media criticism of perceived failures, the impact of globalisation reconfiguring communities, and the rise of managerialism under neo-liberalism's austerity are the contemporary challenges for those engaged with or entering into professions of any sort. Professions in the public, independent and voluntary sectors face particular challenges as the landscape of public sector work is increasingly being reordered by neo-liberalism (Harvey 2005).

The force field of changes to professions increases complexity, uncertainty, undecidability and fluidity across professional practice such as decision making, managing, and planning. Public sector professionals have to manage escalating demand in a period of austerity (Prowle et al. 2014). It is within this landscape that professional experience is currently undergoing a range of contemporary challenges.

Definitions of professions, professionalism and professionalisation

At their simplest, professions are the collective agency and experience of a group of people performing or undertaking a specialised area of activity. Professionals are individual actors who are bearers of the purposeful action of the profession, and who are engaged in everyday practice actions.

The definition of professions needs to recognise the context of professional practice so there are a range of factors that have a determining influence on how we understand professions and 'professions' as a collective activity. For example, in the 1990s there was an increased drive to develop professional activities and practice across a range of social activity such as policing and soldiering. The development of Third Way politics, New Labour's modernisation agenda and new public management provided further impetus for professions (Clarke and Newman 1997) and the age of austerity under the Coalition and later Conservative administrations has produced a range of forces to reconfigure professionalism in a contemporary age. The post-war settlement of the state playing a major role in promoting a more equal society and promoting social justice via state provision and public expenditure is now under threat.

Professions themselves, as an identified group activity, have responded to current changes with increased forms of performance management, reordering of organisational imperatives and increasingly complex demands on the workforce and individuals committed to delivering professional services. For example, actuarial approaches to systems management, increased accountability, globalisation, consumerism, individuation, rights, scrutiny, reviews of performance and managerial demands have provided a contemporary context for professionals with committed values to professionalism. These 'old' and 'new' ways of working in social professions (Seden et al. 2011) are the invitation for those joining professions at the current time. An investigation into the history of professions and reflective practice provides the contours for this book.

Professions

Oakley (1986) suggests that a profession is a 'superior type of occupation' which requires greater formal entry requirements and training. A profession may be characterised as an occupational group which regulates and controls itself and requires advanced education to acquire a specific and exclusively owned body of knowledge and expertise.

Professionalisation is closely linked to professional identity, which is discussed in subsequent chapters. It has also led to the blurring of boundaries between professions. For example, many of health and social care's functions have been appropriated by reconfigured disciplinary areas such as health, psychiatry and psychology (Atwal and Jones 2009).

As society undergoes profound economic, social, political, economic and environmental change, professionals have experienced deep change and the rise of the expert (Brint 1994). Professional identities are framed around efficiency and commerce (Anderson-Gough et al. 1999; Goodrick and Reay 2010) and have replaced the traditional logic and ethos of ethics and public service (Brint 1994). Professions are now multidisciplinary and transnational (Muzio et al. 2013).

Economic rationalism has had a significant impact on many professions in Western society. Much of the neo-liberal agenda has been concerned with targeting professions' capacity to capture domains of service and their funding has fuelled deprofessionalisation (Braverman 1974) or a market rationality (Brown 2006) based on an autonomous and calculating subject, which situates competitive individualism as the central requisite attribute for a citizenry of constantly reinventing entrepreneurs and a new morality of self-development (Lynch 2006).

So how can we understand this shift in professions?

Sociology of the professions

Reports on 'the death of professions as a relevant discipline' (Gorman and Sandefur 2011) and the dominance of conflict-based paradigms (Friedson 1970, 1986, 1994, 2001; Johnson 1972; Larson 1977) have been extremely successful in addressing the limitations of earlier trait-based perspectives and the focus on dominance and monopoly, but have obscured the role that professionals have in constructing, organising and ordering social life (Burrage and Torstendahl 1990; Halliday 1987; Halliday and Karpik 1997; Johnson 1993).

Professions are grounded in Scott's (2008) seminal characterisation of professions as 'Lords of the Dance' who choreograph the broad transformations reconfiguring contemporary political economic systems. As Scott (2008: 219) observes, 'the professions in modern society have assumed leading roles in the creation and tending of institutions. They are the preeminent institutional agents of our time'.

Professions are agentive in that they have the capacity for change, and to drive change they still need to be understood against a backdrop of dominant tendencies and a context of broad change (Abel 1988; Brint 1994; Broadbent et al. 1997; Brock et al. 1999; Cooper and Robson 2006; Hanlon 1999; Krause 1996; Leicht and Fennell 2001; Reed 1996).

Scott's (2008) pillar framework views professions as regulative, normative and cultural-cognitive:

- the regulative pillar stresses rule-setting, monitoring and sanctioning activities, both formal and informal;
- the normative pillar introduces a prescriptive, evaluative and obligatory dimension into social life, stressing 'appropriate' behaviour – given the demands of the situation and the actor's role within it – versus 'instrumental' behaviour, in which attention is focused on the actor's preference and pursuit of self-interest; and
- the cultural-cognitive pillar emphasizes the centrality of symbolic systems: the use of common schemas, frames and other shared symbolic representations that guide behaviour (Scott 2008: 222).

Although professionals might be 'Lords of the Dance' this is not a clear-cut or uncontested terrain. Professions, professionals, professionalisation and deprofessionalisation all have a rich and long history, but we have an emerging definition.

Definitions

Profession/professional: 1) used as a folk concept to signify (a) prestige, respect; (b) full-time work for pay; (c) to perform some task with great skill or proficiency; 2) used as a sociological concept of study: (a) elite classes of occupations with a focus on the characteristics or attributes of such occupations as a taxonomy (the attribute model of professions); (b) a process model, to study the processes through which certain occupations come to acquire power, develop monopolies, and/or lay claim to the status of professional (Leicht and Fennel 2001: 8).

Professional projects: based on the work of Friedson (1986) and Abbot (1988), professional projects are attempts to: 1) enhance the autonomy and freedom of action for occupational incumbents under a set of well-defined professional norms; and 2) defend a specific task domain from encroachment by competing occupational groups or stakeholders (Leicht and Fennel 2001: 8).

Professionalisation: the result of a successful professional project: an occupation is professionalised to the extent that it successfully defines a set of work tasks as its exclusive domain, and successfully defends that domain against competing claims (Leicht and Fennel 2001: 8).

Deprofessionalisation: the process by which professional prerogatives become eroded (Braverman 1974).

Autonomy: the ability of a work group or individual to control their own work behaviour and work conditions.

What does being a professional encompass?

Historically professions have four formative moments. Lester (2007) suggests these are the ancient professions of priesthood, university teaching, law and physicianship; medieval trade occupations of surgery, dentistry and architecture; industrial-era occupations such as engineer; and various groups that have emerged in the twentieth century such as police, social workers, teachers, accountants and personnel managers.

The uneven process of emergent, dominant and residual professions has provided professionalism with different intensity and reach at different times. For example, social work is undergoing an assertive push for professionalism with its protected title, establishment of a learned society such as the (now defunct) College of Social Work, and regulatory bodies such as the Health and Care Professional Council.

There are a range of common-sense, taken-for-granted understandings of what a professional is and an attribute approach that 'begins from the basis assumption that it is possible to draw up a list of fixed criteria for recognizing a profession on which there will be general consensus' (Dingwall 2008: 11). For example, Biestek (1957) attempted this list-type approach for social work:

> Processional activity was basically intellectual, carrying with it great personal responsibility, it was learned, being based on great knowledge and not merely routine; it was practical, rather than academic or theoretic, its technique could be taught, this being the basis of professional education; it was strongly organized internally; and it was motivated by altruism, the professional viewing themselves as working for some aspect of the good of society.
>
> (Becker 1970: 88)

The promotion of a good society and the issue of social justice are the guiding principles of professional practice.

There are alternatives to this approach. Friedson (1970) argues one can distinguish between adopting an ideology of professionalism and the associated characteristics or attribute approach, and the location of a profession within a given social structure or the socio-economic location of professions. Professions here are subject to the process of professionalisation or a collective mobility project similar to professional projects.

Larson (1977: xvi) suggests:

> I see professionalization as the process by which producers of special services sought to constitute and control a market for their expertise. Because marketable expertise is a crucial element in the structure of modern inequality, professionalization appears also as a collective assertion of special social status and as a collective process of upward social mobility.

This collective attempt to control markets for professionalism is extended by Illich (1982) who suggests that the notion of professions is a concept that is used to achieve the successful mystifications of a class interest. This results in professions working to maintain their position in the occupational hierarchy rather than for the benefits of service users or clients.

The interests of professionals, their market position and the mystifications have provided a history to professions for individuals, the context in which they work, the process and the activity of professionals.

Referring to professional regulators, a broad range of behaviours, often distinct from technical ability, are generally termed 'professionalism', although this is not well defined conceptually or methodologically: 'Participants' interpretation of "professionalism" encompass many and varied aspects of behaviour, communication and appearance (including, but not limited to, uniform), as well as being perceived as a holistic concept encompassing all aspects of practice' (HCPC 2014: 3). Professionalism has its basis in individual characteristics and values, but is also largely defined by context. Profiling of professionalism by regulatory bodies suggests a range of baseline behaviour that varies with a number of factors such as organisational support, the workplace, the expectations of others and the specifics of each service user's encounter (HCPC 2014: 3). The key to professional behaviour is an interrelationship between person, context and situational judgement.

The HCPC (2014) suggests that rather than a set of discrete skills, professionalism is better regarded as a 'meta-skill' comprising situational awareness and contextual judgement. 'The true skill of professionalism may be not so much in knowing what to do, but when to do it' (HCPC 2014: 3), that is a dynamic judgement rather than a discrete skill set. The HCPC (2014) examined the interpretation of the term 'professionalism', sources of understanding of professionalism, indicators of being professional or unprofessional, and the point at which people are perceived to become 'a professional', to suggest professionalism is a meta-skill.

Linking professionalism to a 'meta-skill' rather than a set of skills is one of the private troubles and public issues of professionalism. Mills' (1959) The Sociological Imagination refers to the ability to connect individual experiences to societal relationships or to use history, biography and social structure to translate private troubles into public issues. This work is also the process of taking public issues and translating them into an understanding of private troubles. In this way, the private troubles of professionalism and the public issues of professionalism are in a dynamic and fluid relationship.

What are the contours, parameters, shape, form, function and purpose of professions?

Macdonald (2001) calls for a 'professional project' that crystallises or draws together a range of ideas from an array of sources. The Weberian occupational groups draw together classes, status groups and political parties that compete for economic, social and political rewards. Educational qualifications provide an opportunity for increased income. The notion of project carries with it an existential meaning and moral value with a purpose. Macdonald argues for the professional project having four sub-domains or sub-goals of: jurisdiction (Abbot 1988) to establish the cultural work and to establish the legitimacy of practice; producing the producers (Larson 1977) for training and socialisation; monopolisation of professional knowledge; and respectability. The professional project interacts with other actors and audiences and is embedded in a social, political, cultural and economic context (Macdonald 2001: 189).

This embedded nature of projects, with distinct agentic commitment from professionals and goal-orientated activity secured to a set of values, is the pantheon of professionalism. The practice of professionalism has many mediations that detract from this laudable project.

An example drawn from social work is illustrative.

In considering the use of language in relation to the history of social work and demonstrating the correlation between the language of political ideology and the social work profession, Gregory and Holloway (2005) specifically focus upon socio-political and socio-economic contexts. They assert that social work has had three broad phases of development, identified as 'moral enterprise, therapeutic enterprise and managerial enterprise' and the resultant shift in language and the dominant discourse of 'punishment, risk management, consumerism and the market economy' (Gregory and Holloway 2005: 35) – for example, humanistic social work with the 'narratives of disabled activists, black people and women, influencing the current dominant social work discourse of anti-oppressive and anti-discriminatory practice' (Gregory and Holloway 2005: 39). A similar shift in the value base of professionalism can be charted, such as Barnard (2008).

The logic of professions addresses the historicising narrativisation (Larson 1977) and Abbott's (1988) analysis of how occupations gain, maintain, adjust and potentially lose their exclusive jurisprudence over particular tasks.

The 'story' or narrativising of how one becomes a professional is influenced by philosophical works on being and becoming.

Being and becoming

Being is a broad concept that involves the objective and subjective dimensions of reality and existence, and is intimately connected with philosophical reflection from a range of philosophical perspectives. For example, Sartre and existentialism focuses on being, as does Heidegger, and has an application in health and social care (Thompson and Pascal 2012; Koch 1995; Moran 2000; Moran and Mooney 2002; Grbich 2007; Speziale and Carpenter 2007).

Being and becoming, as one of the framing orientations of this discussion, requires an engagement with Heidegger and we now take a 'deep dive' into some philosophy. In *Being and Time* (1962) Heidegger addresses 'the question of being' which he believes philosophers have generally failed to do, focusing on beings as entities (these are 'ontical' questions about the properties of beings, not the ontological questions of their Being). Being, for Heidegger, is 'that which determines entities as entities, that on the basis of which entities are already understood' (Heidegger 1962) or 'there-being' or *Dasein* (or what Sartre calls this 'human reality'). *Dasein* is understood as 'being-in-the-world' as an engaged purposeful agent, not just spatially located, but immersed in a world of meaning. This world is not just a collection of things 'present-to-hand' but is a world of 'equipment' or 'gear' (*Zeug*) of things 'ready-to-hand' (*zuhanden*) that are involved in our purposeful projects. For the professional, much of the training and education is to become proficient in the use of 'ready-to-hand' things, techniques, equipment and gear of the professions. *Dasein* is 'in' a 'relational totality' of 'significance'. This relational totality is what gives things their significance by their relationship to our 'concerns' or 'care' (*Sorge*). For professionals, their relationship of care and concern is to situated 'things' or equipment, gear or the 'ready-to-hand', rather than the 'present-to-hand'. Much discussion about professionals has been caught in the present-to-hand rather than concern over the ready-to-hand.

This book addresses that concern and care to 'light up' or make purposefully 'stand out' the world of everyday engagement in professions. To regard the world as 'present-to-hand' is a result of various 'breakdowns' in our usual, engaged dealings with things (Dreyfus 1991; Cooper 1999). It is to these breakdowns that we now turn.

Scanlon (2011) suggests 'becoming' is the most useful defining concept for a new professional class who understand that their working lives are an open-ended, lifelong process of refinement and learning. The 'ongoingness' of professional development means individual professional identities are constructed throughout professional lives rather than as isolated, rugged, individualistic traditional professionals. This process of becoming is the ongoing journeying of professionalism which is multi-layered and demands engagement and change from the individual.

Becoming has the connotation of flattering dress, of being pretty, handsome, stylish and elegant. However, philosophically, becoming is constant flux and change. There is never an arrival and departure point to becoming a professional, rather a constant process of becoming. It is about a constant flow or movement and evolution, change in time and space and a movement towards. This can uncouple the professional from secure reference points, but it is in the fluidity of movement that change and becoming occurs. As such, this discussion is located in the movement of authors such as philosophers, symbolic interactionists, existentialists and humanists, and how these resources contribute to the understanding of the 'becoming' of a professional journey.

This journey will critically engage with the issues for reflective professionals, and encounter and give air to tensions along the way. For example, 'atrocity stories' are the sorts of account that are common in ethnographic literature on the work of professions (Stimson and Webb 1975). Atrocity stories are the devices whereby users of professional services retrospectively interpret their encounters with professions, negotiate the norms of behaviour, understand the rules of engagement and redress imbalances of power in professional relationships. These stories are dramatic narratives, drawing on shared understanding of the world, casting the teller or user of services as hero and right, against the incompetence and dereliction of others (Dingwall 2008). Through these stories social structures and power relations are rendered rational and comprehensible. The rise of narrative approaches has become significant in professions' narratives; meanings and safety have become watchwords in social work and health and social care practice. The narratives of these professions will be told as we move through the terrain of professionalism and develop reflective accounts of this process.

Professionalism in health and social care

Lester (2007) makes a useful distinction between Model A and Model B professions and professionality.

Table 1.1 Two paradigms of professions and professionality (Lester 2015): Stan Lester's Model A and Model B

	Model A	Model B
Character Capability	technical, logical; problem-solving solvable, convergent problems	creative, interpretive; design congruent futures; 'messes', problematic situations, divergent/'wicked' problems
Approach	solving problems; applying knowledge competently and rationally	understanding problematic situations and resolving conflicts of value; framing and creating desired outcomes
Criteria	logic, efficiency, planned outcomes; cause–effect, proof	values, ethics, congruence of both methods and outcomes; systemic interrelationships, theory, faith
Epistemology	objectivism: knowledge is stable and general; precedes and guides action (pure science, applied science, practice)	constructivism: knowledge is transient, situational and personal; both informs action and is generated by it (cyclic/spiral relationship between theory and practice)
Validation	by reference to others' expectations: standards, accepted wisdom, established discourse; 'truth'	by questioning fitness for purpose, fitness of purpose and systemic validity; 'value'
Thinking	primarily deductive/analytical; sceptical of intuition	inductive, deductive and abductive; uses 'intelligent intuition'
Profession	a bounded, externally-defined role, characterised by norms, values and a knowledge base common to the profession	a portfolio of learningful activity individual to the practitioner, integrated by personal identity, perspectives, values and capability
professionalism	objectivity, rules, codes of practice	exploration of own and others' values, personal ethics, mutual enquiry, shared expectations
professional standards	defined by the employer, professional body or other agency according to its norms and values	negotiated by the participants and other stakeholders in the practice situation in accordance with their values, beliefs and desired outcomes
professional development	initial development concerned with acquiring knowledge, developing competence and enculturation into the profession's value system; continuing development concerned with maintaining competence and updating knowledge	ongoing learning and practice through reflective practice, critical enquiry and creative synthesis and action; continual questioning and refinement of personal knowledge, understanding, practice, values and beliefs

Available at: http://devmts.org.uk/profnal.pdf

This transition from Model A to B characterises the challenge of modern professionalism as a constructive, ongoing negotiated conversation that has lost the security of previous incarnations of professions. Professionals are situated, contextual meaning seekers and creators that work with the demands of professional regulation and the increasing demands of people who use professional services. As professionals become and be, they enact and form professions.

There are also significant levels at which professionalism operates such as the macro, meso and micro scale. The demand for the professional is the constant flux of becoming and continual refinements and adjustments to professional practice within the context and situation of professional regulation and the wider field of neo-liberalism.

What should professional look like?

Phenomenological studies of human learning indicate that for adults there exists a qualitative leap in their learning process from the rule-governed use of analytical rationality in beginners or novices to the fluid performance of tacit skills (Flyvberg 2006: 222). Pierre Bourdieu (1977) called these skilled practitioners *virtuosos* while Dreyfus and Dreyfus (1986) call them *true human experts*.

Flyvberg (2006) suggests that by the procedural analytical rule, following exclusive training individuals would remain at the beginning level in the learning process. It is only with expert activity, intimate knowledge and a move beyond analytical rationality that one becomes a professional.

This book is unified by a social justice approach which suggests equitable access to basic human rights and resources, and health and social care's pivotal role locally and globally in promoting social justice. Injustices tear at the fabric of individuals, groups, communities and society.

For MacIntyre (1984) the human being is a 'story telling animal' and narratives not only give meaningful form to experience already lived but provide us with a forward glance, helping us to anticipate situations even before we encounter them, and allowing us to envision alternative futures (Flyvberg 2006: 240). This holistic meaning making and visioning underlies professionalism.

What should professionals do?

Practice

One of the most central discussions around professionalism is that of professional practice and the day-to-day activity of what professionals do. This is part of the ways of being a professional or the culture of professions.

Definitions of practice revolve around 'the carrying out or exercise of a profession' (OED), 'performance, execution, achievement, working, operation', 'an action or deed', and the action of doing something; the habitual doing or carrying on of something; usual, customary, or constant action or performance; conduct; as a verb or doing word, to pursue or be engaged in a particular profession. Practice then involves doing something.

Mezirow (1997) suggests practice is comprised of 'frames of reference' in terms of: 1) 'habits of mind' – those 'broad, abstract habitual ways of thinking, feeling and acting influenced by assumptions that constitute a set of codes'; and 2) specific 'points of view' – 'the constellation of belief, value judgement, attitude, and feeling that shapes a particular interpretation' (Mezirow 1997: 5–6).

Mezirow (1997: 5) speaks of becoming professional as a 'process of effecting change in a frame of reference'. For Mezirow, 'frames of reference' are the structures of assumptions through which we understand our lived experiences. They shape our thoughts and feelings, expectations, perceptions, cognition and feelings and set 'our line of action'. He argues that 'transformative learners move toward a frame of reference that is more inclusive, discriminating, self-reflective and integrative of experience' (Mezirow 1997: 5).

This movement for an altered frame of reference is a central part of the journey of becoming a professional.

A 'theory of social practices' (Reckwitz 2002) indicates that the 'turn to practices' in social theory seems to be tied to an interest in both the 'everyday' and the 'life-world' or the lived experience of professional practice. With a lived experience focus, vantage point or perspective, the mythology of managerialist cultural constructs dissipates and the actions, thoughts and feelings of professionals come into focus. This is the corporeality and everyday life of becoming a professional.

Reckwitz (2002: 246) suggests 'the vocabularies' of early theorists of practice such as Durkheim and Parsons 'stand opposed to purpose oriented and norm referenced models of explaining actions'. From Reckwitz's (2002: 249) perspective, 'practice theory does not place the social in mental qualities, nor discourse, nor in interaction but in practices'. This adds to the canon of practice theories by changing the location of practice against earlier theorists (such as Bourdieu 1977; Butler 1990; Foucault 1977, 1978, 1985; 2002 [1969]; Garfinkel 1984 [1967]; Giddens 1979, 1984; Latour 2007, Schatzki 1996; Schatski et al. 2001). It also adds a significant element to professional practice by locating it in the practice itself, rather than with reference to imposed or guiding constraints on what professional practice should be according to competences or tick-box performance measures. The practice turn is part of Lester's (2007) Model A and B professionals.

- Reckwitz (2002: 249) suggests 'a practice (*Praktik*) is a routinized type of behaviour consisting of several interconnected elements, including:
- Forms of bodily activities
- Forms of mental activities, things and their use
- A background of knowledge in the form of understanding, knowhow, states of emotion and motivational knowledge'.

Reckwitz (2002: 225) suggests that 'for practice theory bodily and mental patterns are necessary components of practices and are thus social'. This social form of professional practice, deeper and richer than previous theorists', provides a wider field for professional practice beyond simple, superficial reflection.

Schatzki (1996: 89) advocates practice as a 'temporally unfolding dispersed nexus of doings and sayings'. He distinguishes three 'major avenues of linkage' connecting any 'nexus of practice':

1   'Through understandings ... of what to say and do;
2   Through explicit rules, principles, precepts, and instructions; and
3   Through what he identifies as "'teleoaffective" structures embracing ends, projects, tasks, purposes, beliefs, emotions and moods' (Schatzki 2002: 89).

Reading Reckwitz and Schatzki we get a social understanding of practice, with a more embodied notion of 'lived experience'. The tacit dimension of unknown bodily and mental activities and the rule-governed nature of practice provides a richer picture of practice including an ontology of the flesh (Merleau-Ponty 2002).

We also need to understand that any discussion of social action or practice will always take place within a context. This context is highly mediated by a range of forces at many levels and with many voices. However, there is one clear overarching idea that has determinant effects on professional practice – that of neo-liberal capitalism. The theorists of this socio-economic, political and cultural set of forces are discussed in Chapter 2 when read through the lens of philosophical contributions. At this point professionals engaged in practice could make reference to Harvey (2005) for the broad contours of neo-liberalism.

This book is an attempt to foreground the lived experience of professional practice within the context of neo-liberal managerialism.

Performing professionalism

The notion that professionalism and leadership in professionalism is a performance has credence and current interest (Butler 1993; Peck and Dickinson 2009). A distinction can be made between 'professionalism is a performance' and 'professionalism as a performance'. Schechner (2003) proposes that the former relates to actions associated with organisational rituals while the latter is associated with a much broader range of everyday activities and is a more complex phenomenon. Professionalism becomes much more than a list of characteristics of professionals to an efficacious performance in institutional settings. Butler (1993) argues 'the reiterative and citational practice by which discourse produces the effects that it names' (Butler 1993: 2) is the process of perfomativity for professionals.

As Butler (1993: 108) observes:

> [D]iscursive performativity appears to produce that which it names, to enact its own referent, to name and to do, to name and to make. Paradoxically, however, this productive capacity of discourse is derivative, a form of cultural iterability or rearticulation, a practice of resignification ... [W]hat is invoked by the one who speaks or inscribes the law is the fiction of a speaker who wields the authority to make his [sic] words binding, the legal incarnation of the divine utterance.

Indeed, what is delivered through processes of reiteration and citation is nothing less than the organised subject itself:

> [P]erformativity is neither free-play nor theatrical self-presentation; nor can it simply be equated with performance. Performativity cannot be understood outside

a process of iterability, a regularized and constrained repetition of norms. And this repetition is not performed by a subject; this repetition is what enables a subject and constitutes the temporal condition for a subject.

(Butler 1993: 95)

The implication is that possibilities for action, the agency of professionals, are circumscribed by institutional context, and that agency itself arises out of institutional constructions (Hasselbladh and Bejerot 2007). The possibilities of doing something, agency, performativity, contexts and constructions, and institutions are to be discussed in the following chapters as a process of professional reflection.

Reflection

The history of reflection has seminal roots in Dewey (1933), Kolb (1984) and Schön (1983, 1987). Dewey (1933) began to think reflectively to solve problems and developed action-orientated forms of reflection. Mackintosh (1998) suggests the 1980s were a high point in the emergence of reflection for career development. Schön (1983), concerned with professional development of knowledge and skills, makes the distinction between reflection in and on action in a process of ongoing continuous learning, and reflection as immediate (in) or by looking back across practice (on) (Timmins 2015: 75).

The practitioner allows himself [sic] to experience surprise, puzzlement, or confusion in a situation which he finds uncertain or unique. He reflects on the phenomenon before him, and on the prior understandings which have been implicit in his behaviour. He carries out an experiment which serves to generate both a new understanding of the phenomenon and a change in the situation.

(Schön 1983: 68)

Reflection-in-action was the core of 'professional artistry' rather than and contrasted with 'technical-rationality' as the dominant paradigm or way of going on in professionalism. This paradigm, as sets of laws, beliefs, methods and assumptions (Kuhn 1962), has its high point as evidence-based practice valuing quantitative rather than qualitative methods and established protocols rather than intuitive practice.

Schön's work has become part of the 'canon' or 'doxa' in teaching and learning across a spectrum of professional practices. Atkins and Murphy (1993), in health care, identify three stages. The first is Schön's 'experience of surprise' or a trigger for professionals becoming aware of uncomfortable feelings or 'a sense of inner discomfort' or 'unfinished business' (Boyd and Fales 1983). The second stage is critical analysis of feelings and knowledge. The final stage is the development of a new perspective that combines self-awareness, critical analysis, synthesis and evaluation.

In education, Grushka et al. (2005) make a distinction between 'reflection for action', 'reflection in action' and 'reflection on action'. Reflection for action involves the technical (what resources are needed, how long it will take), practical (relevance to different learning styles, previous experience, level of engagement) and critical (why this topic is being taught).

Zeichner and Liston (1996) extend reflection to include five levels:

- Rapid reflection – immediate, ongoing and automatic action by the teacher.
- Repair – a thoughtful teacher makes decisions to alter their behaviour in response to a student's cues.
- Review – when a teacher engages with an element of their teaching.
- Research – when a teacher engages in a more systematic and sustained way, reading research, reviewing literature, conducting research.
- Retheorising and reformulating – a critical examination of practice in light of academic theories.

Broadening reflective practice has been inspired by Schön's work, but it is not without its critics. Eraut (2004) criticises the lack of precision and clarity; Boud and Walker (1998) argue that the context of reflection is ignored; Usher et al. (1997) criticise the unreflective methodology; and Smyth (1989) criticises the theoretical and apolitical nature of his work. Greenwood (1993) requires more reflection-before-action and Moon (1999) suggests reflection-in-action is unachievable. As Ghaye (2000: 7) suggests, 'maybe reflective practices offer us a way of trying to make sense of the uncertainty in our workplaces and the courage to work competently and ethically at the edge of order and chaos'.

Reflective practice is understood as the process of learning through and from experience towards gaining new insights of self and practice (Boud et al. 1985; Boyd and Fales 1983; Mezirow 1981; Jarvis 1992). Brookfield (1990, 1991, 1994, 1995) argues this involves examining assumptions in everyday practice and adopting a critical attitude and self-awareness. The pressures on busy professionals individually neglects a contextual and situated focus on reflection, a critical engagement and a thorough-going self-awarenesss.

Reflective practice is holistic practice, as Johns (2004: xiii) suggests, because:

It focuses on the whole experience and seeks to understand its significance within the whole.

It is grounded in the meanings the individual practitioner gives to the particular experience and seeks to facilitate such understanding.

It acknowledges that the practitioner is ultimately self-determining and responsible for his or her own destiny and seeks to facilitate such growth.

We can add that the reflective practitioner works in a context that is often challenging and conflicted and that practitioners need to be recognised as sentient, corporal humans engaged in a struggle for meaning in a process of becoming.

The centrality of reflection is given by Johns (2004) as:

- practical wisdom
- reflexivity
- becoming mindful
- commitment
- contradiction
- understanding
- empowerment.

Lydia Hall (1964: 151) advocates reflection as a cathartic engagement with creative tensions:

> Anxiety over an extended period is stressful to all the organ functions. It prepares people to fight or flight. In our culture however, it is brutal to fight and cowardly to flee, so we stew in our own juices and cook up malfunction. This energy can be put to use in exploration of feeling through participation in the struggle to face and solve problems underlying the state of anxiety.

As Schön (1987: 1) states:

> In the varied topography of professional practice, there is the high, hard ground overlooking the swamp. On the high ground, manageable problems lend themselves to solution through the application of research-based theory and technique. In the swampy lowland, messy, confusing problems defy technical solution. The irony of this situation is that the problems of the high ground tend to be relatively unimportant to individuals or society at large, however great their technical interest may be, while in the swamp lie the problems of greatest human concern. The practitioner must choose. Shall he [sic] remain on the high ground where he can solve relatively unimportant problems according to prevailing standards or rigor, or shall he [sic] descend into the swamp of important problems and non-rigorous inquiry.

Reflection offers a multi-layered and multi-avenued path to develop the hand, head and heart of professionals into the swampy lowlands. Professional practice, professional cognition and emotional engagement are part of the professional journey of becoming. This journey explores practice, understanding and feelings, a recognition and attention to the corporal situatedness and context of human beings becoming professional.

Reflection also has a philosophical origin from first and second order 'world disclosure' (Heidegger 1962) which refers to how things become meaningful and intelligible by being part of our worldview or the pre-existing, holistically structured background of meaning. Language is the most obvious example of this as we enter a world of language in our everyday life encounters with objects and people. This notion of the disclosure of meaning depends on the context in which we encounter it. These are the conditions of intelligibility. A simple example is a teapot becoming a plant pot; a more contentious example is a prime minister being investigated for historic child sex abuse. Heidegger (1962) suggests we are 'thrown' into this world of pre-existing conditions where activities and qualities are given to us. Building from this, Kompridis (2006) suggests reflective disclosure is a form of social criticism related to practices through which we can imagine and articulate meaningful alternatives to current social and political conditions, by acting back on their conditions of intelligibility.

Timmins (2015: 44) suggests that '[i]n addition to the popularity of *reflection* and *reflective practice* the acknowledged complexity of the world of practice in professional fields such as health and social care means an increasing and recommended use of critical reflection within disciplines'. Reflection has become a watch-word across disciplines and is an analysis of situations and events, but carries with it the danger of a decontextualised and abstract analysis. Critical reflection takes a wider and a contextualised look at the situation within which reflection takes place (Gardner 2014). Critical reflection draws upon the philosophical tradition of the Frankfurt School and critical theory to add the dimension of critical practice that includes a more substantive analysis of personal beliefs, how these fit within social settings and how these social settings influence and affect situations (Fook and Askeland 2006). Fook (2015) and Brookfield (1995) also suggest that power differences in social settings are a necessary component of reflection so it becomes more than an examination of personal experience but is located in social and political structures. Critical reflection extends the reflective project to include assumption hunting (Brookfield 1995), taken-for-granted and common-sense aspects and the power dynamics exercised in reflective situations. As such, critical reflection is both a theory and a process (Gardner 2014) with a deeper look at the underpinning reasons why situations occur and consideration of all the elements that contribute to reflection.

As Gardner (2014) suggests, critical reflection moves beyond the personal of experiences, emotions, thoughts and reactions. It includes the social context, reorganising and affirming differences, opening vistas and horizons, creativity, considering opposing beliefs and thinking about the context in which the experience takes place.

This approach is an appeal to critically reflective practice. Thompson and Pascal suggest critically reflective practice provides a basis for emancipatory practice, to:

- incorporate issues of forethought or planning: reflection-for-practice;
- take greater account of the central role of language, meaning and narrative as key elements in the process of meaning making;
- go beyond individualism or 'atomism' to appreciate the significance of the wider social context;
- take greater account of the emotional dimension of reflection;
- incorporate a greater understanding of the important role of power;
- be clear about the differences between reflection and reflexivity and understand the relationship between the two;
- take account of time considerations, at both individual and organisational levels and, crucially;
- develop a critical approach that addresses the depth and breadth aspects of criticality and the interrelationships between the two.

(Thompson and Pascal 2012: 322)

The final contribution that this reflection on reflection produces is to engage with the temporality of reflection, or when it happens. Most reflection is *a posteriori* or reflection after the event. Significant degrees of reflection take place before the event or *a priori*. This is commonly linked to questions of anticipation or thinking things through before the event takes place. Although this is a beneficial process in a number of ways (to examine what might happen, to prepare, to rehearse, to visualise, to improve performance), too much reflection before an event can become disadvantageous. Focusing too much on the unanticipated or possible future events can cause generalised anxiety disorders, fears or worries. Pre-reflection needs to be used in a productive and protective way to challenge anxiety, and to mitigate against ill-placed or ill-informed pre-reflective concern.

Our reflective engagement is to re-imagine the existing world, propose and explore alternatives and provide an alternative mental landscape or cognitive map of thoughts, concepts, ideas and practice. As such, reflective disclosure becomes a condition for social justice.

Social justice

There is an ongoing debate about whether professionals are practitioners of an art or public servants promoting social justice. Fairness and equality are the two main pillars of social justice. Powers and Faden (2006) suggest social justice is the moral foundation of public health policy and Powell et al. (2012) see it as the idea of creating a society and institutions based on the principles of equality and solidarity that understands and values human rights and dignity for every human being. Social justice is the cornerstone of ethics and is closely linked to equality, fairness, justice, oppression and utilitarianism. Hugman (2014: 139) advises that the principle of justice is widely discussed as one of the common moral values but professional ethics talks specifically about social justice (Banks 2006; Beauchamp and Childress 2009).

Social justice has been considered as a core virtue of professional practice, such as in social work. From the early part of the new millennium, Nussbaum (2003) has led a capabilities definition of justice and identified ten essential capabilities for human flourishing: life; health; play; control over one's own body; control over one's own environment; using one's senses, imagination and thoughts; emotional attachment; use of practical reasoning; ability to live with concern for nature; and freedom to form relationships. These capabilities are seen as irreducible and so unable to be prioritised over each other, and recognising the importance of community and mutual responsibility. The competency or ability to do so is replaced with the capability to develop. This also adds a located, sensuous, embodied sense of capability and the guiding principles for professionals.

Social justice is about groups and a social understanding beyond individuals as the origin of justice and the way that social structures can inhibit, be a barrier to, or confiscate the promotion of justice. Social injustice denies people the potential to live a fully human life, and so denies their humanity and human dignity (Hugman 2014: 140). Social justice demands a refocusing on questions of justice to the social structures and relationships independent of any one individual. Those professions that draw on social theory as part of their knowledge base include health and social care, community work, social work and youth work, nurses and teachers (Carr 2000; Tschudin 2003; Butcher et al. 2007; Sercombe 2010; Banks 2010). Many health and social care professions are seen as directly challenging injustice caused by inequalities and social structures and promoting social justice. For example, ethics is a central part of medicine (Seedhouse 2009). Social justice goes beyond questions of distribution of resources (a form of distributive justice) to challenge oppression (Young 1990). There is an emerging literature on helping professionals and health and social care as philosophically situated, and developing practice as praxis to promote social justice (Kagan et al. 2014).

From the previous discussion we can reflect upon what the role and responsibility of the professional is in an age of austerity. From the vantage point or perspective of the role of the group, professionals are invited to have an articulated set of values that are closely allied and associated with the promotion of social justice. Reflective professionals need to be self-aware of the complex context in which they work, the situated nature of the activity they engage with, and the relationships and alliances they form, and how they themselves fit within this picture. They need resilience, tenacity and maturity to deal with complex situations and competing demands, guided by a beacon of the value, purposefulness and the principal and principle ability to effect change according to social justice.

What follows in this book is an invitation to become a reflective professional and apply this development to complex and challenging situations in everyday life and practice. The rest of this book is an exploration of the swampy lowlands.

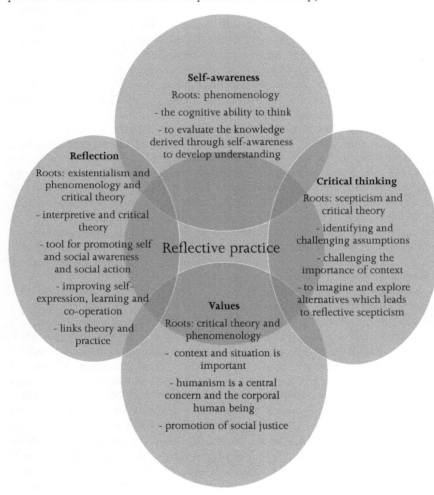

Figure 1.1 Skills underpinning the concept of reflective practice including values (Finlay 2008)

Conclusion

This chapter has discussed professions, professionals, professionalisation and professionalism. The various approaches have moved us to being and becoming professional and the call for social justice. This is shown in diagrammatic form in Figure 1.1. Reflective practice is personal reflection and broader social critique similar to a synthesis of reflection, self-awareness and critical thinking guided by values. In this model of reflection the philosophical roots are in phenomenology (lived experience and consciousness), and critical theory (critical consciousness towards emancipation and challenging discrimination and oppression, promoting social justice with contextual understanding). The existential focus on human beings and their experience in a self-aware reflection challenges inequalities and injustices for social justice.

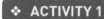

❖ ACTIVITY 1

Professional

Think of a time when you were professional. What did this entail?

Being and becoming

Write a history of being and becoming a professional (this is a self-study or auto-ethnography).

Identify pivotal moments or critical junctures when you can say, 'I was being a professional' or 'I was becoming a professional'. Think about yourself in this context or situation. What where the dominant forces in this field?

How did you feel? Can you arrive at the 'sensuous human activity' of being and becoming a professional?

Reflective disclosure

Can you think of a moment of reflective disclosure? Did you explore alternatives?

References

Abbot, A. (1988) *The System of the Professions*. London: University of Chicago Press.

Abel, R. L. (1988) *The Legal Profession in England and Wales*. New York: Blackwell.

Anderson-Gough, F., Grey, C. and Robson, K. (1999) *Making Up Accountants*. Aldershot: Gower Ashgate.

Atkins, T. W. and Murphy, K. (1993) Reflection: A review of the literature. *Journal of Advanced Nursing*, 18, 1188–92.

Atwal, A. and Jones, M. (eds) (2009) *Preparing for Professional Practice in Health and Social Care*. Oxford: Blackwell.

Banks, S. (2006) *Ethics and Values in Social Work*. Basingstoke: Palgrave Macmillan.

Banks, S. (2010) (4th edn) *Ethics and Values in Social Work*. Basingstoke: Palgrave Macmillan.

Barnard, A. (2008) *The Value Base of Social Work and Social Care: An Active Learning Handbook*. Milton Keynes: Open University Press.

Beauchamp, T. L. and Childress, J. F. (2009) (7th edn) *Principles of Biomedical Ethics*. Oxford: Oxford University Press.

Becker, H. S. (1970) The nature of a profession. In Becker, H. S. (ed.), *Sociological Work*. Chicago: Aldine.

Biestek, F. (1957) *The Casework Relationship*. London: Allen and Unwin.

Boud, D. and Walker, D. (1998) Promoting reflection in professional courses: The challenge of context. *Studies in Higher Education*, 23(2), 191–206.

Boud, D., Keogh, R. and Walker, D. (1985) Promoting reflection in learning: A model. In Boud, D., Keogh, R. and Walker, D. (eds) (1985) *Reflection: Turning Experience into Learning*. London: Kogan Page.

Bourdieu, P. (1977) *Outline for a Theory of Practice*. Cambridge: Cambridge University Press.

Boyd, E. and Fales, A. (1983) Reflective learning: Key to learning from experience. *Journal of Humanistic Psychology*, 23(2), 99–117.

Braverman, H. (1974) *Labor and Monopoly Capital*. New York: Monthly Review.

Brint, S. G. (1994) *In an Age of Experts: The Changing Role of Professionals in Politics and Public Life*. Princeton, NJ: Princeton University Press.

Broadbent, J., Dietrich, M. and Roberts, J. (1997) *The End of the Professions? The Restructuring of Professional Work*. London: Routledge.

Brock, D., Powell, M. and Hinings, C. R. (1999) *Restructuring the Professional Organization: Accounting, Healthcare and Law*. London and New York: Routledge.

Brookfield, S. (1990) Using critical incidents to explore learners' assumptions. In Mezirow, J. (ed.), *Fostering Critical Reflection in Adulthood*. San Francisco: Jossey-Bass.

Brookfield, S. (1991) On ideology, pillage, language and risk: Critical thinking and the tensions of critical practice. *Studies in Continuing Education*, 13(1), 1–14.

Brookfield, S. (1994) Tales from the dark side: A phenomenography of adult critical reflection. *International Journal of Lifelong Education*, 13(3), 203–16.

Brookfield, S. (1995) *Becoming a Critically Reflective Teacher*. San Francisco: Jossey-Bass.

Brown, W. (2006) American nightmare: Neo-liberalism, neoconservativism, and de-moralisation. *Political Theory*, 34(4), 690–714.

Burrage, M. and Torstendahl, R. (eds) (1990) *The Formation of Professions: Knowledge, State and Strategy*. London: Sage.

Butcher, H., Banks, S., Orton, A., and Robertson, J. (2007) *Managing Community Practice: Principles, Policy and Programmes*. Bristol: Policy Press.

Butler, J. (1990) *Gender Trouble*. London: Routledge.

Butler, J. (1993) *Bodies That Matter: On the Discursive Limits Of 'Sex'*. London: Routledge.

Carr, D. (2000) *Professionalism and Ethics in Teaching*. London: Routledge.

Clarke, J. and Newman, J. (1997) *The Managerial State: Power, Politics and Ideology in the Remaking of Social Welfare*. London: Sage.

Cooper, D. E. (1999) *Existentialism: A Reconstruction*. Oxford: Basil Blackwell.

Cooper, D. L. and Robson, K. (2006) Accounting, professions and regulation: Locating the sites of professionalization. *Accounting, Organizations and Society*, 31, 415–44.

Dewey, J. (1933) *How We Think: A Restatement of the Relation of Reflective Thinking to Educative Practice.* Boston, MA: DC Heath.

Dingwall, R. (2008) *Essay on Professions.* Hampshire: Ashgate.

Dreyfus, H. L. (1991) *Being-in-the-World: A Commentary on Heidegger's Being and Time, Division 1.* Cambridge, MA: MIT Press.

Dreyfus, H. and Dreyfus, S. (1986) *Mind over Machine: The Power of Human Intuition and Expertise in the Era of the Computer.* New York: Free Press.

Eraut, M. (2004) Editorial: The practice of reflection. *Learning in Health and Social Care,* 3(2), 47–52.

Finlay, L. (2008) *Reflecting on 'Reflective Practice'.* Practice-based Professional Learning Centre, Open University Press. Available at: www.open.ac.uk/opencetl/resources/pbpl-resources/finlay-l-2008-reflecting-reflective-practice-pbpl-paper-52

Fook, J. (2015) Critical social work practice. In Wright, J. D. (ed.) *International Encyclopaedia of the Social and Behavioural Sciences.* Amsterdam: Elsevier.

Fook, J. and Askeland, G. A. (2006) The 'critical' in critical reflection. In White, S., Fook, J. and Gardner, F. (eds), *Critical Reflection in Context: Applications in Health and Social Care.* Berkshire: Open University Press.

Foucault, M. (1977) *Discipline and Punish: The Birth of a Prison,* trans. Sheridan, A. London: Penguin Books.

Foucault, M. (1978) *History of Sexuality Volume 1: An Introduction,* trans. Hurley, R. New York: Pantheon.

Foucault, M. (1985) *History of Sexuality Volume II: The Use of Pleasure,* trans. Hurley, R. New York: Pantheon.

Foucault, M. (2002 [1969]) *The Archaeology of Knowledge,* trans. Sheridan Smith, A. M. London and New York: Routledge.

Flyvberg, B. (2006) Five misunderstandings about case-study research. *Qualitative Inquiry,* 12(2), April 2006, 219–45.

Friedson, E. (1970) *Profession of Medicine: A Study of the Sociology of Applied Knowledge.* New York: Dodd, Mead & Co.

Friedson, E. (1986) *Professional Powers: A Study of the Institutionalization of Formal Knowledge.* Chicago, IL: University of Chicago Press.

Friedson, E. (1994) *Professionalism Reborn: Theory, Prophecy and Policy.* Cambridge: Polity Press.

Friedson, E. (2001) *Professionalism: The Third Logic.* Cambridge: Polity Press.

Gardner, F. (2014) *Being Critically Reflective.* Basingstoke: Palgrave Macmillan.

Garfinkel, H. (1984 [1967]) *Studies in Ethnomethodology.* Cambridge: Polity Press.

Ghaye, T. (2000) Into the reflective mode: Bridging the stagnant moat. *Reflective Practice,* 1(1), 5–9.

Giddens, A. (1979) *Central Problems in Social Theory: Action, Structure and Contradiction in Social Analysis.* Berkeley, CA: University of California Press.

Giddens, A. (1984) *The Constitution of Society.* Cambridge: Polity Press.

Goodrick, E. and Reay, T. (2010) Florence Nightingale endures: Legitimizing a new professional role identity. *Journal of Management Studies,* 47, 55–84.

Gorman, E. H. and Sandefur, R. L. (2011) 'Golden Age', quiescence, and revival: How the sociology of professions became the study of knowledge-based work. *Work and Occupations,* 38, 275–302.

Grbich, C (2007) *Qualitative Data Analysis: An Introduction.* London: Sage.

Greenwood, J. (1993) Reflective practice: A critique of the work of Argyris and Schön. *Journal of Advanced Nursing,* 19, 1183–87.

Gregory, M. and Holloway, M. (2005) Language and the shaping of social work. *British Journal of Social Work*, 35, 37–53.

Grushka, K., Hinder-McLeod, J. and Reynolds, R. (2005) Reflecting upon reflection: Theory and practice in one Australian university teacher education programme. *Reflective Practice*, 6(1), 239–46.

Hall, L. (1964) Nursing – what is it? *Canadian Nurse*, 60(2), 150–54.

Halliday, T. C. (1987) *Beyond Monopoly: Lawyers, State Crises, and Professional Empowerment*. Chicago, IL: University of Chicago Press.

Halliday, T. C. and Karpik, L. (eds) (1997) *Lawyers and the Rise of Western Political Liberalism: Europe and North America from the Eighteenth to Twentieth Centuries*. Oxford: Oxford University Press.

Hanlon, G. (1999) *Lawyers, the State and the Market: Professionalism Revisited*. Basingstoke: Macmillan Business.

Harvey, D. (2005) *A Brief History of Neo-Liberalism*. Oxford: Oxford University Press.

Hasselbladh, H. and Bejerot, E. (2007) Webs of knowledge and circuits of communication: Constructing rationalized agency in Swedish health care. *Organization* 14(2): 175–200.

HCPC (Health and Care Professionals Council) (2014) *Professionalism in Healthcare Professionals*. London: HCPC.

Heidegger, M. (1962) *Being and Time*, trans. Macquarrie, J. and Robinson, E. New York: Harper and Row.

Hugman, R. (2014) *A–Z Professional Ethics*. Basingstoke: Palgrave Macmillan.

Illich, I. (1982) *Medical Nemesis: The Exploration of Health*. New York: Pantheon Press.

Jarvis, P. (1992) Reflective practice in nursing. *Nurse Education Today*, 12(3), 174–81.

Johns, C. (2004) (2nd edn) *Becoming a Reflective Practitioner*. Oxford: Blackwell.

Johnson, T. J. (1972) *Professions and Power*. London: Macmillan.

Johnson, T. (1993) Expertise and the state. In Johnson, T. and Gane, M. (eds), *Foucault's New Domains*. London: Routledge, pp. 139–52.

Kagan, P. N., Smith, M. C. and Chinn, P. L. (2014) *Philosophies and Practice of Emancipatory Nursing: Social Justice as Praxis*. London: Routledge.

Koch, T. (1995) Interpretive approaches in nursing research: The influence of Husserl and Heidegger. *Journal of Advanced Nursing*, 21(5), 827–36.

Kolb, D. A. (1984) *Experimental Learning*. London: Prentice Hall.

Kompridis, N. (2006) *Critique and Disclosure: Critical Theory between Past and Future*. Cambridge, MA: MIT Press.

Krause, E. A. (1996) *The Death of the Guilds: Professions, States and the Advance of Capitalism: 1930 to the Present*. New Haven, CT: Yale University Press.

Kuhn, T. (1962) *The Structure of Scientific Revolutions*. Chicago, IL: Chicago University Press.

Larson, M. S. (1977) *The Rise of Professionalism: A Sociological Analysis*. Berkeley, CA: University of California Press.

Latour, B. (2007) *Reassembling the Social: An Introduction to Actor-Network-Theory*. Oxford: Oxford University Press.

Leicht, K. and Fennell, M. (2001) *Professional Work: A Sociological Approach*. Oxford: Blackwell.

Lester, S. (2015) *On Professions and Being Professional*, Available at: www.devmts.org.uk/profnal.pdf

Lynch, K. (2006) Neo-liberalism and marketization: The implications for higher education. *European Educational Research Journal*, 5(1): 1–17.

Macdonald, K. (2001) *The Sociology of the Professions*. London: Sage.

MacIntyre, A. (1984) (2nd edn) *After Virtue: A study in Moral Theory.* Notre Dame, IN: University of Notre Dame Press.

Mackintosh, C. (1998) Reflection: A flawed strategy for the nursing profession. *Nursing Education Today,* 18(7), 325–39.

Merleau-Ponty, M. (2002) *Phenomenology of Perception: An Introduction.* London: Routledge Classics.

Mezirow, J. (1981) A critical theory of adult learning and education. *Adult Education* 32(1), 3–24.

Mezirow, J. (1997) Transformative learning: Theory to practice. *New Directions for Adult and Continuing Education,* 74, Summer, 5–12.

Mills, C. W. (1959) *The Sociological Imagination.* Oxford: Oxford University Press.

Moon, J. (1999) *Reflection in Learning and Professional Development: Theory and Practice.* London: Kogan Page.

Moran, D. (2000) *Introduction to Phenomenology.* New York: Routledge.

Moran, D. and Mooney, T. (eds) (2002) *The Phenomenology Reader.* New York: Routledge.

Muzio, D., Brock, D. M. and Suddaby, R. (2013) Professions and institutional change: Towards an institutionalist sociology of the professions. *Journal of Management Studies,* 50(5), July, 700–721.

Nussbaum, M. (2003) Capabilities as fundamental elements: Sen and social justice. *Feminist Economics,* 9(2/3), 33–59.

Oakley, A. (1986) Feminism, motherhood and medicine – who cares? In Mitchell, J. and Oakley, A. (eds), *What is Feminism?* Oxford: Basil Blackwell, pp. 127–50.

Peck, E. and Dickinson, H. (2009) *Performing Leadership.* Basingstoke: Palgrave.

Powell, M., Johns, N. and Green, A. (2012) *Social Justice in Social Policy.* Available at: www.social-policy.org.uk/lincoln2011/PowellJohnsGreen%20P7.pdf (accessed 25 April 2014).

Powers, M. and Faden, R. (2006) *Social Justice: The Foundations of Public Health and Health Policy.* Oxford: Oxford University Press.

Prowle, A., Murphey, P. and Prowle, M. (2014) Managing escalating demand at a time of financial austerity. *Journal of Finance and Management in Public Services,* 12(1), 1–14.

Reckwitz, A. (2002) Toward a theory of social practices: A development in culturalist theorizing. *European Journal of Social Theory,* 5(2), 243–63.

Reed, M. I. (1996) Expert power and control in late modernity: An empirical review and theoretical synthesis. *Organisation Studies,* 17, 573–97.

Scanlon, L. (2011) *'Becoming' a Professional.* Berlin: Springer Verlag.

Schatzki, T. (1996) *Social Practices: A Wittgensteinian Approach to Human Activity and the Social.* Cambridge: Cambridge University Press.

Schatzki, T. R. (2002) Social science in society. *Inquiry,* 45(1), 119–38.

Schatzki, T., Cetina, K. K. and von Savigny, E. (2001) *The Practice Turn in Contemporary Theory.* Abingdon, Oxon: Routledge.

Schechner, R. (2003) *Performance Studies: An Introduction.* London: Routledge.

Schön, D. (1983) *The Reflective Practitioner.* Avebury: Aldershot.

Schön, D. (1987) *Educating the Reflective Practitioner.* San Francisco, CA: Jossey-Bass.

Scott, W. R. (2008) Lords of the dance: Professionals as institutional agents. *Organization Studies,* 29, 219–38.

Seden, J., Matthews, S., McCormick, M. and Morgan, A. (eds) (2011) *Professional Development in Social Work.* London: Routledge.

Seedhouse, D. (2009) (3rd edn) *Ethics: The Heart of Health Care.* Chichester: Wiley.

Sercombe, H. (2010) *Youth Work Ethics.* London: Sage.

Smyth, J. (1989) Teachers' work and the politics of reflection. *American Educational Research Journal*, 29, 267–300.

Speziale, H. S. and Carpenter, D. R. (2007) (4th edn) *Qualitative Research in Nursing: Advancing the Humanistic Imperative.* Philadelphia: Lippincott Williams & Wilkins.

Stimson, G. V. and Webb, B. (1975) *Going to See the Doctor.* London: Routledge, Kegan and Paul.

Thompson, N. and Pascal, J. (2012) Developing critically reflective practice. *Reflective Practice: International and Multidisciplinary Perspectives*, 13(2), 311–25.

Timmins, F. (2015) *Reflective Practice.* London: Palgrave.

Tschudin, V. (2003) *Ethics in Nursing: The Caring Relationship.* Cambridge: Butterworth-Heinemann.

Usher, R., Bryant, I. and Johnston, R. (1997) *Adult Education and the Postmodern Challenge: Learning Beyond the Limits.* London: Routledge.

Young, I. M. (1990) *Justice and the Politics of Difference.* Princeton, NJ: Princeton University Press.

Zeichner, K. M. and Liston, D. P. (1996) *Reflective Teaching: An Introduction.* Mahwah, NJ: Lawrence Erlbaum Associates Publishers.

Chapter 2
Philosophy for professionals

The practice of philosophy

Adam Barnard and Hannah Sawtell

Chapter outline

This chapter will:

- introduce philosophical traditions of thought
- help you to understand key thinkers in philosophy
- help you to understand the contribution they make to professional practice.

This chapter will examine philosophical traditions of thought and the contribution they make to professional practice. The traditions of critical theory, phenomenology, pragmatism, postmodernism and feminism will be considered, to provide an orientation to professional practice. The provision of philosophy for professionals is a unique and distinctive engagement that is often neglected in developing reflective practitioners and professionals.

It is time for philosophy to be recognised for the contribution it can make areas of social life but particularly to becoming a reflective professional. Philosophy contributes to the critical thinking of professionals and practitioners, examines the value base of everyday practice and decision making and enhances self-awareness and reflection. Philosophers have only interpreted the world in various ways; the point, however, is to change it. Philosophy can rejuvenate practice (Seedhouse 2009: viii); it can be a guide to ideas, morals and practice. To engage with philosophy is to increase your bandwidth of curiosity and cross the threshold into an adventurous world.

The practice of philosophy for professionals has some distinct benefits for practitioners. This chapter charts the major intellectual movements, the classical writings and the major figures of European philosophy. As each intellectual movement is reviewed, the contribution made to professional practice is considered.

There are many ways to carve a cake but to make a manageable journey through European philosophy we can start with four sections. The first is from phenomenology to hermeneutics. The second from Marxism to critical theory. The third from structuralism to deconstruction. The fourth from feminism through its various waves. Each major tradition of thought is supported by a thumbnail sketch of the contribution of each of the selected classical writings and major individuals in this tradition. This is one narrative amongst many and there are different ways of presenting and interpreting the ideas put forward. The hope is that at the end of the chapter you will have a workable knowledge of broad philosophical ideas, their contribution to practice and how each thinker contributes to social justice.

The context for this discussion is that each thinker, tradition and intellectual movement provides material for reflective development. It opens the 'horizon of possibilities' and invites, if not demands, a reflexive and critical engagement. The energy and time given to reflective consideration of each thinker and tradition will provide fruitful results and provide resources and directions for practice and for promoting social justice.

The use of visual methodologies intends to stimulate a different register and provoke thought and reflection from a different standpoint.

1. Jacques Derrida

(15 July 1930, El Biar, France – 9 October 2004, Paris, France)

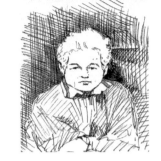

French philosopher

Impact: Across the humanities and social sciences.

Contribution: Différance, deconstruction, the trace, arche-writing, text, spacing, the supplement, undecidability, iteration.

Criticism: Challenge of nihilism, incomprehensibility.

Key works

Derrida, J. (1978) *Writing and Difference*. London: Johns Hopkins University Press.
Derrida, J. (1976) *Of Grammatology*. London: Johns Hopkins University Press.
Derrida, J. (1982) *Margins of Philosophy*. Chicago: University of Chicago Press.
Derrida, J. (1994) *Spectres of Marx: The State of the Debt, The Work of Mourning, and The New International*. New York: Routledge.

Introductory text

Royle, N. (2003) *Jacques Derrida*. London: Routledge.

2. Martin Heidegger

(26 September 1889, Barden, Germany – 26 May 1976, Freiburg, Germany)

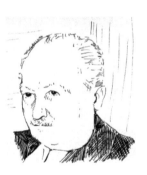

German philosopher

Impact: Across philosophy and informing subsequent theorists.

Contribution: Dwelling, throwness, temporality, enframing.

Criticism: Irrationalism, political implications, difficult to read.

Key works

Heidegger, M. (1967) *Being and Time*. Oxford: Blackwell.
Heidegger, M. (1992) *The Concept of Time*. Bloomington, IN: Indiana University Press.
Heidegger, M. (2013) *The Question Concerning Technology and Other Essays*. New York: Harper Torchbooks.

Introductory text

Caputo, J. D. (1986) *Mystical Element in Heidegger's Thought*. New York: Fordham University Press.

3. Claude Levi-Strauss

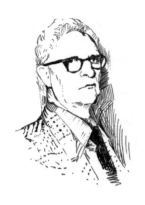

(28 November 1908, Brussels, Belgium – 30 October 2009, Paris, France)

French anthropologist and ethnologist

Impact: Across the humanities and social sciences.

Contribution: Structuralism and structural anthropology, binary oppositions, myths.

Criticism: Difficult to understand, artificial separation of opposites.

Key works

Levi-Strauss, C. (1961) *Tristes Tropiques*. London: Hutchinson and Co.

Levi-Strauss, C. (1964) *Mythologies I–IV*. Paris: Plon.

Levi-Strauss, C. (1969 [1948]) *The Elementary Structures of Kinship*. London: Eyre & Spottiswoode.

Levi-Strauss, C. (1978) *Myth and Meaning*. London: Routledge, Kegan and Paul.

Introductory text

Simons, J. (2002) *From Kant to Levi-Strauss: The Background to Contemporary Critical Theory*. Edinburgh: Edinburgh University Press.

4. Pierre Bourdieu

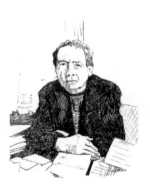

(1 August 1930, Denguin, France – 23 January 2002, Paris, France)

French sociologist, anthropologist and philosopher

Impact: Reflexive sociology, and across the humanities and social sciences.

Contribution: Cultural, social symbolic capital, habitus, field, symbolic violence, doxa.

Criticism: Separation of object (field) and subject (habitus), too cultural.

Key works

Bourdieu, P. (1977) *Outline of a Theory of Practice*. Cambridge: Cambridge University Press.

Bourdieu, P. (1987) *Distinction: A Social Critique of Taste*. Harvard: Harvard University Press.

Bourdieu, P. (1993) *Language and Symbolic Power*. Harvard: Harvard University Press.

Bourdieu, P. (2000) *The Weight of the World: Social Suffering in Contemporary Society*. Stanford: Stanford University Press.

Introductory text

Swartz, D. (1998) *Culture and Power: The Sociology of Pierre Bourdieu*. Chicago: Chicago University Press.

5. Michel Foucault

(15 October 1926, Poitiers, France – 25 June 1984,
Paris, France)

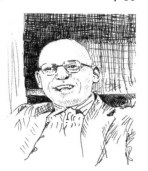

French philosopher and historical researcher

Impact: Social construction.

Contribution: Early structuralist work and dividing
practices, social and discursive practices, self-regulating
epistemes, archaeology, regimes of truth, discourses,
rules of formation.

Criticism: Too cultural, little ability to resist power and knowledge.

Key works

Foucault, M. (1966 [1965]) *Madness and Civilization*. New York: Pantheon.
Foucault, M. (1972 [1969]) *The Archaeology of Knowledge*, translated by A. Sheridan Smith.
    New York: Harper and Row.
Foucault, M. (1973 [1963]) *The Birth of the Clinic*, translated by A. Sheridan Smith. New
    York: Pantheon.
Foucault, M. (1973 [1966]) *The Order of Things*. New York: Vintage.
Foucault, M. (1988) *History of Sexuality*, 3 volumes: *Introduction, The Uses of Pleasure*, and *Care
    of the Self*, translated by Robert Hurley. New York: Vintage Books.

Introductory text

Rabinow, P. and Dreyfus, H. L. (1982) *Michel Foucault: Beyond Structuralism and Hermeneutics*.
    Chicago: Chicago University Press.

6. Anthony Giddens

(8 January 1938, London, UK –)

British sociologist

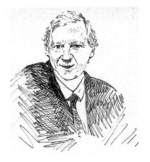

Impact: Sociologist with policy impact.

Contribution: Early career sociologist, structure and agency, translators of founding fathers Marx and Weber, structure and agency, capitalism and modernity, structuration, reflexivity.

Criticism: Syncretic loosing original criticality, too focused on structure and agency.

Key works

Giddens, A. (1971) *Capitalism and Modern Social Theory*. Cambridge: Polity.
Giddens, A. (1973) *The Class Structure of the Advanced Societies*. London: Macmillan.
Giddens, A. (1976) *New Rules of Sociological Method*. London: Hutchinson.
Giddens, A. (1979) *Central Problems in Social Theory*. London: Macmillan.
Giddens, A. (1984) *The Constitution of Society*. Cambridge: Polity.
Giddens, A. (1990) *Consequences of Modernity*. Cambridge: Polity.
Giddens, A. (1991) *Modernity and Self-Identity*. Cambridge: Polity.
Giddens, A. (1992) *The Transformation of Intimacy*. Cambridge: Polity.
Giddens, A. (1994) *Beyond Left and Right*. Cambridge: Polity.
Giddens, A. (1998) *The Third Way: The Renewal of Social Democracy*. Cambridge: Polity.

Introductory text

Halpin, D. (2003) *Hope and Education: The Role of the Utopian Imagination*. London: Routledge.

7. Hans-George Gadamer

(11 February 1900, Marburg, Germany – 13 March 2002, Heidelberg, Germany)

German philosopher

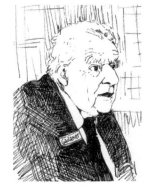

Impact: Continental philosophy and hermeneutics.

Contribution: Metaphysics, epistemology, ontology, language, practical philosophy and fusion of horizons.

Criticism: Syncretic loosing original criticality, too focused on structure and agency.

Key works

Gadamer, A. (1981) *Reason in the Age of Science*. Cambridge, MA: MIT Press.
Gadamer, A. (1976) *Philosophical Hermeneutics*. Berkeley, CA: University of California.
Gadamer, A. (2004) *Truth and Method*. New York: Crossroad.

Introductory text

Palmer, R. E. (ed.) (2007) *The Gadamer Reader: A Bouquet of the Later Writings*. Evanston, IL: Northwestern University Press.

8. Wilhelm Dilthey

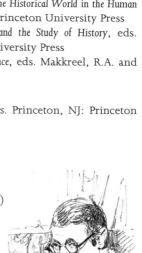

(19 November 1833, Wiesbaden-Bierich, Germany –
1 October 1911, Seis am Schlem, Austria)

German philosopher, psychologist and sociologist

Impact: Continental philosophy, literary criticism and
hermeneutics.

Contribution: *Verstehen*, intellectual history, hermeneutic
circle, human sciences.

Criticism: Syncretic loosing original criticality, too focused o

Key works

Dilthey, W. (1960) *Truth and Method*. Cambridge, MA: MIT Press.

Dilthey, W. (1991) *Selected Works, Volume I: Introduction to the Human Sciences*, eds. Makkreel, R.A. and Rodi, F. Princeton, NJ: Princeton University Press

Dilthey, W. (2010) *Selected Works, Volume II: Understanding the Human World*, eds. Makkreel, R.A. and Rodi, F. Princeton, NJ: Princeton University Press

Dilthey, W. (2002) *Selected Works, Volume III: The Formation of the Historical World in the Human Sciences*, eds. Makkreel, R.A. and Rodi, F. Princeton, NJ: Princeton University Press

Dilthey, W. (2010) *Selected Works, Volume IV: Hermeneutics and the Study of History*, eds. Makkreel, R.A. and Rodi, F. Princeton, NJ: Princeton University Press

Dilthey, W. (1996) *Selected Works, Volume V: Poetry and Experience*, eds. Makkreel, R.A. and Rodi, F. Princeton, NJ: Princeton University Press

Introductory text

Makkreel, R. A. (1993) *Dilthey: Philosopher of the Human Studies*. Princeton, NJ: Princeton University Press.

9. Jean-Paul Sartre

(21 June 1905, Paris, France – 15 April 1980, Paris, France)

French philosopher, playwright and activist

Impact: Continental philosophy, literary criticism and
hermeneutics.

Contribution: Existentialism, existence precedes essence,
freewill, ontology, authenticity, bad faith.

Criticism: Too free, not politically engaged enough,
fusion of existentialism and Marxism.

Key works

Sartre, J.-P. (1943) *Being and Nothingness: An Essay on Phenomenological Ontology*. New York: Washington Square Press.

Sartre, J.-P. (1948) *Existentialism and Humanism*, translated by Philip Mairet. London: Greener Books.

Introductory text

Aronson, R. (1980) *Jean-Paul Sartre – Philosophy in the World*. London: NLB.

10. Friedrich Nietzsche

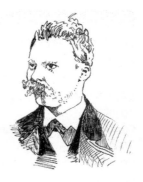

(15 October 1844, Röcken, Germany – 25 August 1900, Weimar, Germany)

German philosopher and poet

Impact: Metaphysics, nihilism, 'death of god'.

Contribution: Übermensch, Apollonian and Dionysian, 'school of suspicion'.

Criticism: Nihilism, political interpretation.

Key works
Nietzsche, F. (1872) *The Birth of Tragedy*. London: Allen Unwin.
Nietzsche, F. (1876) *Untimely Meditations*. Cambridge: Cambridge University Press.
Nietzsche, F. (1878) *Human, All Too Human*. Cambridge: Cambridge University Press.
Nietzsche, F. (1882) *The Gay Science*. Leipzig: E. W. Fritzsche.
Nietzsche, F. (1883) *Thus Spoke Zarathustra*. London: Random House.
Nietzsche, F. (1886) *Beyond Good and Evil*. Leipzig: Verlag von Naumann.
Nietzsche, F. (1887) *On the Genealogy of Morality*. Leipzig: Verlag von Naumann.
Nietzsche, F. (1888) *Twilight of the Idols*. Leipzig: Verlag von Naumann.

Introductory text
Kaufmann, W. (1974) *Nietzsche: Philosopher, Psychologist, Antichrist*. Princeton, NJ: Princeton University Press.

11. Ludwig Wittgenstein

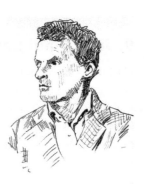

(26 April 1889, Vienna – 29 April 1951, Cambridge, UK)

Austrian-British philosopher

Impact: Language, metaphysics, nihilism, 'death of god'.

Contribution: Centrality of language, language games.

Criticism: Self-undermining later work.

Key works
Wittgenstein, L. (1921) *Tractatus Logico-Philosophicus*. London: Kegan Paul.
Wittgenstein, L. (1953) *Philosophical Investigations*. Oxford: Blackwell.

Introductory text
Monk, R. (1990) *Ludwig Wittgenstein: The Duty of Genius*. London: Free Press.

12. Jürgen Habermas

(18 June 1929, Düssledorf, Germany –)

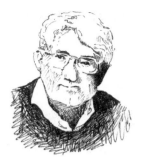

German sociologist and philosopher

Impact: Across the social sciences, social theory, and third-generation critical theorist.

Contribution: Communicative rationality, ethics, system-lifeworld.

Criticism: Demands too much of agents to have clear access to reason.

Key works
Habermas, J. (1971) *Knowledge and Human Interests*. Boston, MA: Beacon Press.
Habermas, J. (1975) *Legitimation Crisis*. Boston, MA: Beacon Press.
Habermas, J. (1981) *The Theory of Communicative Action*. Boston, MA: Beacon Press.

Introductory text
McCarthy, T. (1978) *The Critical Theory of Jürgen Habermas*. Cambridge, MA: MIT Press.

13. Thomas Kuhn

(18 June 1922, Cincinnati, Ohio – 17 June 1999, Cambridge, Massachussetts, USA)

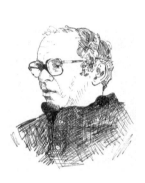

American physicist, philosopher and historian

Impact: Across the natural and social sciences, epistemology, philosophy of science.

Contribution: Scientific knowledge, 'shifts', paradigms, social context of knowledge.

Criticism: Unchallenging of science, or vested interests in knowledge production.

Key work
Kuhn, T. (1964) *The Structure of Scientific Revolutions*. Chicago: Chicago University Press.

Introductory text
Bird, A. (2000) *Thomas Kuhn*. Princeton, NJ and London: Princeton University Press and Acumen Press.

14. John Rawls

(21 February 1922, Baltimore, MD – 24 November 2002,
Lexington, MA, USA).

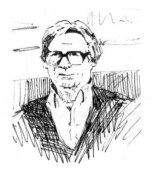

American philosopher

Impact: Across the social sciences and humanities,
analytical and political philosophy.

Contribution: Justice as fairness, original position,
veil of ignorance, reflective equilibrium.

Criticism: Too liberal, does not challenge inequalities.

Key works
Rawls, J. (1971) *Justice as Fairness*. Cambridge, MA: Cambridge University Press.
Rawls, J. (1993) *Political Liberalism: The John Dewey Essays in Philosophy*, 4. New York: Columbia
University Press.

Introductory text
Freeman, S. (2007) *Rawls*. Abingdon: Routledge.

15. Maurice Merleau-Ponty

(14 March 1908, Rochefort-sur-le-mer, France –
3 May 1961, Paris, France)

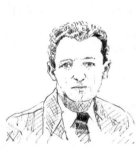

French philosopher

Impact: Existential phenomenology, continental
philosophy.

Contribution: Consciousness, ontology of 'flesh in the world', corporality.

Criticism: Too liberal, does not challenge inequalities.

Key works
Merleau-Ponty, M. (1962) *Phenomenology of Perception*. New York: Humanities Press.
Merleau-Ponty, M. (1968) *The Visible and the Invisible*. Evanston, IL: Northwestern
University Press.
Merleau-Ponty, M. (1973) *Adventures in the Dialectic*. Evanston, IL: Northwestern University
Press.

Introductory text
Toadvine, T. and Lawlor, L. (2007) *The Merleau-Ponty Reader*. Evanston, IL: Northwestern
University Press.

16. Max Horkheimer

(14 February 1895, Zuffenhausen, Germany –
7 July 1973, Nuremberg, Germany)

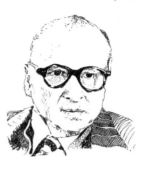

German Jewish philosopher

Impact: Philosophy and social sciences, Frankfurt School.

Contribution: Critical theory, authoritarian personality,
instrumental reason.

Criticism: Impenetrable writing, agents too determined.

Key works
Horkheimer, M. (1941) *Eclipse of Reason.* New York: Humanities Press.
Horkheimer, M. (1944) *Dialectic of the Enlightenment.* New York: Humanities Press.

Introductory text
Jay, M. (1996) *The Dialectical Imagination: A History of the Frankfurt School and the Institute of Social
Research, 1923–1950* (2nd edn). Berkeley, CA: University of California Press.

17. Gilles Deleuze

(18 January 1925, Paris, France – 4 November 1995,
Paris, France)

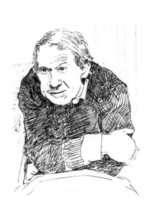

French philosopher

Impact: Literature, film, continental philosophy.

Contribution: Affect, assemblage, body without organs,
deterritorialisation, line of flight, plane of immanence,
rhizome, schizoanalysis, univocity of being.

Criticism: Selective reading of authors he critiques.

Key works
Deleuze, G. (1962) *Capitalism and Schizophrenia: Anti-Oedipus.* New York: Viking.
Deleuze, G. (1968) *Difference and Repetition.* New York: Columbia University Press.
Deleuze, G. (1973) *A Thousand Plateaus.* Paris: Les Editions de Minuit.
Deleuze, G. and Guattari, F. (1976) Rhizome, in *A Thousand Plateaus.* London: Continuum.

Introductory text
Badiou, A. (1999) *Deleuze: The Clamour of Being.* Minneapolis, MN: Minesota Press.

18. Herbert Marcuse

(19 July 1898, Berlin, Germany – 29 July 1979,
Starnberg, Germany)

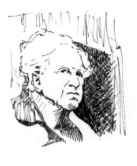

German-American sociologist and philosopher

Impact: Philosophy and social sciences, Frankfurt School.

Contribution: Critical theory, one-dimensional man,
technical reason, repressive desublimation, critique of
capitalism of advanced industrial society.

Criticism: Criticism from orthodox Marxism, too Freudian, passive view of
consumers.

Key works
Marcuse, H. (1955) *Eros and Civilisation: A Philosophical Inquiry into Freud.* New York: Beacon
    Press.
Marcuse, H. (1964) *One-Dimensional Man.* New York: Beacon Press.

Introductory text
Jay, M. (1996) *The Dialectical Imagination: A History of the Frankfurt School and the Institute of Social
    Research, 1923–1950* (2nd edn). Berkeley, CA: University of California Press.

19. Louis Althusser

(October 1918, Birmendreïs, French Algeria –
22 October 1990, Paris, France)

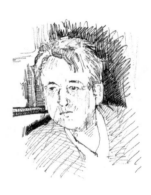

French philosopher

Impact: Structural Marxism.

Contribution: Epistemological break, overdetermination,
ideological state apparatus, interpellation.

Criticism: Complex, neologisms, vague and ambiguous,
historical inaccuracies.

Key works
Althusser, L. (1965) *For Marx.* London: Verso.
Althusser, L. (1965) *Reading Capital.* London: Verso.
Althusser, L. (1968) *Lenin and Philosophy and Other Essays.* New York, NY: Monthly Review
    Press.

Introductory text
Callinicos, A. (1976) *Althusser's Marxism.* London: Pluto Press.

20. Jean-François Lyotard

(10 August 1924, Versailles, France –
21 April 1998, Paris, France)

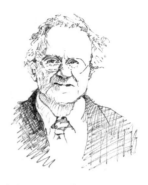

French philosopher and social theorist

Impact: Postmodern thought.

Contribution: The 'postmodern condition', language games, the collapse of the 'grand narrative', the sublime, libidinal economy.

Criticism: Defined groups in language games, destructive nihilism, complex.

Key works

Lyotard, J.-F. (1984) *The Postmodern Condition: A Report on Knowledge*. Manchester: Manchester University Press.

Lyotard, J.-F. (1993) *Libidinal Economy*. London: Athlone.

Lyotard, J.-F. (2011) *Discourse, Figure*. Minneapolis, MN: University of Minnesota Press.

Introductory text

Harvey, R. and Roberts, M. S. (eds) (1993) *Toward the Postmodern*. Atlantic Highlands, NJ: Humanities Press.

21. Richard Rorty

(4 October 1931, New York City, USA – 8 June 2007, Palo Alto, California, USA)

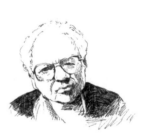

American philosopher

Impact: Epistemology, pragmatism.

Contribution: Post-philosophy, final vocabulary, ironism.

Criticism: Inaccurate readings of others.

Key works

Rorty, R. (1979) *Philosophy and the Mirror of Nature*. Princeton, NJ: Princeton University Press

Rorty, R. (1982) *Consequences of Pragmatism*. Minneapolis, MN: University of Minnesota Press.

Introductory text

Gross, N. (2008) *Richard Rorty: The Making of an American Philosopher*. Chicago: Chicago University Press.

22. Immanuel Kant

(22 April 1724, Königsberg, Prussia – 12 February 1804,
Königsberg, Prussia)

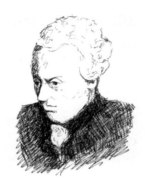

German philosopher

Impact: Kantianism, Western philosophy.

Contribution: Categorical imperative, transcendental
philosophy, synthetic a priori, noumenon.

Criticism: Inaccurate readings of others.

Key works
Kant, I. (1785) *Ground Work for the Metaphysics of Morals*. Riga: Johann Friedrich Hartnoch.
Kant, I. (1787) *Critique of Pure Reason*. Riga: Johann Friedrich Hartnoch.
Kant, I. (1788) *Critique of Practical Reason*. Riga: Johann Friedrich Hartnoch.

Introductory text
Scruton, R. (2001) *Kant: A Very Short Introduction*. Oxford: Oxford University Press.

23. Georg Wilhelm Friedrich Hegel

(27 August 1770, Stuttgart, Germany – 14 November 1831,
Berlin, Germany)

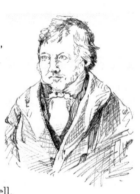

German philosopher

Impact: Hegelianism, German idealism.

Contribution: Absolute idealism, master–slave dialectic,
'sublation' (Aufheben), geist ('mind-spirit'), thesis,
anti-thesis synthesis.

Criticism: Idealism, the rational kernel in a metaphysical shell.

Key works
Hegel, G. W. F. (1910) *Phenomenology of Mind*. Mineola, NY: Dover Publications.
Hegel, G. W. F. (1977) *Phenomenology of Spirit*. Mineola, NY: Dover Publications.

Introductory text
Houlgate, S. (2005) *An Introduction to Hegel: Freedom, Truth and History*. Oxford: Blackwell.

24. Plato

(428/427 BCE, Athens, Greece – 348/347 BCE, Athens, Greece)

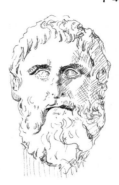

Ancient Greek philosopher

Impact: Platonism, Western philosophy.

Contribution: Rhetoric, art, literature, epistemology, theory of the forms, the cave, ethics and virtue.

Criticism: Aristotle's response.

Key works

Plato (1966) *Phaedo*. Cambridge, MA: Harvard University Press.
Plato (2004) *Republic*. Indianapolis, IN: Hackett.
Plato (1997) *Complete Works*. London: Hackett.

Introductory text

Blackburn, S. (1996) *The Oxford Dictionary of Philosophy*. Oxford: Oxford University Press.

25. Aristotle

(384 BCE, Stagira, Northern Greece – 322 BCE, Euboea, Greece)

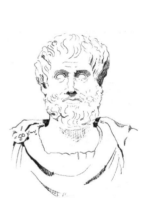

Greek philosopher

Impact: Platonism, Western philosophy.

Contribution: Golden mean, Aristotelian logic, politics, epistemology, ethics.

Criticism: Misogyny and sexism.

Key works

Aristotle (1933) *Metaphysics*. Cambridge, MA: Harvard University Press.
Aristotle (1975) *Nicomachean Ethics*. Grinnell, IA: The Peripatetic Press.
Aristotle (2011) *Eudmenian Ethics*. Oxford: Oxford World Classics.

Introductory text

Cantor, N. F. and Klein, P. L. (eds) (1969) *Ancient Thought: Plato and Aristotle. Monuments of Western Thought 1*. Waltham, MA: Blaisdell Publishing Co.

26. Julia Kristeva

(24 June 1941, Sliven, Bulgaria –)

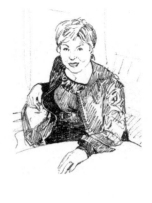

Bulgarian-French philosopher

Impact: Psychoanalysis, sociology and feminism.

Contribution: Literary criticism, semiotics and the pre-mirror stage, abjection.

Criticism: Ethnocentrism, reactionary and persecutory, misogyny and sexism.

Key works

Kristeva, J. (1989) *Black Sun: Depression and Melancholia.* New York: Columbia University Press.

Kristeva, J. (2000) *Crisis of the European Subject.* New York: Other Press.

Introductory text

Moi, T. (ed.) (1986) *The Kristeva Reader.* Oxford: Basil Blackwell.

27. Luce Irigaray

(3 May 1930, Blaton, Bernissart, Wallonia, Belgium –)

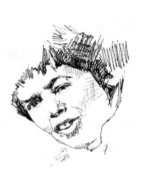

Belgian philosopher

Impact: Psychoanalysis, sociology and feminism.

Contribution: 'Women on the market'.

Criticism: Essentialism.

Key works

Irigaray, L. (1974) *Speculum of the Other Woman.* Ithaca: Cornell University Press.

Irigaray, L. (1977) *This Sex Which Is Not One.* Ithaca: Cornell University Press.

Introductory text

Whitford, M. (ed.) (1992) *The Luce Irigaray Reader.* Oxford: Basil Blackwell.

28. Simone de Beauvoir

(9 January 1908, Paris, France – 14 April 1986, Paris, France)

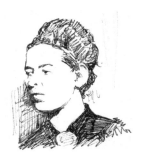

French feminist philosopher

Impact: Feminism.

Contribution: Ethics of ambiguity, feminist ethics, gender studies.

Criticism: Uses patriarchal assumptions.

Key works
de Beauvoir, S. (1949) *The Second Sex*. Oxford: Blackwell.
de Beauvoir, S. (1977) *The Ethics of Ambiguity*. New York, NY: Citadel Press.
de Beauvoir, S. (1981) *Adieux: A Farewell to Sartre*. New York, NY: Pantheon.

Introductory text
Appignanesi, L. (2005) *Simone de Beauvoir*. London: Haus.

29. Auguste Comte

(19 January 1798, Montpellier, France – 5 September 1857, Paris, France)

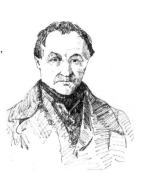

French sociologist

Impact: Sociology.

Contribution: Positivism.

Criticism: Uses crude distinctions.

Key works
Comte, A. (1853) *The Positive Philosophy of Auguste Comte*. Cambridge: Cambridge University Press.
Comte, A. (1865) *A General View of Positivism*. Cambridge: Cambridge University Press.

Introductory text
Macherey, P. (1989) *Comte: La philosophie et les sciences*. Paris: PUF.

30. Ferdinand de Saussure

(26 November 1857, Geneva, Switzerland – 22 February
1913, Vufflens-le-Château, Vaud, Switzerland)

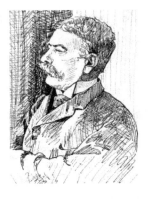

Swiss linguist

Impact: Structuralism and semiotics.

Contribution: Semiology, langue and parole, synchronic
analysis, arbitrariness of the linguistic sign.

Criticism: Outdated.

Key work
de Saussure, F. (1977 [1916]) *Course in General Linguistics*. Glasgow: Fontana/Collins.

Introductory text
Culler, J. (1976) *Saussure*. Glasgow: Fontana/Collins.

31. John Dewey

(20 October 1859, Burlington, Vermont, USA –
1 June 1952, New York City, New York, USA)

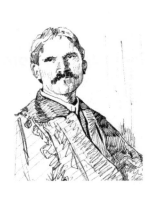

American philosopher, psychologist and educational
reformer

Impact: Pragmatism.

Contribution: Philosophy of education, reflective
thinking, progressive education.

Criticism: Too liberal, uncritical of education.

Key work
Dewey, J. (1909) *Moral Principles in Education*. Cambridge: The Riverside Press.

Introductory text
Hickman, L. and Alexander, T. (1998) *The Essential Dewey: Volumes 1 and 2*. Bloomington,
IN: Indiana University Press.

32. Walter Benjamin

(15 July 1892, Berlin, Germany – 26 September 1940,
Portbou, Spain)

German philosopher

Impact: Western philosophy and humanities.

Contribution: Literary theory, aesthetics, philosophy of
language and history, Arcades project.

Criticism: Challenging writing.

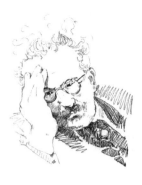

Key works
Benjamin, W. (1936) *The Work of Art in the Age of Mechanical Reproduction*. London: Penguin.
Benjamin, W. (1940) *On the Concept of History/Theses on the Philosophy of History*. New York,
NY: Classic House Books.
Benjamin, W. (2006) *The Writer of Modern Life: Essays on Charles Baudelaire*. Cambridge, MA:
Harvard University Press.

Introductory text
Eiland, H. and Jennings, M. W. (2014) *Walter Benjamin: A Critical Life*. Cambridge, MA and
London: Harvard University Press.

33. Edward Said

(1 November 1935, Jerusalem – 25 September 2003,
New York, USA)

Palestinian-American literary theorist

Impact: Postcolonialism.

Contribution: Occidentalism, Orientalism, the other.

Criticism: Overbearing concept, political propaganda.

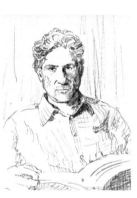

Key works
Said, E. (1993) *Culture and Imperialism*. London: Random House.
Said, E. (1994) *The Politics of Dispossession: The Struggle for Palestinian Self-Determination, 1969–
1994*. London: Random House.

Introductory text
McCarthy, C. (2010) *The Cambridge Introduction to Edward Said*. Cambridge: Cambridge
University Press.

34. Frantz Fanon

(20 July 1925, Fort-de-France, Martinique – 6 December 1961, Bethesda, MD, USA)

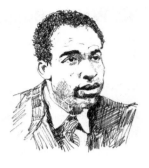

Philosopher

Impact: Postcolonialism and philosophy.

Contribution: Double consciousness, anti-oppressive struggle.

Criticism: Violence and politics.

Key works
Fanon, F. (1952) *Black Skin, White Masks*. New York: Grove Press.
Fanon, F. (1959) *A Dying Colonialism*. New York: Grove Press.
Fanon, F. (1961) *The Wretched of the Earth*. New York: Grove Weidenfeld.

Introductory text
Gendzier, I. (1974) *Frantz Fanon: A Critical Study*. London: Wildwood House.

35. Hannah Arendt

(14 October 1906, Hanover, Germany – 4 December 1975, New York City, USA)

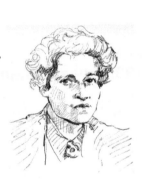

Western philosopher

Impact: Continental philosophy.

Contribution: *Homo faber*, praxis, banality of evil.

Criticism: Too liberal, uncritical of education.

Key works
Arendt, H. (1951) *The Origins of Totalitarianism*. New York: Schocken.
Arendt, H. (1958) *The Human Condition*. Chicago: University of Chicago Press.
Arendt, H. (1963) *Eichmann in Jerusalem: A Report on the Banality of Evil*. New York: Viking.

Introductory text
Young-Bruehl, E. (1982) *Hannah Arendt: For Love of the World*. New York: Yale University Press.

36. Homi Bhabha

(1949, Mumbai, India –)

Indian philosopher

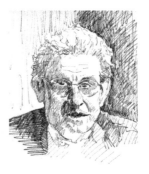

Impact: Post-colonial theory.

Contribution: Third space, enunciatory present.

Criticism: Indecipherable jargon.

Key work
Bhabha, H. (1994) *The Location of Culture*. London: Routledge.

Introductory text
Huddart, D. (2006) *Homi K. Bhabha*. London: Routledge.

37. Guy Debord

(28 December 1931, Paris, France – 30 November 1994,
Bellevue-la-Montagne, Haute-Loire, France)

French situationist philosopher

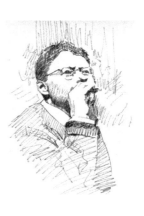

Impact: Situationism.

Contribution: Spectacle, détournement, psychogeography,
derive, recuperation.

Criticism: Indecipherable jargon.

Key work
Debord, G. (1991) *The Society of the Spectacle*. Paris: Plon.

Introductory text
Hussy, A. (2001) *The Game of War: The Life and Death of Guy Debord*. London: Cape.

38. Edmund Husserl

(8 April 1859, Prostějov, Czech Republic – 27 April 1938, Freiburg, Germany)

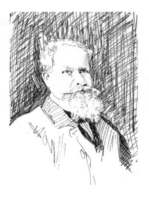

German phenomenological philosopher

Impact: Phenomenology, epistemology.

Contribution: Phenomenology, epoché, reduction.

Criticism: Indecipherable jargon.

Key works

Husserl, E. (1973) *Logical Investigations*. London: Routledge.
Husserl, E. (1965) *Phenomenology and the Crisis of Philosophy*. New York: Harper & Row.
Husserl, E. (1960 [1931]) *Cartesian Meditations*. Dordrecht: Kluwer.

Introductory text

Bernet, R., Kern, I. and Marbach, E. (1993) *Introduction to Husserlian Phenomenology*. Evanston, IL: Northwestern University Press.

39. Francis Bacon

(22 January 1561, Strand, London – 9 April 1626, Highgate, Middlesex, UK)

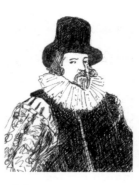

English empiricist philosopher

Impact: Empiricism, epistemology.

Contribution: Baconian method, scientific method, knowledge comes from sense experience, Novum Organum (new method).

Criticism: One-dimensional view of the development of knowledge.

Key works

Bacon, F. (1597) (1st edn) *Essays*. London: William Pickering.
Bacon, F. (1605) *The Advancement and Proficiency of Learning Divine and Human*. London: Cassell and Company.
Bacon, F. (1612) (2nd edn – 38 essays) *Essays*. London: William Pickering.
Bacon, F. (1620) *Novum Organum Scientiarum* [New Method]. Boston, MA: Taggard and Thompson.

Introductory text

Rossi, P. (1978) *Francis Bacon: From Magic to Science*. London: Taylor & Francis.

40. Isaac Newton

(25 December 1642, Woolsthorpe, Lincolnshire –
20 March 1726, Kensington, UK)

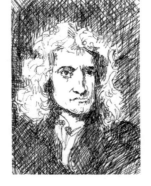

English founding father of scientific method

Impact: Enlightenment philosopher, scientific revolution, epistemology.

Contribution: Laws of motion, gravitation, Newtonian mechanics.

Criticism: Sets the standard for future scientific research.

Key works

Newton, I. (1999) *The Principia: Mathematical Principles of Natural Philosophy.* California: University of California Press.

Newton, I. (1728) *De mundi systemate.* London: J. Tonson, J. Osborn and T. Longman.

Introductory text

Andrade, E. N. De C. (1950) *Isaac Newton.* New York: Chanticleer Press.

41. John Locke

(23 August 1632, Somerset, UK – 28 October 1704, Essex, UK)

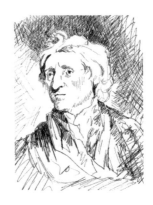

British philosopher

Impact: Enlightenment philosophy, epistemology.

Contribution: Social contract, table rasa (blank slate), natural law.

Criticism: Sets the standard for future scientific research.

Key works

Locke, J. (1689) *Two Treatises of Government.* London: Forgotten Books.

Locke, J. (1690) *An Essay Concerning Human Understanding.* Ware, UK: Wordsworth Editions.

Locke, J. (1693) *Some Thoughts Concerning Education.* Cambridge: Cambridge University Press.

Introductory text

Yolton, J. W. (1969) *John Locke: Problems and Perspectives.* Cambridge: Cambridge University Press.

42. Socrates

(469 BCE – 399 BCE, Greece)

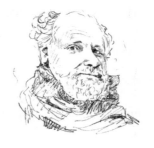

Ancient Greek philosopher

Impact: Founder of Western philosophy.

Contribution: Socratic method, Socratic irony.

Criticism: Oral tradition.

Key works
Through the accounts of classical writers

Introductory text
Rudebusch, G. (2009) *Socrates*. Oxford: Wiley-Blackwell.

43. George Berkeley

(12 March 1685, Kilkenny, Ireland – 14 January 1753,
Oxford, UK)

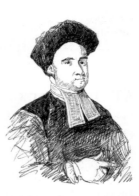

Anglo-Irish philosopher

Impact: Enlightenment philosopher, epistemology.

Contribution: Subjective idealism, master argument.

Criticism: Too idealistic.

Key works
Berkeley, G. (1709) *An Essay towards a New Theory of Vision*. Ann Arbor, MI: University of
    Michigan Library.
Berkeley, G. (1710) *A Treatise Concerning the Principles of Human Knowledge*, Part I. Cambridge,
    MA: Hackett Classics.

Introductory text
Daniel, S. H. (ed.) (2007) *Re-examining Berkeley's Philosophy*. Toronto: University of Toronto
    Press.

44. Gayatri Chakravorty Spivak

(24 February 1942, Calcutta, India –)

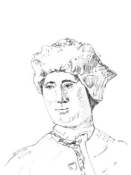

Indian scholar and translator

Impact: Postcolonial philosopher.

Contribution: Subaltern, strategic essentialism, epistemological performance, deconstruction.

Criticism: Style over substance.

Key works
Spivak, G. C. (2007) *Can the Subaltern Speak*. Austria: Turia and Kant.
Spivak, G. C. (1976) *Of Grammatology*. Baltimore: Johns Hopkins University Press.
Spivak, G. C. (1987) *In Other Worlds: Essays in Cultural Politics*. London: Routledge.
Spivak, G. C. (1988) *Selected Subaltern Studies*. Oxford: Oxford University Press.
Spivak, G. C. (1990) *The Post-Colonial Critic – Interviews, Strategies, Dialogues*. London: Routledge.
Spivak, G. C. (1993) *Outside in the Teaching Machine*. London: Routledge.
Spivak, G. C. (1999) *A Critique of Postcolonial Reason: Towards a History of the Vanishing Present*. Cambridge, MA: Harvard University Press.

Introductory text
Morton, S. (2007) *Gayatri Spivak: Ethics, Subalternity and the Critique of Postcolonial Reason*. Cambridge: Polity.

45. David Hume

(7 May 1711, Edinburgh, Scotland – 25 August 1776, Edinburgh, Scotland)

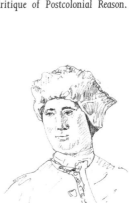

Scottish enlightenment philosopher

Impact: Empiricism.

Contribution: Problem of causation, induction, is-ought problem, epistemology.

Criticism: Hesitant realist.

Key works
Hume, D. (1777 [1748]) *An Enquiry Concerning Human Understanding*. London: A. Millar.
Hume, D. (1739) *A Treatise of Human Nature*. London: John Noon.
Hume, D. (1779) *Dialogues Concerning Natural Religion*. Cambridge, MA: Hackett Classics.
Hume, D. (1741) *Essays, Moral and Political*. Edinburgh: A. Kincaid.

Introductory text
Ardal, P. (1966) *Passion and Value in Hume's Treatise*. Edinburgh: Edinburgh University Press.

46. Karl Popper

(28 July 1902, Vienna, Austria – 17 September 1994, London, UK)

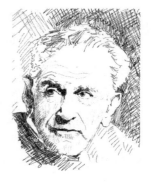

Austrian philosopher of science

Impact: Empiricism.

Contribution: Problem of induction, falsification, tyranny of totalitarianism.

Criticism: Too liberal.

Key works
Popper, K. (1934) *The Logic of Scientific Discovery*. London: Routledge.
Popper, K. (1945) *The Open Society and Its Enemies*. London: Routledge and Kegan Paul.
Popper, K. (1963) *Conjectures and Refutations: The Growth of Scientific Knowledge*. London: Routledge and Kegan Paul.

Introductory text
Magee, B. (1977) *Popper*. London: Fontana.

47. Thomas Aquinas

(28 January 1225, Sicily, Italy – 7 March 1274, Fassonova, Italy)

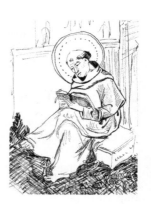

Italian theologian and scholar

Impact: Epistemology and ethics.

Contribution: Problem of induction, falsification, tyranny of totalitarianism.

Criticism: Confusion of faith and reason.

Key works
Aquinas, T. (1254) *On Being and Essence*. Cambridge, MA: Hackett Classics.
Aquinas, T. (1257) *Disputed Questions on Truth*. London: Sage.

Introductory text
Grabmann, M. and Virgil, M. (2006) *Thomas Aquinas: His Personality and Thought*. Montana: Kessinger.

48. Erving Goffman

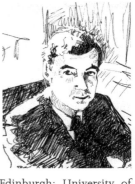

(11 June 1922, Mannville, Alberta, Canada – 19 November 1982, Philadelphia, Pennsylvania, USA)

Canadian sociologist

Impact: Everyday life, interactionism.

Contribution: Sociology of everyday life, symbolic interactionism, dramaturgy.

Criticism: Confusion of faith and reason.

Key works

Goffman, E. (1959) *The Presentation of Self in Everyday Life.* Edinburgh: University of Edinburgh Social Sciences Research Centre.

Goffman, E. (1961) *Asylums: Essays on the Social Situation of Mental Patients and Other Inmates.* New York: Doubleday.

Goffman, E. (1963) *Stigma: Notes on the Management of Spoiled Identity.* London: Penguin.

Goffman, E. (1974) *Frame Analysis: An Essay on the Organization of Experience.* London: Harper and Row.

Introductory text

Burns, T. (1992) *Erving Goffman.* London and New York: Routledge.

49. Sigmund Freud

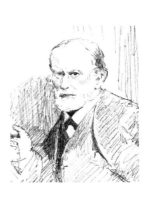

(6 May 1856, Freiberg, Austria – 23 September 1939, Hampstead, London, UK)

Austrian psychoanalyst

Impact: Psychoanalysis.

Contribution: Unconscious, Id, ego, super ego, dreams as the royal road to the unconscious, Eros and Thanatos.

Criticism: From feminism.

Key works

Freud, S. (1900) *The Interpretation of Dreams.* New York, NY: Basic Books.

Freud, S. (1904) *The Psychopathology of Everyday Life.* New York, NY: Dover Publications.

Freud, S. (1913) *Totem and Taboo: Resemblances between the Psychic Lives of Savages and Neurotics.* Boston, MA: Random House.

Freud, S. (1915–17) *Introductory Lectures on Psycho-Analysis.* London: Penguin.

Freud, S. (1920) *Beyond the Pleasure Principle.* New York, NY: Liverights Publishing.

Freud, S. (1923) *The Ego and the Id.* London: W.W. Norton and Co.

Freud, S. (1926) *Inhibitions, Symptoms and Anxiety.* London: W.W. Norton and Co.

Freud, S. (1930) *Civilization and Its Discontents.* London: Hogarth Press.

Introductory text

Brown, N. O. (1985) *Life Against Death: The Psychoanalytic Meaning of History.* Hanover, NH: Wesleyan University Press.

50. Karl Marx

(5 May 1818, Trier, Germany – 14 March 1883, London, UK).

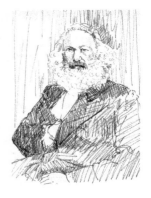

German philosopher

Impact: Marxism.

Contribution: Surplus value, theory of labour, class struggle, false consciousness, materialist conception of history.

Criticism: Utopian.

Key works

Marx, K. (1844) *Economic and Philosophic Manuscripts.* New York, NY: Prometheus Books.
Marx, K. (1848) *The Manifesto of the Communist Party.* New Haven, CT: Yale University Press.
Marx, K. (1857) *Grundrisse.* London: Penguin.
Marx, K. (1867) *Kapital.* Ware: Wordsworth Editions.

Introductory text
McLellan, D. (2006) *Karl Marx: A Biography.* Hampshire: Palgrave MacMillan.

51. Giorgio Agamben

(22 April 1942, Rome, Italy –)

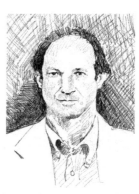

Italian philosopher

Impact: Continental philosophy.

Contribution: State of exception, from of life, homo sacer, biopolitics, the coming community.

Criticism: Utopian.

Key works

Agamben, G. (1995) *Homo Sacer: Sovereign Power and Bare Life.* Stanford, CA: Stanford University Press.
Agamben, G. (2003) *State of Exception.* Chicago: Chicago University Press.
Agamben, G. (2013) *Opus Dei: An Archeology of Duty.* Stanford, CA: Stanford University Press.
Agamben, G. (1998) *Remnants of Auschwitz: The Witness and the Archive.* Cambridge, MA: MIT Press.

Introductory text
Mills, C. (2006) *The Philosophy of Giorgio Agamben.* Montreal: McGill-Queen's University Press.

52. Susan Bordo

(24 January 1947, Newark, New Jersey, USA –)

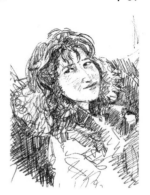

American feminist

Impact: Gender and women's studies.

Contribution: Surplus value, theory of labour, class struggle, false consciousness, materialist conception of history.

Criticism: Utopian.

Key works

Bordo, S. (1987) *The Flight to Objectivity: Cartesianism and Culture.* Albany, NY: State University of New York Press.

Bordo, S. (1993) *Unbearable Weight: Feminism, Western Culture and the Body.* Oakland, CA: University of California Press.

Bordo, S. (1997) *Twilight Zones: The Hidden Life of Cultural Images from Plato to O.J.* Oakland, CA: University of California Press.

Introductory text

Welton, D. (ed.) (1998) *Body and Flesh: A Philosophical Reader.* Malden, MA: Blackwell.

Conclusion

The philosophical traditions of thought contribute to the resources available for critical reflective practice and are an introduction to the ideas, morals and practice that informs reflection.

Having charted the major philosophers, a note of caution is worth introducing. A story has many interpretations and this is one way of presenting the history of ideas and the sources or resources available for the reflective practitioner to put into practice. The use of visual presentations of each philosopher provides a different cognitive register into which the philosophical contribution can be located. The order and presentation of each philosopher is from one vantage point or can be an arbitrary choice and it remains for the reader to impose their own order on the contributions of each philosopher.

The philosophers can help; for example, Foucault on *The Order of Things* and *The Archaeology of Knowledge* provides ways to locate ideas in dominant discourses and to examine and explore the rules of formation or regimes of truth that surround different philosophical systems. The presentation allows for a 'cut out and keep' resource of philosophers that can contribute to a 'top trumps' of philosophy to explore and expound the relative merits and criticism of each individual. Played like a game of cards, individuals can be grouped together to form 'schools of thought' or traditions or histories of ideas to add dynamism and playfulness to learning about philosophy. It also addresses that age old comment of 'whether the book has pictures'.

Reference

Seedhouse, D. (2009) (3rd edn) *Ethics: The Heart of Health Care.* Chichester: Wiley.

Chapter 3
Values and ethics for professionals

Adam Barnard

Chapter outline

This chapter will introduce:

- the field of values and ethics in health and social care
- traditions or schools of thought in ethics
- the distinction between ethical issues and ethical dilemmas
- the call for a contextual, embodied critically reflective ethics.

The ethics of professionalism is a murky terrain of swampy lowlands and this discussion will provide a navigable chart through value-based perspectives and the ethics of professionalism. Taking a historical approach, the shifts in values and ethics are mapped to arrive at a horizon of possibilities for ethical practice. Illustrative examples allow engagement with ethical debate in practice and provide fertile ground to explore the ethics of professionalism.

It has long been argued that health and social care is a value-based form of professional activity. In the field of a professional ethics, 'values' usually take the form of general ethical principles relating to how professionals should treat the people they work with and what sorts of actions are regarded as right or wrong. Vigilante (1974) calls values the 'fulcrum of practice', Bernstein (1970) suggests they offer 'vision and discernment' and Younghusband (1967) suggests they are 'everywhere in practice'. Timms (1983) pleaded for 'value-talk' to be central to health and social work. Values have a rich and detailed history and an exploration of the historical emergence of those values allows us to gain some purchase on the present, and to explore contemporary controversies and dilemmas.

There are four spheres in health and social care values and ethics. The first area is the more abstract field of moral philosophy that forms a backdrop to ethical debates in health and social care. The second area is the distinct forms of legislation that have created the context for health and social care practice alongside providing legal responses to particular health and social care issues and cases. The third area is the domain of political ideologies and the way that these have shaped and sculpted health and social care models, methods and practices. The final area is the historical emergence of health and social care as a profession and the struggle for a professional identity that has engaged health and social care workers. Broad reviews of ethics and moral philosophy can be found in Hamlyn (1987), Rachel (2003) and Grayling (2004).

Firstly, a word on how we can understand the change in ideas about values and ethics. Thomas Kuhn's The Structure of Scientific Revolutions became one of the most influential books of the twentieth century. Kuhn, as a physicist turned philosopher of science, conducted research to teach a course on the history of science to humanities students at Harvard in the 1960s (Holloway 2005: 63). Kuhn's picture of the development of scientific ideas, and by extension ideas in general, did not fit with the 'common-sense' or 'customary' view. This would suggest that ideas develop in a piecemeal, evolutionary and cumulative way, each idea building on the contribution of previous generations.

Kuhn's work revolutionised this common-sense or customary view by suggesting that ideas develop in a much more dramatic and interruptive process. He used the term 'paradigm' to express the 'constellation of beliefs, assumptions and techniques' that hold sway at a given point in time. People are socialised into a paradigm and it becomes the accepted 'world view' or 'received idea' (Rojeck et al. 1988) of a particular community. Paradigms dominate a period of 'normal science' where a community engages in simple puzzle solving rather than raising any challenging or difficult questions about the paradigm itself. There is a high degree of social control in the adherence to the paradigm. The growth of anomalies, which do not fit this paradigm or received idea stand out due to the strong attachment to a paradigm. Kuhn argues when these anomalies become unbearable, science enters a period of crisis when a more far-reaching and speculative acceptance of a new paradigm emerges. This process results in a 'paradigm shift' or scientific revolution that overthrows the previous world of knowledge and replaces it with a new world view.

The classic paradigm shift in science is the move from Aristotelian to Copernican astronomy. The classical world view saw the cosmos as a series of concentric circles with the Earth fixed at the centre. The planets moved around the Earth with nothing beyond them except the realm of God (Holloway 2005: 65). This was the big story throughout Europe for centuries until the anomalies identified by Copernicus prompted the search for a new paradigm that could accommodate the troublesome anomalies. The Copernican revolution shifted the paradigm of the universe to locate the Sun at the centre of our system and develop a 'helio-centric' world view. We could suggest Einstein overturned the world of Newton and brought about a new paradigm in physics. It is now widely accepted that a vision of 'flat Earth' is discredited and we accept the shifting ground of plate tectonics as the composition of the world.

We can provide a further example of the power of the paradigm drawn from child-care policy. Lorraine Fox Harding (1997) has identified four paradigms or value positions in child-care policy. The first paradigm is laissez faire and patriarchy up to the mid-nineteenth century that sought to preserve family privacy, and by which parents, particularly fathers, had power over children with minimal state intervention. The image of a disciplinarian Victorian patriarch holds sway. This is 'the view that power in the family should not be disturbed except in extreme circumstances, and the role of the state should be a minimal one' (Fox Harding 1997: 9). By the end of the nineteenth century 'state paternalism and child protection' emerged. This saw the protection of children by an emerging group of (female) professionals. This is associated with the growth of state intervention in the late nineteenth and early twentieth centuries. State intervention is often authoritarian, biological family bonds undervalued and good-quality care substituted. The criticism of state paternalism in the post–Second World War period attempted to defend families from heavy-handed state intervention and offer greater levels of help and support. This saw 'kinship defenders or defence of the birth family' emerge as a dominant paradigm. The final paradigm in relation to child protection is the 'children's rights and child liberation' perspective. Children are now seen as the bearers of rights and able to participate in decision-making processes.

Fox Harding's work shows the historic paradigmatic shifts of value positions in relation to child-care policy in social work theory and practice. Having examined the way in which ideas develop, we can turn our attention to the paradigm shifts that are evident in social work and social care values. We have provided a flavour of this process with Fox Harding above but will extend this argument.

The following discussion examines the broad historical changes in values within health and social care. Further reading is provided at the end of the chapter for those wanting to examine the philosophical basis to values, ethics and social work. There have been a multitude of varied value systems that could have been selected. For example, the Arab world, Africa and China have all contributed philosophical discussion to questions of values. Similarly, the rich and varied sets of values that can be derived from various religious systems will not be explored nor will we explore the policy implications of these key values.

Values at work and the values of professions

In a working context it is necessary to have agreed standards of behaviour. For example, some behaviour and action in a non-work environment is unacceptable in a professional working environment. A sexual or romantic relationship is not acceptable between a professional such as a social worker, teacher or doctor and a service user, patient or pupil, even when both parties are consenting adults (Beckett and Maynard 2013).

❖ ACTIVITY 1

When you visit a doctor, what expectations would you have of him or her in terms of standards of conduct? How do these expectations differ from those you would have of a friend?

You would expect your doctor not to pass on information to others without your express permission and consent. With a friend you might work on the assumption that you can pass on news unless you made it clear that you did not want this to happen (Beckett and Maynard 2013: 81).

You would expect doctors to keep themselves up to date with the health problems you present with and possess a level of knowledge and skill about recognising and treating your illness (Beckett and Maynard 2013: 81). You would want a doctor to have contemporary and current knowledge on their recommendations for treatment, not to have dreamt how to treat you.

You would expect your doctor to be able to examine intimate parts of your body without it being sexual or altering the relationship with the doctor (Beckett and Maynard 2013: 81).

You would expect your doctor to provide you with a service regardless of personal feelings for you as a person (Beckett and Maynard 2013: 81).

You would expect uniform and consistent standards of behaviour between professionals.

Ethics

Ethics is a word that has several meanings but is narrower and more specific than values. Ethics relates to our overall stance on life or our general notions of what is important (Beckett and Maynard 2013: 20), our moral compass or the traditions of thought or philosophical schools we draw upon to inform how we 'go on' in everyday life. Beckett and Maynard (2013: 20) also suggest that ethics refer to actual rules and principles of conduct and ethics are the practical application of values. Dubois and Miley (2008: 111) recommend that 'whereas values are the implicit or explicit beliefs about what people consider good, ethics relates to what people consider correct or right'.

There are a number of approaches, or traditions, or schools or histories of ideas that underpin ethics and values. These are utilitarianism, deontology, virtue and an ethics of care.

Utilitarianism – consequentialism

Consequentialism, based strongly on the political tradition of liberalism and utilitarianism, is concerned with the outcomes, results or consequences of actions and how far actions promote intrinsic goods like happiness or pleasure. Actions are right in as far as they promote happiness for utilitarians. The strength of consequentialism is its intuitive appeal. It makes sense to say those things are good that promote happiness. There are problems with this approach. For example, what counts as happiness; how can you measure it; it uses a crude calculation that does not allow for individual differences or preferences; is this the same between peoples, cultures and societies; what duration do you count; it is an unrealistic ethics; and are there other motivations for ethics? Most difficult, the idea of consequences promoting happiness can lead to atrocities rather than the greater good. Finally, consequentialism considers individuals as moral saints who do not have a moral obligation or special responsibilities to others. For example, should we give all our money to charity or do we have a special responsibility to family? For example, if you are given a test of your courage to execute one of your party so the rest can go free, consequentialism would suggest you should on a simple calculation, but most people would consider individuals have 'integrity' (Smart and Williams 1973: 98–117) or a special responsibility to the group (Sidgwick 1981).

Utilitarianism and consequentialism have been used to promote the idea of public welfare. Actions that lead to an overall aggregate of happiness are morally right actions (Goodin 1995; Bailey 1997). This moral perspective is often contrasted with deontology and Kantian ethics.

Deontology

Deontologists such as Kant (1991) reject consequentialism and utilitarianism, arguing it is principles that justify certain actions, that is those things that come before or precede actions, not the consequences. Kant's ethics have received sustained examination (O'Neill 1989; Baron 1995) and he provides a different basis for ethics. '[T]he ground of obligation must be looked for, not in the nature of man nor in the circumstances of the world in which he is placed, but solely *a priori* in the concepts of pure reason' (Kant 1991: 55).

With reason as the capacity to make decisions, people make moral laws from ethical principles or maxims. A hypothetical imperative is when you do something to achieve something else, or 'if ... then' decisions (Fitzpatrick 2008: 46), such as work hard to succeed. These are instrumental goods or using one thing to achieve another. Intrinsic goods are those that are good in themselves such as human well-being or flourishing or happiness. This leads to Kant's famous formulation of the categorical imperative in *Groundwork*: 'I ought never to act except in such a way that I can also will that my maxim should become a universal law' (Kant 1991: 67). As such, Kant provides a universal ethical theory that the way we act should be generalised to everyone, and everyone should have a duty to uphold this universal moral law.

Fitzpatrick (2008: 46) argues that Kant identifying the capacity to reason, and the demand to recognise others' rationality, leads him to a second formulation of the categorical imperative to 'act in such a way that you always treat humanity, whether in your own person or in the person of any other, never simply as a means, but always at the same time as an end' (Kant 1991: 9). In a 'kingdom of ends' we would all recognise each other's ability to reason, act according to universal laws of morality and treat each other with respect (for our reason and duty to laws). This has the derived principle of 'respect for others' that has become central to health and social care. Commentators, such as Fitzpatrick (2008: 47) argue this 'is the core of what for many is the most persuasive model of liberalism: one based on the freedom of rational being to observe the laws and duties of universal reason in a moral and social system of mutual respect'.

There are many criticisms levelled at Kant's ethics (MacIntyre 1967: ch. 14). It is too formal and rigid; it is abstract and too distant from everyday life; it is emotionless, treating individuals as moral robots; it requires an unquestioning duty to morality rather than being moral; and it excludes consequences. Kant is also seen as too universalist, too rational, too Western (Fitzpatrick 2008: 86). Deontology is strong on individual autonomy, but poor on social justice. It is an atomistic ethics that requires a reasoning subject or individual who has an emotionless obedience to the rules. Focusing on universal laws ignores consequences to try to militate against certain undesirable effects. Kant's emphasis on the kingdom of ends means that there will always be a presumption in favour of the individual's sovereignty, their inherent moral worth, an important point whenever the actual consent of agents is difficult to obtain (Fitzpatrick 2008: 87), such as in end-of-life decisions.

Virtue

Driver (2007: 136) suggests dissatisfaction with utility and Kant over their abstract and emotionless ethics has led commentators to consider the agent or actor rather than their actions or principles. Aristotle sees virtue as leading to *eudaimonia* or human well-being. Aristotle's virtue ethics have been characterised as the 'doctrine of the mean' where virtues lie between two vices or extremes. For example, bravery lies between cowardice and foolhardiness, and temperance lies between gluttony and abstinence. For Aristotle, the ends of actions are moral if they fulfil the functions of human nature, the good being a flourishing of human potential, and virtue ethics updates this position. MacIntyre (1985) has made a significant contribution to contemporary virtue ethics.

It has been argued that virtue ethicists overemphasise common humanity, do not provide a guide for action and deny contemporary findings in psychology (Driver 2007: 150). The relationship of social justice can also be problematic for virtuists. Virtues change over time and place. The strength of virtue ethics is in the indeterminancy of moral decisions against the calculus of utilitarians and the moral imperatives of Kantians.

Ethics of care

Emotional responsiveness is a key element of an ethics of care which is associated with feminism (Banks 2012: 77). An ethics of care has refocused ethical considerations to connections, relationships and practice rather than a virtue, or quality or characteristic.

Tronto (1993) and Sevenhuijsen (1998) characterise care as a social practice or a collective human activity with a distinct purpose based on shared values or an ethics of care. It 'focuses on social relations and the social practices and value that sustain them' (Held 2006: 20).

Gilligan (1982) identified two 'moral voices' in interviews she conducted, suggesting an ethics of justice and an ethics of care. An ethics of justice is the principle base of utilitarian and Kantian moralities emphasising rights and duties, abstract moral principles impartiality and rationality. This is compared to a feminist emphasis on responsibility rather than duty and consequences, relationships rather than principles.

An ethics of care has been extended to include five phases (Tronto 1993: 127–36):

1   Attentiveness: noticing the need for care in the first place – actively seeking awareness of others and their needs and points of view (of caring about).
2   Responsibility: assuming responsibility for care – with responsibility being embedded in a set of implicit cultural practices, rather than a set of formal rules (taking care of).
3   Competency: the actual work of care that needs to be done – one's ability to do something about another's needs (care giving).
4   Responsiveness: the response of a person who is cared for to the care giving – remaining alert to the possibilities of abuse that arise from the care receiver's vulnerability.
5   Integrity of care: the four phases fitting together as a whole, involving knowledge of the context of the care process and making judgements about conflicting needs and strategies. These judgements require assessment of need in social and political and personal contexts.

Banks (2011) speaks of a 'situated ethics of social justice' that takes social justice as its starting point and qualifies it by its situatedness. She provides a six-point plan:

1   Radical social justice. A base line of equality of opportunities but an engagement with oppression and injustice for individuals, groups and cultures.
2   Empathic solidarity. Involves abilities of critical analysis and critical thinking in the context of professional activity.
3   Relational autonomy. Power as moral agents to work for 'power with' others, including service users.
4   Collective responsibility for resistance. Good and just practice and resisting bad practice. Autonomy is relational in the context of oppressive and constraining structures. Constructive alliances of professionals, workers, service users and sharing responsibility to promote social justice.
5   Moral courage. The disposition to act in difficult, challenging and uncomfortable situations.
6   Working in complexity and contradictions. Working in space of care and control, prevention and enforcement, empathy and equity (Banks 2011).

The various traditions or schools of thought provide guidance on the attempt to resolve ethical issues in practice and current extensions have added a more situated, virtue-based move towards social justice. For health and social care practitioners, medical ethics adds to the context of ethical issues.

Medical ethics

Medical ethics is a system of moral principles that applies to values, judgement and decision making in medicine. It is also the practical application in clinical settings of medical ethics.

The BMA suggests there are different approaches used in medicine such as giving priority to the principles that should guide decisions, focusing more on the outcomes or consequences of decisions and giving priority to the inner dispositions or virtues of the decision maker (BMA 2015). Although not advocating a particular approach, there are key concepts in ethical decision making in health and medicine that need to be considered.

Self-determination

The ability to decide and to act for oneself is referred to as 'autonomy'. The most obvious expression of self-determination is the right of competent adults to refuse any proposed medical intervention, even where the decision may result in death. The only exception is compulsory treatment under mental health legislation such as the Mental Capacity Act.

Capacity or competence

This is not a principle itself but a key concept in medical ethics. The capacity or competence to make a decision is ordinarily a prerequisite for a decision to be respected. A decision by someone lacking capacity to refuse life-sustaining treatment can be overridden.

Confidentiality

A respect for the confidences of patients is central to good medical practice. The right of adult patients to control their private information is linked to the principle of self-determination. The consequences of not respecting confidences could include patients withholding relevant information and a loss of trust in the medical profession.

Honesty and truth-telling

This is the communication of information in ways that are believed to be truthful and that are not intended to deceive the recipient. It can be thought of as a virtue in health professionals and also as a prerequisite for a respect for patient self-determination.

Benefit and harm

To do good and avoid harm are among the oldest exhortations in medicine. Often in medicine though the good can only be achieved at the risk of harm. Medical interventions are ordinarily justified where the anticipated benefits exceed the harms. There can be disagreement about how benefit and harm are interpreted. A patient can be harmed for example by having life-saving treatment that she rejects being imposed upon her.

Fairness or equity

There are a range of issues here. People should be treated fairly – people with equal needs should be given equal consideration – and should not be discriminated against in the provision of health services. On a wider level, health services should also be distributed according to good moral reasons and not arbitrarily or because of resources.

Rights

In addition to relevant legal rights, such as the right to refuse treatment, these also point to the idea that human beings have certain moral rights which relate to basic human interests or entitlements that simply cannot be taken from them, irrespective of how much benefit may accrue to others.

Medical ethics have received sustained treatment from, for example, Seedhouse (2009). Beauchamp and Childress (2001) suggest respect for autonomy, beneficence or doing good, non-maleficence or doing no harm, and justice of distributing benefits and risks are the founding principles of medical ethics.

In considering ethical dilemmas, there is often an acute sense of confusion, anxiety, guilt and regret about ethical judgements and decisions. Banks (2011) suggests 'developing a capacity of critical reflection and reflexivity is much more than simply learning procedures or demonstrating competencies'. Ethical problems that have a resolution (Thompson et al. 2000) and ethical problems that do not require a critical and reflective engagement with the situation, and the various stakeholders, demand a consideration of the options available.

Limitations of cases and codes

Banks (2009: 57) expresses concerns at the overuse of 'ethical dilemmas' and case studies when teaching professional ethics as 'the focus in professional ethics textbooks on difficult cases makes it seem as if "ethical issues" only arise when a problematic or difficult case arises'.

Banks (2009) outlines three traditional approaches to professional ethics. The first approach is the tendency to associate both the study and practice of 'professional ethics' with professional codes. Ethics becomes conformity to rules, procedures and standards such as filling out an ethics form before conducting research or working within a crude set of procedural rules. The second approach is focused upon conduct or the actions of professional practitioner and make reference to codes of conduct. The third approach is to abstract cases from their context, remove character, emotion or circumstance from ethical consideration. This focuses on clinical case studies or decision-making processes in resolving ethical dilemmas.

Banks (2009) suggests that ethics is embedded in everyday life as well as professional life and the scope of professional ethics should be broadened from codes, conduct and cases to include commitment, character and context. This would include ethics as situated, and address contemporary issues of ethics such as moral phenomenology, care ethics and virtue ethics.

We could approach ethics in professional life following models such as Gallagher's ETHICS framework: Enquire about facts, Think through options, Hear views, Identify principles, Clarify meaning, Select action (Gallagher and Sykes 2008). Alternatively, we could follow Banks and Gallagher (2009):

1 Seeing ethics everywhere. Rather than separating ethics as a discrete area of study and abstracting ethical issues from practice learning, we can see ethics as embedded in practice learning and across the curriculum.

2 Working with contextualised living stories/accounts. In addition to working with short cases framed as dilemmas or involving difficult decisions, students and practitioners can be encouraged to give longer, more personal narrative accounts of their everyday professional lives, including their feelings, imaginings, hopes and fears.

3 Balancing logic (analysis) with passion (feelings, emotions, imagination). While recognising the importance in professional work of being able to justify decisions, reason logically and argue coherently, it is equally important to develop the capacities of students and practitioners to be morally perceptive, sensitive and compassionate.

4 Use of role plays, simulation, literature, poetry, drama. In education and training for the social professions the use of role play and other creative methods is well established, especially in teaching communication skills. These approaches are equally valuable in learning and teaching about ethics.

5 Focusing on developing the capacities of practitioners to do 'ethics work'. The idea of 'ethics work' is a development of Hochschild's (1983) concept of 'emotion work', which she introduced in relation to her study of flight attendants to encapsulate the work that goes into being caring, attentive and compassionate in situations where this would not be our natural response. We could characterise as 'ethics work' the hospice social worker's use of her imagination and moral sensitivity. Ethics work involves emotion work, but has added dimensions of:
- moral perception or attentiveness to the salient moral features of situations
- recognition of the political context of practice and the practitioner's own professional power (reflexivity)
- the moral struggle to be a good practitioner – maintaining personal and professional integrity while carrying out the requirements of the agency role. This would include handling the moral distress that comes from seeing what ought to be done but not being able to do it. It involves developing the moral qualities of courage and professional wisdom.

The development of a situated and philosophically informed consideration of ethics is a significant step forward in teaching and learning and doing ethics work. It returns ethical dilemmas to everyday life and situated understanding of what it means to be an ethical practitioner. Reflecting ethically or the ethical reflective practitioner is part of the becoming professional in health and social care.

Banks (2009) calls for an extension of ethics in professional life as a broadened philosophical project to move beyond rational, principle-based action to include virtues, relationships and emotions. We could extend this call to include a situated, contextual and corporeal consideration of ethics. Reflection is the vehicle or mechanism or way to improve these considerations and an interpretive phenomenological approach (Benner 1994) the way to put flesh on the bones of reflective ethical concerns.

❖ ACTIVITY 2

Consider what it means to be unprofessional? Think of instances of behaviour on the part of a health and social care worker – or another professional – which you would regard as unprofessional.

What does unprofessional mean?

What do we mean by acting in an unprofessional way (Beckett and Maynard 2013: 83)?

❖ ACTIVITY 3

Draw up a list of contracting ground rules that will lead to ethical activities. The table below shows examples of how previous groups have responded to the activity.

Issues raised	Issues raised previously	Suggested ground rules
Confidentiality and its limits	Avoid conflict	● Acceptance
Respect for others/ people not behaviour	Elegant and legitimate challenging	● Confidentiality
Challenging tactfully	Difficulty of being 'put on the spot'	● Trust
Participation, contribution, involvement	Competition versus cooperation and help	● Respect
Listening	Respect for others (others' opinions)	● Acknowledge and respect difference
Punctuality and habits (e.g. phones)	Respect for differences	● Positive feedback
Preparation and organisation	Non-judgemental	● Constructive criticism
'Turn taking'	'Turn taking'	● Listen
Allowing space and time to express	Encouragement	● Honesty
Non-judgementalism	'Ice breaking'	● Understanding
Skilled working	'Language' (use of)	● Allow space
Sensitivity to others but not avoiding issues	Responsive to all needs	● Allow silence
Informed, appropriate and relevant discussion	Values direction of tasks	● Acknowledge personal experience(s) and pain (without judgement or expectation of explanation)
Awareness of others	Punctuality	
Things we might have included:	Professional	● Allow expression of emotion
Have fun	Playfulness	● But no violence, aggression or threats
Mistakes	Enjoyment	

Remember to reflect on those things you have learned from each activity and/or the issues the work presented for you.

References

Bailey, J. (1997) *Utilitarianism, Institutions, and Justice.* Oxford: Oxford University Press.

Banks, A. (2012) *Ethics and Values in Social Work.* Basingstoke: Palgrave Macmillan.

Banks, S. (2009) From professional ethics to ethics in professional life: Implications for learning and teaching and study. *Ethics and Social Welfare,* 3(1), 55–63.

Banks, S. (2011) Ethics in an age of austerity: Social work and the evolving new public management. *Journal of Social Intervention: Theory and Practice,* 20(2), 5–23.

Banks, S. and Gallagher, A. (2009) *Ethics in Professional Life: Virtues for Health and Social Care.* Basingstoke: Palgrave Macmillan.

Baron, M. (1995) *Kantian Ethics Almost Without Apology.* Ithaca, NY: Cornell University Press.

Beauchamp, T. and Childress, J. (2001) (5th edn) *Principles of Biomedical Ethics.* Milton Keynes: Open University Press.

Beckett, C. and Maynard, A. (2013) (2nd edn) *Values and Ethics in Social Work.* London: Sage.

Benner, P. (ed.) (1994) *Interpretive Phenomenology: Embodiment, Caring and Ethics in Health and Illness.* Thousand Oaks, CA: Sage.

Bernstein, S. (1970) *Further Explorations in Groupwork.* London: Bookstall.

BMA (British Medical Association) (2015) *Ethics Took Kit for Students.* Available at: www.bma.org.uk/support-at-work/ethics/medical-students-ethics-tool-kit/key-concepts (accessed 15/2/16)

Driver, J. (2007) *Ethics: The Fundamentals.* Oxford: Blackwell.

Dubois, B. and Miley, K. (2008) (6th edn) *Social Work: An Empowering Profession.* London: Pearson.

Fitzpatrick, T. (2008) *Applied Ethics and Social Problems: Moral Questions of Birth, Society and Death.* Bristol: Policy Press.

Fox Harding, L. (1997) (2nd edn) *Perspectives in Child Care Policy.* London: Longman.

Gallagher, A. and Sykes, N. (2008) A little bit of heaven for a few? A case analysis. *Ethics and Social Welfare,* 2(3), 299–307.

Gilligan, C. (1982) *In a Different Voice: Psychological Theory and Women's Development.* Cambridge, MA: Harvard University Press.

Goodin, R. (1995) *Utilitarianism as Public Policy.* Cambridge: Cambridge University Press.

Grayling, A. C. (2004) *What is Good? The Search for the Best Way to Live.* London: Phoenix.

Hamlyn, D. W. (1987) *The Penguin History of Western Philosophy.* Harmondsworth: Penguin.

Held, V. (2006) *The Ethics of Care: Personal, Political, Global.* Oxford: Oxford University Press.

Hochschild, A. (1983) *The Managed Heart: Commercialisation of Human Feeling.* Berkeley: University of California Press.

Holloway, R. (2005) *Looking in the Distance: The Human Search for Meaning.* Edinburgh: Canongate.

Kant, I. (1991) *Groundwork of the Metaphysics of Morals.* London: Routledge.

MacIntyre, A. (1967) *A Short History of Ethics: A History of Moral Philosophy from the Homeric Age to the Twentieth Century.* London: Routledge, Kegan Paul.

MacIntyre, A. (1985) *After Virtue: A Study in Moral Theory.* London: Duckworth.

O'Neill, O. (1989) *Constructions of Reason: Exploration of Kant's Practical Philosophy.* Cambridge: Cambridge University Press.

Rachel, J. (2003) *The Elements of Philosophy.* London: McGraw Hill.

Rojeck, C., Peacock, G. and Collins, S. (1988) *Social Work and Received Ideas*. London: Routledge.

Seedhouse, D. (2009) *Ethics: The Heart of Health Care*. Chichester: Wiley.

Sevenhuijsen, S. (1998) *Citizenship and the Ethics of Care: Feminist Considerations on Justice, Morality and Politics*. London: Routledge.

Sidgwick, H. (1981) *The Methods of Ethics*. Indianapolis, IN: Hackett.

Smart, J. J. C. and Williams, R. (1973) *Utilitarianism: For and Against*. Cambridge: Cambridge University Press.

Thompson, I., Melia, K. and Boyd, K. (2000) (4th edn) *Nursing Ethics*. Edinburgh: Churchill Livingston.

Timms, N. (1983) *Social Work Values: An Enquiry*. London: Routledge and Kegan Paul.

Tronto, J. (1993) *Moral Boundaries: A Political Argument for an Ethics of Care*. London: Routledge.

Vigilante, J. (1974) Between values and science: Education for the professional during a moral crisis or is proof truth? *Journal of Education for Social Work*, 10(3), 107–15.

Younghusband, E. (1967) *Social Work and Social Values*. London: Allen and Unwin.

Chapter 4
Professional identity

Nick Hartop, Adam Barnard and Mick Wilkinson

Chapter outline

This chapter will introduce:

- professionalism, identity and the self
- the formulation of professional identities
- professions: social work, health and social care, youth justice (to include multi-agency working)
- reflective practice and social justice
- a vignette, questions and further reading.

Professionalism

So what does it mean to be a 'professional'? A brief literature search produces suggestions as to what the make-up of a professional might involve. Current contemporary themes include (but are not limited to) ideas around: accountability; integrity; competency; knowledge and qualifications. However, clarity around a definitive ideal of what it means to be a 'professional' may not be clearly outlined in organizational settings. Many professions are subject to legislative changes, shifts in occupational standards, practices and requirements. The concept, therefore, of the construction of what it is to be a 'professional' is subject to change throughout time. What may have been considered 'good practice' in the fields of 'health, social care and justice' ten years ago may, due to advances in scientific developments and changes in policy, practice and cultural approaches, be framed in contemporary climates as 'unprofessional' and in a further ten years even 'negligent'. Evetts (2003: 397) provides some helpful clarity for defining 'professions' in her work surrounding 'The Sociological Analysis of Professionalism':

> Professions are essentially the knowledge-based category of occupations which usually follow a period of tertiary education and vocational training and experience. A different way of categorizing these occupations is to see professions as the structural, occupational and institutional arrangements for dealing with work associated with the uncertainties of modern lives in risk societies.

Evetts (2003) further comments upon 'professionalism', suggesting that the concept can be comprehended as symbolic processes, during which advocates make representations associated with status and authority in relation to occupational values. Holdaway (2016) notes the harmony of this symbolic process in relation to Becker and Hughes' perspectives of symbolic interactionism (Becker 1970; Hughes 1958; Hughes 1994). Ritzer and Walczak (1986) describe much of the historical sociological discourse surrounding what it is to be professional or a member of a profession as stemming from two main themes, *functionalist* and *trait models*. The former has its foundations in Durkheimian theory relating to order, consensus and moral communities based on occupational membership, and *processual models* rooted in the works of Marx and Weber which include the relationships of power domains and social action (Parsons 1951).

Pavalko's (1971: 4) eight-point outline of professional or occupational criteria provides a framework to position work-based activity:

1   Specialized theory and intellectual technique required.
2   Relevance to basic social values and processes.
3   Nature of preparation in terms of amount and specialization of training and degree of symbolization and ideation required.
4   Motivation for work meaning service to society as opposed to self-interest.
5   Autonomy of practice.
6   Sense of commitment or strength of calling to the profession.
7   Sense of professional community and culture.
8   Strength of codes of ethics.

Pavalko's offering enables all genres of work to be made subject to the criteria, placing the concept of profession as dependent upon the 'placements and the social constructions of the placements, in the context of labour markets and, the place of higher education in preparation for the occupation' (Carpenter and Stimpson 2007: 268). Friedson (2001: 34–35) continues the theme raised by Pavalko in relation to service to society as opposed to self-interest, in that professionalism and processes of professionalization are relative to the concept of the role's importance to society (Friedson 2001: 214). Friedson also suggests that 'the ideal-typical position of professionalism is founded upon the official belief that the knowledge and skill of a particular specialization requires a foundation in abstract concepts and formal learning' (Friedson 2001: 34–35). The lure of students and practitioners to be engaged in socially recognized or accredited professional activity, owning the power, skills and freedom to problem solve and make decisions in the interests of others, ensures that the topic of professionalism within sociological discourse will remain a crucial theme.

Self

The self has had contemporary expression from ancient Hellenistic and Roman thought (Gill 2006) to a technologically mediated self (Jones 2006), to being mirrored in the home (Marcus 2006). There is a wide and varied literature on the self that reflects the rise and concern with identity, self-identity and its relationship to self (Elliott 2007; du Gay 2007; Elliott and du Gay 2009).

The seminal works on the self, with rich, detailed and extended reflections of the self, are found in Seigel (2005) and Taylor (1989). The self is anchored in conflicting discourses and competing dialogues and is shaped and formed in the discursive apparatus in which it is evoked. Indeed, contemporary deconstructive readings of the idea of the self in works such as Seigel's (2005) comprehensive guide certainly mitigate against any finality of definition.

Western notions of the self have emerged from diverse and contradictory social, political and cultural strands from Roman legal theory, Greco-Roman Stoic philosophy, Christian theology and the metaphysical soul as a kind of self-substance to the advent of industrial capitalism (Burkitt 2008: 25). Taylor (1989) has argued that the 'expressivist' Romantic movement in eighteenth-century European society understood the self as something to be made through an individual's creative expression in his history of the self.

The intersection of self and social relations has been ably demonstrated and charted by Rose (1990), who provides a history of the self to conclude that we have a current regime of the self, in part constructed by psychology's rise of profoundly ambiguous relations between the ethics of subjectivity, the truth of psychology and the exercise of power. Psychology as a form of knowledge, a type of expertise and a ground for ethics governs subjectivity and self in the contemporary era. The conception of self has changed from autonomous, atomized self to a new individualized or enterprising self.

For Rose (1990) the image of an 'enterprising self' was so potent because it was not an idiosyncratic obsession of the right of the political spectrum; to the contrary, it resonated with basic presuppositions concerning human beings that remain to this day widely distributed amongst all political persuasions. Rose (1990: 151) sums up these presuppositions as follows; that the self will:

- be a subjective being
- aspire to autonomy
- strive for personal fulfilment in its earthly life
- interpret its reality and destiny as a matter of individual responsibility
- find meaning in its existence by shaping its life through acts of choice.

Rose (1990: 3) argues the image of the self has come under question both practically and conceptually. The self is 'coherent, bounded individualized, intentional, the locus of thought, action, and belief, the origin of its own actions, the beneficiary of a unique biography'. This fixed and frozen entity of identity of our history, heritage and experience, characterized by a profound inwardness of a regulatory ideal of an 'internal universe of the self', has undergone contemporary challenge. For example, the self has been technologically invaded, turned outwards and inwards, supplemented and amended.

The 'individualized self' under modernization and the emergent discourse of the twentieth century is captured by Geertz (1979: 229) who states:

[t]he Western conception of the person as a bounded, unique, more or less integrated motivational and cognitive universe, a dynamic center of awareness, emotion, judgement and action, organized into a distinctive whole and set contrastively against other such wholes and against a social and natural background is, however incorrigible it may seem to us, a rather peculiar idea within the context of world's cultures.

There is a wealth of localized, specific, culturally diverse and contested notions of the self. The rigidity and lack of temporal understanding of the self is, as Charles Taylor suggests:

a function of a historically limited mode of self interpretation, one which has become dominant in the modern West and which may indeed spread thence to other parts of the globe, but which has a beginning in time and space and may have an end.

(Taylor 1989: 111)

Reflexively, we can recognize that the individual self is located within a number of technological discourses derived from education, social psychology, and professional practice. Reflection on the historical development of this idea such as in the work of Foucault (2007, 2002, 1988, 1984a, 1984b, 1984c, 1981) examines and explores the competing and conflicting technologies at work on the self.

Development of the self therefore embodies two inter-related dimensions of means–ends structured technologies of the self: the first stage is already predicated upon an ordering of human beings involved in accordance with the rationality of its own particular protocols. Second, in agreement with the ordering of theoretical reason (Heidegger 1962), the precise locus for the human being is found to be one of a multiplicity of possible technological 'inventions' we call the self, mediated by the discourses in which it may have been thrown in practice. These technological inventions in a professional field are constituted by the notion of identity.

The relationship between self and identity has historically aroused much debate. The self has a notion of self-concept, our whole selves including our self-esteem (or self-confidence as the link between self-identity and ideal self), self-image (how we define ourselves) and ideal self (of what we would like to be).

Identity

A person's identity is answering the question 'who am I?' with the competing and conflicting identities of others. Jenkins (2008) suggests there are three central parts to an identity: an individual or personal element; a collective or social element, and the embodiment of identity. The rich detail or sensual experience is necessary to understand the sources and multi-layered identity. Constraint and agency in taking up an identity are also contested. Sociologists suggest primary identities are formed early in life, such as gender, ethnicity, class, and secondary identities that people are socialized into such as social roles, occupations and status positions.

Identity is defined as the 'distinctive aspects of an individual's character or the character of a group which relates to their sense of self' (Giddens and Sutton 2014: 138). The concept originated with the work of Cooley (1902) and Mead (1934) and is related to self and social identity. Cooley's 'looking glass' self suggests others' evaluation of an individual has an effect on a person's view of themselves. Mead (1934) argued that an individual's sense of self is formed by social interaction and cannot be dislocated from the study of society, culture and ideology. A sense of self is a necessary condition for personal identity and takes place in consumerism, individualization and privatization.

Despite multiple psycho-social approaches in the field of 'identity studies', Tajfel's 'Social Identity Theory' (SIT) arguably produced a framework of underpinning theoretical coherence that made the topic of social identity a crucial concept of the discipline of social psychology (Worchel et al. 1998).

For Tajfel, self-identity is constructed by the groups to which we associate or attach ourselves. The feelings of belonging and projections of self-image and in turn self-esteem are enhanced by the groups we associate our self-identity with. This is described as the perception of oneness with or belongingness to some human aggregate (Tajfel and Turner 1985). Social Identity Theory promotes that belonging to a group (for example, family, supporting or participating in a sports team, social class, political party) becomes a vital part of the fabric of a person's make-up, and these attachments should not be considered to be abstract associations that have an insignificant impact upon the construction of an individual's self-identity.

This process, however, does not take place without its complications as whilst attaching oneself towards what Tajfel (1979) describes as an 'in group', individuals attempt to enhance the standing of that group in order to boost self-image (for example, Leicester City Football Club is the finest team to grace the League ...). We may do this not solely by giving this outward impression of superiority but also by demonstrating our disdain for other groups (which in this case might be to express a dislike for other football teams), which Tajfel (1979) describes as 'out-groups' due to being rejected by an individual as part of their self-identity. Social Identity Theory considers this process as a positive form of discrimination, which helps an individual separate and construct a self-image that distinguishes themselves from other groups – though arguably does so with prejudicial undertones.

Social Identity Theory promotes a three-stage rationale which individuals undertake in the form of a cognitive process when considering adopting group membership attachments: categorization, social identification and social comparison (Tajfel and Turner 1979).

The process of categorization is how we as individuals frame our own interpretations of our surroundings (this psychological/mental process will of course differ between individuals), helping us to distinguish difference and classify the surroundings to which we are subject and thus inform judgements on how we wish to interact with our environments. Some simplistic examples of this process may relate to categorization on the basis of religion, nationality, occupation, political allegiance, ethnicity and so on. Although this may seem a stereotypical process, essentially, on a social level, 'stereotypes are the expression of the attribution of features shared by different members of a group without taking into account the inter-individual differences' (Worchel et al. 1998: 4). Tajfel offers the following definition of categorization: 'Categorization refers to psychological processes which tend to organize the environment into categories or groups of persons, objects, events (or groups of some of their characteristics) according to their similarities, their equivalences concerning their actions, their intentions or behavior' (Tajfel 1972: 272).

Stage 2 of the rationale, social identification, refers to the process of an individual taking on a group identity post-categorization. Social Identity Theory promotes the notion that as individuals we initially take on and behave within the parameters of our own understanding and beliefs that we have categorized as pertaining to the group identity. An example of this may be that an individual wishing to join a new friendship circle is likely to conform and act in similar manners to how that individual perceives the group in relation to their own categorization processes.

Stage 3 of the process (social comparison) relates to the comparative process of measuring 'in-group' identities against 'out-groups'. This process takes place in order to evaluate ourselves against similar others (Festinger 1954). The impact of this evaluation has multiple outcomes, including competition between groups for favourability in social standing in order to compete for economic, political or social resources and may cause further divisions and polarization between similar groups as prejudices begin to manifest in order that group members retain favourable emotional attachment to their in-group.

How are professional identities formulated?

Upon the commencement of engaging in a professional role, as individuals, each of us arrives with our own, unique personal identity. Our social identities, however, are arguably shaped not by personal identity but by the labels that others attach to us through collectively observing, processing and interpreting our behaviours. Arguably, this collision of personal and social identity in organizational settings has consequences which impact on how we see ourselves and how colleagues see us. After all, what we consider we 'bring to the party' and how our behaviour 'at the party' is interpreted, may involve multiple perspectives! Fortunately, the concepts of 'self' and 'identity' should be considered to be dynamic factors that we have the ability to influence and change throughout our professional careers as we engage in reflective practices and develop new approaches to situations, re-inventing how we see ourselves and attempting to outwardly demonstrate practice that influences how others perceive us. Niemi (1997) describes this process of self-reflection as reshaping identity due to questioning the personal view and, in turn, students of a profession may be viewed as active participants in forming their professional identities. The workplace, therefore, might be viewed as a melting pot which impacts upon the construction of both 'self' and 'identity' (Haslam 2001).

As a student embarking upon a career in a professionally recognized arena or as an existing professional entering a new role, the process requires the learning and delivery of new skills to be applied in the workplace in accordance with the social boundaries and rules which regulate or steer behaviour in the particular work-based setting. Van Maanen and Schein (1979: 226) describe these social rules as 'appropriate mannerisms, attitudes and social rituals' to which a subject must outwardly give the impression of compliance or potentially risk a lack of effectiveness – or worse, the removal of the opportunity to fulfil the role (Ibarra 1999; Leary and Kowalski 1990; Goffman 1959). Thus, Van Maanen and Schein (1979) propose that those who appear to conform, comply or 'act out' such behaviours are accepted 'into the fold', having been granted inclusion through demonstrating their ability to formulate corresponding identities to those of their colleagues.

Professional identities have a conflicting mix of self-identity, self-concepts, self-esteem and ideal self. Professional identity is defined as one's professional self-concept based on attributes, beliefs, values, motives and experiences (Ibarra 1999; Schein 1978). Bleakley (2004) notes that professional identity is shaped by discourse between individuals, which is a continuous process, impacting on the social construction of professional identities. Social Identity Theory (SIT) (Tajfel and Turner 1986) and Self Categorization Theory (SCT) (Turner et al. 1987) do not entertain the notion that professional groups differ from other group identities – post-categorization processes, professionals will become members of the most favourable in-group(s), which may also enhance their personal identity if their attachments and relationships within the group grow stronger, leading to self-verification, self-gratification and a greater sense of self-esteem (Tajfel 1978).

Colby and Sullivan (2008) identify a 'four-dimensional framework' that defines professionalism through: intellectual training (graduate programme); skill-based practice (work-based learning); certain values and ethical standards (defined professional values); and existence of regulatory bodies (HCPC) (Colby and Sullivan 2008: 405), whilst recognizing standardization across professions necessitates prescribed notions of minimum standards of proficiency and expectations of continued professional development.

Social work

Social work as a profession has undergone significant scrutiny and change over the last decade. For example, professional registration and a new Code of Practice are being enshrined in legislation and there have been important debates in an attempt to identity, clarify and explore the role of social work and its value in society (Bogg 2010; CSIP/ NIMHE 2006; Merchant 2007; Parrot 2006; Ray et al. 2008; Scottish Executive 2006; Department of Health 2007).

Within the social work profession, a body of literature exists that seeks to define professionalism through an established expert knowledge base and theoretical perspectives (Evans 2013; May and Buck 1998; Trevithick 2007), whilst recognizing the importance of the professions' need to reconcile its values and professional role with service-user trust and public perceptions (Beddoe 2010).

This importance of professional role with service-user trust and public perceptions was recently identified within allied professions with the stated 'scandal' of Mid Staffs NHS Foundation Trust: Public Inquiry (Francis 2013) that resulted in damaging media and professional status coverage. It is suggested that professional bodies such as the College of Social Work and the Nursing and Midwifery Council utilize notions of profession/ professionalism within these circumstances to reiterate standards and regulatory function (for example, graduate profession/adherence to regulatory function/evidence-informed practice) as mitigating factors when considering public perception and trust (Andrew 2012; TCSW 2012). A preference in identification of individual accountability over professional status is often used as a defence mechanism within these circumstances, for example 'eighteen social workers struck off or suspended in England' (Community Care 2013), thereby blame is attributed to individual deficit rather than structural or ideological influences.

In contemplating the political impact upon the definition of professionalism within social work (and many other professions), New Labour's defined 'third way' implemented managerialist approaches and target-driven cultures from 2001–10 in order to demonstrate perceived transparency and accountability of individuals and organizations (Clarke and Newman 1997; McDonald et al. 2008; Dickens 2012), leading to many professions becoming heavily regulated in order to demonstrate effectiveness and accountability (Batmanghelidjh 2008; Dickens 2012). A growing body of evidence suggests that the present government approach of neo-liberalist notions of 'profession/professionalism' moves away from collective responsibility, reinforcing the perception of individual responsibility, and thereby contributing to a 'blame culture' within professions (McInnes and Lawson-Brown 2007; McLaughlin 2010; Bondi et al. 2011; Parker and Doel 2013).

When considering the challenges for professional identity within current political ideologies and practice, social work academics highlight the importance of practitioners balancing professional wisdom and effective judgement in order to attain measureable outcomes (Banks 2013: abstract; Bondi et al. 2011; Masocha 2013). Taking a more directive stance, others suggest a radical approach to addressing the challenges of managerialist practices to professionalism within social work, adopting 'deviant social work' practice that includes 'resistance, subterfuge and deception' as methods of regaining previously held philosophical beliefs and identities (Carey and Foster 2011; Gilbert and Powell 2010; Ferguson 2008).

Health and social care

The Quality Assurance Agency's subject benchmarking for health and social care describes the nature and characteristics of programmes and training and the general expectations or standards for qualification awards. They are an external source of reference, internal quality assurance and general guidance for articulating learning outcomes, and provide flexibility and variety in an overall conceptual framework. The client, patient or service users' perspectives are included, as are inter-professional learning and work-based and practice settings.

The statement of common purpose is the common feature that overall subject benchmarks what health and social care is. The common purpose develops an emerging framework under three main headings: values in health and social care practice; the practice of health and social care; the knowledge and understanding of health and social care.

The values of health and social care include: accountability, explanation and justification for actions and decisions: respect for clients' and patients' (individuals, groups or populations) individuality, dignity and privacy; the clients' and patients' right to be involved in decisions about their health and social care; justification of public trust and confidence; high standards of practice; protection from risk or harm; cooperation and collaboration with colleagues; and education.

The practice of health and social care informs decisions and judgements in a variety of contexts and problem solving. This includes: the identification and assessment of health and social care needs; the development of plans to meet these needs; the implementation of these plans; and evaluation of this implementation.

The knowledge and understanding of health and social care is shared across the structure, function and dysfunction of the human body; physical and psychological human growth and development; psychology applied to health and social care; sociology and social policy; public health principles, practice and education; legislation and professional and statutory codes of conduct; ethics; and evidence-based practice.

These combined overarching frameworks of values, practice, knowledge and understanding form the educational and theoretical basis for health and social care professions. Although separate professions will draw on disciplinary knowledges, they are unified by a statement of common purpose. In the current state of austerity, the growth of applied professions in a variety of health and social care roles forms the context for professionalism.

Youth justice

In the wake of the 1998 Crime and Disorder Act, youth justice provision, formerly provided by social work staff, gradually became the domain of not only social workers but also probation officers, police officers, education, health, accommodation, substance misuse and youth and community work staff.

> The formal separation of the team from Social Services was experienced as removing the legitimating authority of their professional body. The removal of these

clarifying and legitimating supports of their professional identity brought about a consequent loss of occupational belonging.

(Souhami 2007: 184)

Applying Tajfel's (1979) Social Identity Theory, this seemingly created tensions in relation to self-identity and in-group and out-group categorization processes, arguably triggering an impact on social identity and social comparison stages of SIT.

> First, the absorption of practitioners from partner agencies into the team blurred the boundaries between 'them' and 'us'. Practitioners were suddenly deprived of a clear demonstration of what was distinct about their occupational identity. Second, the formation of the YOT (Youth Offending Team) required the development of new multi-agency practice and administrative routines.

(Souhami 2007:184)

The standardization of assessment and the introduction of evidence-based monitoring and evaluation of activities invoked a change in approach which brought into question the ethos of what it meant to be a youth justice practitioner and the professional skills and value base that should be applied to the role. Pycroft and Gough (2010: 218) raises the implication that despite some limited guidance from the Home Office (1999) in respect of roles for differing agency staff, 'research suggested that YOT personnel were carrying out the same tasks despite differences in professional background, training and qualifications' (Ellis and Boden 2005: 1). Studies in differing YOTs by Burnett and Appleton (2004) and Ellis and Boden (2005) both concluded that the dominant practitioner ethos within the teams studied, regardless of professional background, remained that of social work. Robinson (2011) also notes that at 'practice level' youth justice still holds elements of 'traditional' social services intervention. Power processes in team-based work are processes of meaning and identity formation (Bleakley 2004). These induce the team members to consent to dominant organizational views, even if these pose potential disadvantages (Dooreward and Brouns 2003). For students and practitioners planning a career or secondment in youth justice work, Edwards et al. (2009) encourage the notion of inter-professional education, noting the benefits for practitioners in becoming 'professionally multi-lingual' in their understanding and ability to communicate across agencies in the professional acronyms and glossaries of a range of agency backgrounds.

Morgan (2007), Burnett and Appleton (2004: 35) and Crawford (1994: 505) collectively agree in the principle of the potential benefits to be reaped by multi-agency youth justice teams; however, Pycroft and Gough (2010) suggest that despite the good intentions underpinning multi-agency narratives, YOTs are failing in their targets and lacking in any realistic achievements, whilst noting the complexities of joint working and citing examples of prior multi-agency failings, notably in relation to re-offending rates and child abuse. Murphy et al. (2006) propose a framework for success in terms of inter-agency practices that place particular emphasis on the clarity of roles and responsibilities and clear lines of communication and consultation. It is notable that for many commentators, the responsibility of inter-professional success appears to have shifted away from strategic and managerial responsibility and into the hands of operational staff:

Murphy cautions against inter-agency efforts being dominated by a particularly powerful perspective (2004), and Leadbetter (2008) against guarding particular elements of practice. A challenge for all staff therefore is to foster professional efficacy, while also remaining open to the expertise of others (Edwards et al. 2008). Practitioners who are most secure in their skill base should arguably be the most likely to recognise the skills of others without feeling threatened. It is important instead to know what other practitioners can offer, how to access their expertise and then how to co-ordinate and bring together different elements of practice.

(Baker et al. 2011: 131)

In relation to an identified professionally qualified status, tensions in YOTs arguably exist between those deemed as having a professional qualification and correlating pay scales and those who do not. In February 2016 the Youth Justice Board released a bulletin containing a consultation document, announcing proposal plans for a Youth Justice National Qualification Framework pitched at level 5 of academic study stating that, 'The YJB is committed to supporting the development of a professionally qualified youth justice workforce' (YJB 2016). However, previous accredited qualifications at level 5 of study have not necessarily entitled individuals who have successfully completed the award to eligibility to apply for positions of qualified status and correlating pay conditions, opportunities and responsibilities. Even this should be the case with the introduction of the new framework, professional tensions around educational parity potentially may remain, considering the historical trend for professionally qualified 'youth justice staff' to be educated to level 6 of study, usually incorporating an assessed practice-based placement requirement (for example, BA Hons Social Work, BA Hons Youth and Community Work – JNC accredited).

Identity and social justice

The literature around social justice in relation specifically to 'professional identities' is limited. Much of the rhetoric surrounding the principles of social justice in the context of identity relates to concepts of distribution and redistribution and comparative studies highlighting cultural differences. Fraser (1998: 1) describes the conflict around these polarized themes and proposes a more integrated approach: 'As a result, we are asked to choose between class politics and identity politics, social democracy and multiculturalism, redistribution and recognition. These, however, are false antitheses. Justice today requires both redistribution and recognition. Neither alone is sufficient.'

The concept of distributive justice is sometimes understood as the moral assessment of distributions, or as the moral assessment of individual or collective decisions in light of how they affect distributions. Since the publication of Rawls's 'Theory of Justice', however, discussions of distributive justice have tended to focus more narrowly on the moral assessment of systems of social rules in light of how they affect distributions.

(Barry 2014: 1)

A contemporary example of a requirement for redistributive justice and recognition in relation to professional identity might be a company structure that culturally rewards staff (through economic, role and title-related progression) who earn fees for selling goods which, in turn, profits the organization, yet overlooks or fails to consider equal recompense for staff employed in areas of the business which save costs, resulting in similar profits, through efficiently managing and reducing expenditure relating to company resources, administration, marketing and policy development. It is notable that the latter-described roles may also often incorporate a gender bias in terms of workforce numbers, thus adding further tensions to in-group and out-group attachments and barriers in developing professional parity and recognition.

Baldry and Hallier (2010) have examined attempts to 'humanise' workplaces by having 'fun' activities to smooth the private home and public work life. They suggest these management attempts to change identities rather than 'oiling the wheels' of production may alienate workers. Similarly, Saunders (2008), looking at collective identities in ecological social movements based around a central idea or ideological preference, examines how identities are formed and maintained.

The struggle for identity has been engaged within professional fields such as the Mental Health Service Users' Movement (Pilgrim 2014).

The United Nations Department for Economic and Social Affairs (DESA) (United Nations 2006) considers the terms 'social justice' and 'distributive justice' to be interchangeable, outlining six important areas of inequality relating to the distribution of: income; assets; opportunities for work and remunerated employment; access to knowledge; health services, employment, social security and safe environment; and opportunities for civic and political participation.

Chapter summary, reflective practice and professional identity vignette

This chapter summary introduces approaches to professional reflection and facilitates the opportunity to critically consider the application of the knowledge, skills and understanding progressively gained from the chapter to an applied vignette, utilizing structured reflective models.

In order that our professional behaviours consciously develop, critiquing ourselves both during and post experiences relating to identity and practice should be deemed an essential part of professional development. Models of reflection provide practitioners and students with frameworks facilitating review of professional experiences. The effectiveness of incorporating reflective processes to one's experience is likely to be dependent on the depth of reflection applied. Students and professionals should be prepared to develop their engagement with critically reflective cognitive processes, prompting analysis, evaluation and comparative considerations in relation to personal, social and political values, structures and agency which impact upon their own professional behaviours.

Atkins and Schutz (2008: 26) describe the skills involved as relating to processes of 'self-awareness, description and factual reporting, critical analysis, synthesis and evaluation'. In relation to depth of reflection, Goodman (1984) provides a three-tier framework which outlines levels of reflective engagement: level one is being primarily descriptive, giving consideration to practical concepts; level 2 is the application of theory to practice and considerations relating to issues and values; and level 3 is the act of framing the implications in wider contexts, considering ethical, political and social significances.

The principle structure of a reflective model is to essentially engage in the following basic processes geared around 'experience, reflection and action', which are broadly described as ERA models:

1 Outlining the event or experience – What happened?
2 Engaging in reflective processes upon the experience – How did it go? How do I know this?
3 Taking action, moving forward as a result of the reflective process – How might I do it differently next time to improve outcomes or sustain performance levels?

An array of options exists when deciding which reflective model to employ. Established offerings include but are not limited to Borton's (1970) succinct three-stage ERA questioning model: 'What? So what? Now what?'; Johns' (2000) model of structured reflection; Gibbs' (1988) reflective cycle; Atkins and Murphy's (1993) cyclical model; and Schön's (1983) consideration of reflective processes during experience 'on and in action'.

The aforementioned reflective models offer the opportunity for differing approaches in relation to structure, process and questioning prompts. It is recommended that students new to employing reflective processes begin with the arguably more simplistic ERA models and as their reflective abilities progress, engage with models containing more demanding structural requirements. Particular reflective models have their origins in experiential learning theories such as Kolb's (1984) Experiential Learning Cycle. Students and practitioners should, without question, explore such approaches to experience-related learning, but consider the differences between reflective models and not necessarily use or apply them as interchangeable concepts.

Parisha has been employed within the social care services sector for six years. She is a registered social worker who has spent the entirety of her post-qualifying career working with vulnerable young people. Her previous working environment was culturally diverse, consisting mainly of newly qualified social workers, some of whom Parisha mentored, supported and line-managed.

She has recently taken on a new senior role working in a multi-agency team tasked with safeguarding vulnerable adults. As the sole social worker in the team, she has found that the existing policies and procedures operate in established standardized processes and do not reflect the aims and values from her previous professional experience and educational background.

Parisha has attempted in the past week to influence and challenge her colleagues in relation to these matters, though she feels that the culture of the workplace remains rigid and her suggestions and recommendations have been ignored. Although having only worked in the organization for six weeks, she is beginning to become frustrated with her colleagues and on occasion this has been apparent to all, especially in team meetings. Parisha is currently questioning her decision to change jobs, though remains determined to turn things around in her new role.

Parisha is the only non-white team member and the youngest practitioner in an established team of five male members.

Using an ERA (Experience, Reflection, Action)-structured reflective model for each area, consider Parisha's predicament in relation to the chapter content. What processes might be occurring in relation to the below categories and how might Parisha approach some of the barriers she finds herself facing in her new professional environment:

- professionalism
- self
- identity
- the formation of new professional identities
- social justice and professional identity.

📖 Further reading

Fraser, N. (1998) Social justice in the age of identity politics: Redistribution, recognition, participation. *WZB Discussion Paper*, No. FS I 98–108.

Moon, J. (1999) *Reflection in Learning and Professional Development – Theory and Practice*. London: Kogan Page.

Morales, J. F., Paez, D. and Worchel, S. (1998) *Social Identity – International Perspectives*. London: Sage Publications.

Pycroft, A. and Gough, D. (2010) *Multi-Agency Working in Criminal Justice: Control and Care in Contemporary Correctional Practice*. Portland, OR and Bristol: Policy Press.

Souhami, A (2007) *Transforming Youth Justice: Occupational Identity and Cultural Change*. Cullompton: Willan.

References

Andrew, N. (2012) Professional identity: Are we there yet? *Nurse Education Today*, 32(8), 846–49.

Atkins, S. and Murphy, K. (1993) Reflection: A review of the literature. *Journal of Advanced Nursing*, 18, 1188–92.

Atkins, S. and Schutz, S. (2008) (4th edn) Developing the skills for reflective practice. In Bulman, C. and Schutz, S. (eds) *Reflective Practice in Nursing*. Chichester: Blackwell Publishing, pp. 25–54.

Baker, K., Kelly, G. and Wilkinson, B. (2011) *Assessment in Youth Justice*. Bristol: Policy Press.

Baldry, C. and Hallier, J. (2010) Welcome to the House of Fun: Work space and social identity. *Economic and Industrial Democracy*, 31(1), 150–72.

Banks, S. (2013) Negotiating personal engagement and professional accountability: Professional wisdom and ethics work. *European Journal of Social Work*, 16(5), 587–604.

Barry, C. (2014) Redistribution. In Zalta, E. N. (ed.), *The Stanford Encyclopedia of Philosophy* (Spring 2014 Edition) http://plato.stanford.edu/archives/spr2014/entries/redistribution/ (accessed 6 March 2016).

Batmanghelidjh, C. (2008) Preface. In Barnard, A., Horner, N. and Wild, J. (eds), *The Value Base of Social Work and Social Care*. Maidenhead: Open University Press.

Becker, H. (1970) *Sociological Work – Method and Substance*. Chicago: Alan Lane / The Chicago Press.

Beddoe, L. (2010) Health social work: Professional identity and knowledge. *Qualitative Social Work*, 2013(12), 24. Originally published online 9 August 2011. http://qsw.sagepub.com/ (accessed 21 April 2014).

Bleakley, A. (2004) Better dead than red? What Soviet psychology taught us about learning that saved our skins – a case study of multi-professional teamwork in operating theatres. Paper presented to Discourse, Power, Resistance Conference, University of Plymouth, April 2004.

Bogg, D. (2010) *Values and Ethics in Mental Health Practice: Post-Qualifying Social Work Practice*. Exeter: Learning Matters.

Bondi, L., Carr, D., Clark, C. and Clegg, C. (eds) (2011) *Towards Professional Wisdom: Practical Deliberation in the People Professions*. Farnham: Ashgate.

Borton, T. (1970) *Reach, Touch and Teach*. London: Hutchinson.

Burkitt, I. (2008) *Social Selves*. London: Sage.

Burnett, R. and Appleton, C. (2004) Joined up services to tackle youth crime: A case-study in England. *British Journal of Criminology*, 44(1), 34–55.

CSIP/NIMHE (Care Standards Improvement Partnership / National Institute for Mental Health England) (2006) *The Social Work Contribution to Mental Health Services*. London: TSO.

Carey, M. and Foster, V. (2011) Introducing 'deviant' social work: Contextualising the limits of radical social work whilst understanding (fragmented) resistance within social work labour process. *British Journal of Social Work* 41(3), 576–93. First published online 2 February 2011.

Carpenter, S. and Stimpson, M. T. (2007) Professionalism, scholarly practice, and professional development in student affairs. *NASPA Journal*, 44(2), 265–84. http://dx.doi.org/10.2202/1949-6605.1795

Clarke, J. and Newman, J. (1997) *The Managerial State: Power, Politics and Ideology in the Remaking of Social Welfare*. London: Sage.

Colby, A. and Sullivan, W. M. (2008) Formation of professionalism and purpose: Perspectives from the preparation for professions programme. *University of Saint Thomas Law Journal*, 404.

Community Care, (2013) Eighteen social workers struck off or suspended in England since January. http://www.communitycare.co.uk/2013/05/14/eighteen-social-workers-struck-off-or-suspended-in-england-since-january/#.U8JmlvldWSo (accessed 12 July 2014).

Cooley, C. H. (1902) *Human Nature and the Social Order*. New York: Scribner's.

Crawford, A. (1994) The partnership approach: Corporatism at the local level? *Social and Legal Studies*, 3(4), 497–519.

Department of Health (2007) *New Ways of Working for Everyone*. London: TSO.

Dickens, J. (2012) The definition of social work in the United Kingdom, 2000–2010. *International Journal of Social Welfare*, 21, 34–43.

Dooreward, H. and Brouns, B. (2003) Hegemonic power processes in team-based work. *Applied Psychology: An International Review*, 51(1), 414–22.

du Gay, P. (2007) *Organising Identity: Persons And Organisations 'After Theory'*. London: Sage.

Edwards, A., Apostolov, A., Dooher, I. and Popova, A. (2008) Working with extended schools to prevent social exclusion. In Morris, K. (ed.), *Social Work and Multi-Agency Working*. Bristol: Policy Press, pp. 47–66.

Edwards, A., Daniels, H., Gallagher, T., Leadbetter, J. and Warmington, P. (2009) *Improving Inter-Professional Collaborations: Multi-Agency Working for Children's Well Being*. London: Routledge.

Elliott, A. (2007) (2nd edn) *Concepts of the Self*. Cambridge: Polity Press.

Elliott, A. and du Gay, P. (2009) *Identity in Question*. London: Sage.

Ellis, T. and Boden, I. (2005) Is there a unifying professional culture in Youth Justice Teams? Papers from British Criminology Conference, Vol. 7.

Evans, T. (2013) Organisational rules and discretion in adult social work. *British Journal of Social Work*, 43(4), 739–58.

Evetts, J. (2003) The sociological analysis of professionalism: Occupational change in the modern world. *International Sociology*, 18(2), 395–415.

Ferguson, I. (2008) *Reclaiming Social Work: Challenging Neo-Liberalism and Promoting Social Justice*. London: Sage.

Festinger, L. (1954) A theory of social comparison processes. *Human Relations*, 7, 117–40.

Foucault, M. (1981 [1976]) *The History of Sexuality: Volume 1: The Will to Knowledge*. London: Penguin Books.

Foucault, M. (1984a) *Power: Essential Works of Foucault 1954–1984, Volume 3*, trans. R. Hurley and others, J. D. Faubion (ed.). New York: The New Press.

Foucault, M. (1984b) *The History of Sexuality, Volume 2: The Use of Pleasure*. London: Penguin Books.

Foucault, M. (1984c) *The History of Sexuality, Volume 3: The Care of the Self*. London: Penguin Books.

Foucault, M. (1988) *Technologies of the Self: A Seminar with Michel Foucault*, ed. L. H. Martin, H. Gutman, P. H. Hutton. Amherst, MA: University of Massachusetts Press.

Foucault, M. (2002 [1966]) *The Order of Things*. London and New York: Routledge.

Foucault, M. (2007) *Security, Territory, Population*. London: Palgrave.

Francis, R. (2013) *Mid Staffordshire NHS Foundation Trust Public Inquiry*. www.midstaffspublicinquiry.com/report (accessed 23 April 2014).

Fraser, N. (1998) Social justice in the age of identity politics: Redistribution, recognition, participation. *WZB Discussion Paper*, No. FS I 98–108.

Friedson, E. (2001) *Professionalism: The Third Logic*. Cambridge: Polity Press.

Geertz, C. (1979) From the native's point of view: On the nature of anthropological understanding. In Rabinow, P. and Sullivan, W. M. (eds), *Interpretive Social Science*. Berkeley, CA: University of California Press, pp. 225–42.

Gibbs, G. (1988) *Learning by Doing: A Guide to Teaching and Learning Methods*. Oxford: Further Education Unit, Oxford Polytechnic.

Giddens, A. and Sutton, P. W. (2014) *Essential Concepts in Sociology*. Cambridge: Polity Press.

Gilbert, T. and Powell, J. L. (2010) Power and social work in the United Kingdom: A Foucauldian excursion. *Journal of Social Work*, 10(1), 3–22.

Gill, C. (2006) *The Structured Self in Hellenistic and Roman Thought*. Oxford: Oxford University Press.

Goffman, E. (1959) *The Presentation of Self in Everyday Life*. Garden City, NY: Doubleday.

Goodman, J. (1984) Reflection and teacher education: A case study and theoretical analysis. *Interchanges*, 15, 9–26.

Haslam, S. A. (2001) *Psychology in Organizations: The Social Identity Approach*. London: Sage.

Heidegger, M. (1962) *Being and Time*. Oxford: Blackwell.

Holdaway, S. (2016) *The Re-Professionalisation of the Police in England and Wales: Professionalism and Regulation*. Unpublished paper.

Home Office (1999) *Inter-Departmental Circular on Establishing Youth Offending Teams*. London: Home Office.

Hughes, E. (1958) *Men and Their Work*. Glencoe, IL: Free Press.

Hughes, E. (1994) *On Work, Race, and the Sociological Imagination*. Chicago: University of Chicago Press.

Ibarra, H. (1999) Provisional selves: Experimenting with image and identity in professional adaptation. *Administrative Science Quarterly*, 44(4), 764–91.

Jenkins, R. (2008) (3rd edn) *Social Identity*. Oxford: Routledge.

Johns, C. (2000) *Becoming a Reflective Practitioner*. Oxford: Blackwell Science.

Jones, A. (2006) *Self/Image: Technology, Representation and the Contemporary Subject*. London: Routledge.

Kolb, D. (1984) *Experiential Learning as the Science of Learning and Development*. Englewood Cliffs, NJ: Prentice Hall.

Leadbetter, J. (2008) Learning in and for interagency working: Making links between practice development and structured relationships. *Learning in Health and Social Care*, 7(4), 198–208.

Leary, M. R. and Kowalski, R. M. (1990) Impression management: A literature review and two-component model. *Psychological Bulletin*, 107(1), 34–47.

Marcus, C. C. (2006) *House as Mirror of Self: Exploring the Deeper Meaning of Home*. Berwick, ME: Nicolas-Hays.

Masocha, S. (2013) We do the best we can: Accounting practices in social work discourses of asylum seekers. *British Journal of Social Work* (2013), 1–16.

May, T. and Buck, M. (1998) Power, professionalism and organisational transformation. *Sociological Research Online*, 3(2). http://www.socresonline.org.uk/3/2/5.html (accessed 21 April 2014).

McDonald, A., Postle, K. and Dawson, C. (2008) Barriers to retaining and using professional knowledge in local authority social work practice with adults in the UK. *British Journal of Social Work*, 38(7), 1370–87 (first published online 25 April 2007).

McInnes, A. and Lawson-Brown, V. (2007) 'God' and other 'do-gooders': A comparison of the regulation of services provided by general practitioners and social workers in England. *Journal of Social Work*, 7, 341.

McLaughlin, K. (2010) The social worker versus the General Social Care Council: An analysis of care standards tribunal hearings and decisions. *British Journal of Social Work*, 40(1), 311–27 (first published online 4 October 2008).

Mead, G. H. (1934) *Mind, Self and Society*. Chicago: Chicago University Press.

Merchant, C. (2007) Matching skills to need. *Mental Health Today*, April 2007, 23–25.

Morgan, R. (2007) Letter to all YJB staff, YOT managers, YOI governors, STC and LASCH managers and selected others, 26 January. Unpublished.

Murphy, M., Shardlow S., Davis, C. and Race, D. (2006) Standards – a new baseline for interagency training and education to safeguard children? *Child Abuse Review*, 15(2), 138–51.

Niemi, P. (1997) Medical students' professional identity: self-reflection during the preclinical years. *Medical Education*, 31, 408–15.

Parker, J. and Doel, M. (eds) (2013) *Professional Social Work*. London: Sage/Learning Matters.

Parrot, L. (2006) (1st edn) *Values and Ethics in Social Work Practice*. Exeter: Learning Matters.

Parsons, T. (1951) *The Social System*. Chicago: Free Press.

Pavalko, R. M. (1971) *Sociology of Occupations and Professions*. Itasca, IL: F. E. Peacock Publishers.

Pilgrim, D. (2014) (3rd edn) *Key Concepts in Mental Health*. London: Sage.

Pycroft, A. and Gough, D. (2010) *Multi-Agency Working in Criminal Justice: Control and Care in Contemporary Correctional Practice*. Portland, OR and Bristol: Policy Press.

Ray, M., Pugh, R., Roberts, D. and Beech, B. (2008) *Mental Health and Social Work*. SCIE Research Briefing 26. London: SCIE.

Ritzer, G. and Walczak, D. (1986) *Working: Conflict and Change*. Englewood Cliffs, NJ: Prentice Hall.

Robinson, A. (2011) *Foundations for Offender Management: Theory, Law and Policy for Contemporary Practice*. Bristol: Policy Press.

Rose, N. (1990) *Governing the Soul: The Shaping of the Private Self*. London: Routledge.

Saunders, C. (2008) 'Double-edged swords? Collective identity and solidarity in the environmental movement. *British Journal of Sociology*, 59(2), 227–53.

Schein, E. H. (1978) *Career Dynamics. Matching Individual and Organizational Needs*. Reading, MA: Addison-Wesley.

Schön, D. (1983) *The Reflective Practitioner: How Professionals Think In Action*. London: Temple Smith

Scottish Executive (2006) *Changing Lives: Report of the 21st Century Social Work Review*. Available at: http://www.scotland.gov.uk/Publications/2009/04/07112629/6 (accessed 1 February 2012).

Seigel, J. (2005) *The Idea of the Self: Thought and Experience in Western Europe since the Seventh Century*. Cambridge: Cambridge University Press.

Souhami, A. (2007) *Transforming Youth Justice: Occupational Identity and Cultural Change*. Cullompton: Willan.

Tajfel, H. (1972) La categorisation sociale. In S. Moscovici (ed.), *Introduction a la psychologie sociale*, Vol 1. Paris: Larousse.

Tajfel, H. (1978) Interindividual behaviour and intergroup behaviour. In H. Tajfel (ed.), *Differentiation between Social Groups: Studies in the Social Psychology of Intergroup Behaviour*. London: Academic Press.

Tajfel, H. (1979) Individuals and groups in social psychology. *British Journal of Social Psychology*, 18, 183–90.

Tajfel, H. and Turner, J. C. (1979) An integrative theory of inter-group conflict. In W. G. Austin and S. Worchel (eds), *The Social Psychology of Intergroup Relations*. Monterey, CA: Brooks/Cole.

Tajfel, H. and Turner, J. C. (1985) The social identity theory of intergroup behavior. In S. Worchel and W. G. Austin (eds), *The Psychology of Intergroup Relations*. Chicago: Nelson-Hall, pp. 6–24.

Tajfel, H. and Turner J. C. (1986) The social identity theory of intergroup behaviour. In Worchel, S. and Austin, W. G. (eds), *The Psychology of Intergroup Relations*. Chicago: Nelson-Hall.

Taylor, C. (1989) *Sources of the Self: The Making of Modern Identity*. Cambridge: Cambridge University Press.

TCSW (The College of Social Work) (2012) *Professional Capabilities Framework*. http://www.collegeofsocialwork.org/pcf.aspx (accessed 9 December 2013).

Trevithick, P. (2007) Revisiting the knowledge base of social work: A framework for practice. *British Journal of Social Work*, 38(6), 1212–37.

Turner, J. C., Hogg, M. A., Oakes, P. J., Reicher, S. D. and Wetherell, M. (1987) *Rediscovering the Social Groups: A Self-Categorization Theory*. Cambridge, MA: Basil Blackwell.

United Nations (2006) *Social Justice In An Open World – The Role Of The United Nations*. New York: United Nations. www.un.org/esa/socdev/documents/ifsd/SocialJustice.pdf (accessed 6 March 2016).

Van Maanen, J. and Schein, E. G. (1979) Toward a theory of organizational socialization. In Staw, B. M. and Cummings, L. L. (eds), *Research in Organizational Behavior*, 1, 209–64. Greenwich, CT: JAI Press.

Worchel, S., Rothgerber, H., Day, E. A., Hart, D. and Butemeyer, J. (1998) Social identity and individual productivity within groups. *British Journal of Social Psychology*, 37(4), 389–413.

YJB (2016) YJBulletin, Issue 50. http://youthjusticeboard.newsweaver.co.uk/yots2/6d6nq6otsjh18y2wai8wwk? (accessed 6 March 2016).

Chapter 5
Working in organisational systems
Current challenges and dilemmas

Simon Howard

Chapter outline

This chapter will introduce:

- the importance of organisational culture
- an understanding of contemporary organisational challenges
- leadership and management perspectives
- the importance of reflective practice and supervision
- the learning organisation.

This chapter explores the nature of contemporary English social work and related organisational systems from a generic perspective, with examples from adult and child care practice, reflecting on current workplace culture and values. This discourse is also useful and relevant for health care practitioners within their organisations where working environments are shaped and influenced by similar phenomena, discussed within the chapter, which overlap with social work. The chapter also enables the reader to reflect on their own current or future organisational and professional role in their working systems, in general, within the United Kingdom or abroad. Using practical reflective activities, the chapter illustrates how practitioners could promote service-user-focused values and social justice within their own (or other) organisations, even in the fluid and changing working circumstances created by the externalities of new public management and managerialism.

Importance of organisational culture

There is a moral philosophy at the heart of social work practice, a Kantian 'categorical imperative', that social work is a relationship-based and human activity (Ruch 2005; Trevithick 2014). This is underpinned by social justice and a commitment to support and empower service users to make positive changes despite structural oppression and disadvantage (Beckett and Maynard 2013; Dalrymple and Burke 2006).

However, practitioner success when working in organisations is not solely determined by the 'reciprocity' and progress of social worker and service-user interactions (Rogowski 2011). There is often a tension between internal cases based on 'service-user-focused' decision making and wider organisational and central government interests (Hughes and Wearing 2013). With organisational culture providing the vital dialogue and language, this allows organisations to frame competing demands and develop practice to lead workplace initiatives for the benefit of staff and service users alike. Indeed, Lawler and Bilson (2010: 146) define organisational culture as: 'Factors such as beliefs, behaviour, values and practices, which together establish the environment for professional practice and service delivery'.

In principle, this sounds straightforward. One would assume that social work and social care organisations would foster the co-production of services with the important resource of service users and be authentic about the values and approaches of a service, for example timely help and consistent services, to achieve good holistic outcomes and social justice. Many an organisational service plan follows these or similar lines. On this basis, we should all know a good organisation 'when we see one' (Baum and Rowley 2002: 2) and recognise the value of their social construct of human activity (Aldrich 1999) to a common good, for example with social work empowering service users to access their rights, obtain justice and reduce discrimination and poverty to promote economic well-being (BASW 2016).

However, Ayre and Preston-Shoot (2010) note that the assumption that all social work employers and practitioners are 'rational social justice actors' in children's social care provision needs closer scrutiny due to managerialism. Indeed, within adult care social work Evans (2012) notes that organisations can be 'rule saturated', reducing practitioner discretion and empowerment with service users and impairing service delivery. Organisations providing social work can be 'Janus faced' and have a 'shadow side' (and culture) defined by Egan (1993: 4) as:

> All those things that substantially and consistently affect the productivity and quality of the working life of a business, for better or worse, but which are not found on organisation charts, in company manuals or in the discussions that take place in formal meetings.

Effectively, a hidden ideology and culture can emerge, in relation to seen or unforeseen external pressures, which constructs the informal bottom of the organisational iceberg 'below the waterline' (French and Bell 1999), directing practice behind an operational 'public face' that creates the formal top of the iceberg above 'the waterline' (see Figure 5.1).

This was the case with the Mid Staffordshire NHS Trust (Francis 2013), where the public face of adult health care was defended by the trust as at least 'adequate', amongst a mass of positive patient output data from target- not patient-centred care, which actively hid malpractice, and a system under serious pressure for both patients and staff. Francis (2013: 4) noted that there was: '[a] culture focused on doing the system's business – not that of the patients' and '[a]n institutional culture which ascribed more weight to positive information about the service than to information capable of implying cause for concern'.

Furthermore, the Casey Report (Casey 2015a, 2015b) and her reflection on the Child Sexual Exploitation (CSE) in Rotherham noted similar organisational issues in child care services to the Francis Report above on the failings at Mid Staffs. Children were being harmed due to an unhealthy organisational culture in Rotherham which included senior management and elected members above the line of their organisational iceberg. This denied the scope of the CSE problem and set some very questionable priorities to vulnerable children at risk of CSE, even after the damning Jay Report (Jay 2014) on CSE in Rotherham the previous year. The real voices of children involved in CSE were obscured in a negligent 'top-down' system that allowed and condoned CSE, framing CSE as a marginal chid protection issue (after Melrose and Pearce 2013) while actively obscuring dissenting practitioner warnings about the scale and harm of CSE in

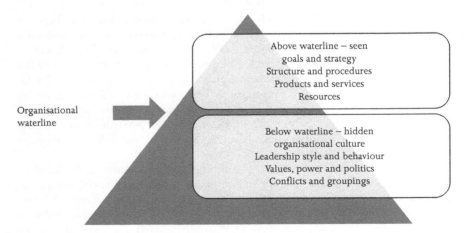

Organisational waterline

Above waterline – seen
goals and strategy
Structure and procedures
Products and services
Resources

Below waterline – hidden
organisational culture
Leadership style and behaviour
Values, power and politics
Conflicts and groupings

Figure 5.1 Organisational iceberg

Rotherham. Casey (2015b) illustrated an example of the power politics and conflicts that can lie beneath the waterline in any organisations that wish to work for a common good but unfortunately and tragically do not.

Therefore, there is a real need for a transparent service-user-focused organisational culture within our health, social work and social care agencies to make adult services personal and reduce harm (Lawson et al. 2014) and allow child protection services to be a humane setting for practitioners to promote change (Featherstone et al. 2014) and social justice with their families. A positive 'just culture' (Featherstone et al. 2014: 75) from employers is a key feature in promoting and maintaining coherent service provision, i.e. 'the way things are done', with culture being a vital 'social glue' that holds the organisation together during change (Hawkins and Shohet 2006: 168).

This has been developed further recently by Bevan and Fairman (2014: 24) asking leaders of health and social care agencies to create an organisational culture at work that radically changes thinking and practice, as 'more of the same' in services will not be creative enough to meet future demand. They note that organisational leaders are not 'out-of-the-box' thinkers or initiative takers as they spend too much time on operational delivery, 'creating an unconscious bias towards the status quo'. There is a need to activate the change agents who are often at the edge of organisations, for example front-line practitioners, service users etc., to change mind-sets and build bridges to new resources, including service-user-led provision reflecting social justice principles. This approach brings us back to relationship-based practice with humanity and co-creation in service provision (Ruch 2005; Trevithick 2014).

The recent developments in personalisation and self-directed support in adult care social work (Gardner 2014) fall into the latter category. This is dependent on organisational cultures supporting a shift to social workers being brokers of services working with service users' needs and narratives. However, there has been research and comment (Mencap 2012; Needham 2014) that the personalisation agenda has been used by organisations to change and close services, for example day centres, to meet budget requirements rather than use 'income generation' to drive innovative service-user provision, for example community hubs for adults with learning difficulties. Mencap (2012) indicates that services have been summarily closed without reference to service-user needs and wishes. It could be surmised here that the 'shadow side[s]' of organisations (Egan 1993) have effectively used an enabling initiative to promote changes that meet organisational monetary needs rather than service-user needs. Needham (2014: 104) notes that the inclusive service-user narrative of personalisation is difficult to implement in practice and its very ambiguity (and flexibility) for service users means that organisations can use a neo-liberal agenda for 'the community hub story-line simply as cover for retrenchment of the welfare state' with its cutbacks in care and managerialism.

❖ REFLECTIVE ACTIVITY

- To what extent does the organisation you work in or organisations you know have a 'shadow side'?
- Could you map an organisational iceberg from your findings?

Understanding contemporary organisational challenges

'Human service organisations are faced today with many of the market based dilemmas and problems that beset private sector and corporate organisations' (Hughes and Wearing 2013: 162). This can be seen to be a legacy of new public management in organisations (Hood 1991; Dunleavy and Hood 1994; Pollitt 1993), which can be paraphrased as a quest for frugality informed by the market. This developed as an organisational response to a backdrop of budget cuts stemming from the Thatcher administration in the 1980s. There is a requirement for an output-led organisational approach, developing prompt even speedy timescale-led practice, supported by a disciplined, focused and managed workforce. Organisational agility is the key to success – being able to commission services from the private (or any) sector, and manage organisational structures flexibly, for example by devolving budgets and organisational unbundling to create structures and services that offer best value and effectiveness. In contrast, governance is often simplified and rigid (Lawler and Bilson 2010; Practice Governance Group 2011; Simmons 2007), being a framework for organisations with explicit management and accountability structures implemented as 'top-down' hierarchical structures. In shorthand, organisations have to be agile and 'do more with less' but are always fearful of falling foul of governance that is linear and one-dimensional.

Therefore, new public management approaches can be seen as a rational necessity in times of continuous change due to the ongoing challenges of changing legislation and policy from successive governments. The number of contentious issues between the state, organisations and social work and care seems to continually grow and outputs have to be reconciled innovatively and sensibly within finite public sector resources. In this context, Hamel (in Bevan and Fairman 2014) concludes: 'The organisations that survive the future will be those that are capable of changing as fast as change itself'.

New public management can be viewed as being part of an entrepreneurial neo-liberal 'common-sense' approach (Harvey 2005) to building organisations. However, commentators, such as Harlow (2003) and Rogowski (2011, 2013), see recent new public management as a hegemonic mode of organisational discourse in social work and care, creating managerialism which is counterproductive to value-led organisational practice, staff welfare and service-user needs. Managerialism focuses on the controlling (rather than developmental) aspects of management and supervision, for example the procedure, timescale and tick box. It is linear 'businessology' (Harris 2003) divorced from the human complexity of practice. As a consequence of the latter, practice becomes focused on speed (Virilio 2012a, 2012b) and technology rather than the substance of performance as a professional, with social workers (BASW 2012), as with many public sector employees, worrying about the pace of their work and their interaction with organisational systems such as information technology.

There are concerns that managerialism curtails professional judgement and creative thinking by output 'rule-based' methodologies (Morrison 2010) linked to performance targets to ensure services are effective and efficient, within an increasingly finite resource-based operating system. Practitioners become 'technical rational' practitioners (Munro 2011, 2012) within positivist organisational cultures that promote predictability, accountability and standardisation in social work. Indeed, similar issues are seen within professions across health and social care where organisations are managerialist focused (Kirkpatrick et al. 2005).

The fact that practitioners are following agreed procedures and/or paperwork is no guarantee that need will be assessed properly (Rogowski 2010, 2013) nor that service users will be safeguarded, especially when due process reduces practice time with service users (Hardy 2015a). If practitioners spend less time with service users due to the externalities of the paperwork and due process, the service outcomes may be of a lower standard and even rushed. Therefore, external practitioner regulation in the form of new procedures stemming from child care serious case reviews (Rawlings et al. 2014) has arguably confused practitioners and agencies more than it has enlightened them. White et al.'s (2009) research on the Common Assessment Framework (CAF), a vital outcome of New Labour's *Every Child Matters* early intervention programme and a vehicle to promote 'respectful curiosity' in practice (Laming 2003) after the death of Victoria Climbié, concluded that: 'The CAF constrains professional practice in particular ways – it is indeed designed to exert its own "descriptive demands" which are intended to help and inform professional sense making, but which can feel tyrannical to the form completers'.

Families' narratives and needs are commodified for a digitised form and the information technology system around the form becomes the practitioner's focus, as well as the timescale for completion. Information technology systems such as the Integrated Children's System (ICS) can be deficient and contrary to the core functions of social work in listening to children and provisioning effective support and safeguarding to families (Ince and Griffiths 2011; Munro 2011), thereby serving an organisational managerialist demand for business data rather than securing the right outcomes for children and families. As Broadhurst et al. (2010) note, social work at the 'front door' with families is increasingly focused on procedures being technology driven by extrinsic monitoring, with the result that social work visits become an event and risk management process according to criteria rather than an autonomous interaction with service users guided by professional values and practice such as the HCPC's standards of conduct, performance and ethics (HCPC 2016).

The Victoria Climbié Foundation (VCF 2014: 14) and British Association of Social Workers (BASW 2012) have found that social workers feel they are becoming demoralised and deprofessionalised (Munro 2011) and at risk of being 'crowded out' of their profession by the very organisational structures that should support them, for example supervision led by performance management rather than critical reflection about practice (Lawler 2015). The VCF (2014) note that at a time when the profession should be supported and optimistic, for example with the establishment of chief social workers in adult and children and families social work (DfE and DOH 2013), it was disheartened to hear that 'less than a quarter of respondents feel optimistic about their future in the current system'. Howe (2014: 48) is intuitive when he says, 'today it is very difficult to think about child abuse and neglect in any other way except in terms of improved systems, more guidelines, better communication, tighter supervision and less optimism'.

Therefore, the current challenge for all social work and care organisations is to work positively with the current troika of governance, markets and managerialism (after Lawler and Bilson 2010) without alienating employees further and being service-user focused when commissioning effective services. Goodman and Trowler (2011) in

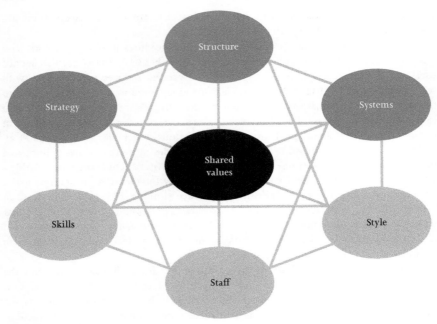

Figure 5.2 The McKinsey 7S model
Source: Adapted from: www.nwacademy.nhs.uk/developingtogether/mckinsey-7ss-model

their reclaiming social work (Hackney) model achieved the latter when they used the McKinsey 7S model (Figure 5.2) to redefine their organisation's conceptual map into hard and soft elements.

They understood that the hard elements of their practice system, i.e. strategy, structure and systems, needed to be aligned with the soft elements, i.e. skills, staff and style, and that these elements were co-dependent. To reinforce a workplace operating system with shared human social work values at its core, i.e. where families were experts in their own needs, practitioners needed to be supported through the soft elements of workforce planning, to be reflective and open about risk in an organisational culture that understood mistakes could be made when dealing with complexity. The results in an inner-city area were astonishing, with 40 per cent less children in care and staff sick leave halved (Rix 2011) and this model was adopted widely by other employers (Forrester et al. 2013). Indeed, Forrester et al. (2013) also note that managerialist hierarchical *hard-element-led* organisations (Francis 2013; Thorlby et al. 2014) in health and social care are 'brittle' due to their lack of ability to invest successfully in practitioners' soft elements, such as skills and style, to enable them through supervision to manage risk and need at the front line in partnership with families (or adults).

Munro (2012), along similar lines, has been very critical of managerialism and targets and her findings informed a recent relaxation of timescale speeds (Munro and Stone 2014) within child care assessments to ensure less time is spent on relentless electronic recording. She (2012: 14) concludes:

One painful lesson that some have reported is that they found timescales had been operating as a smokescreen and, once removed, they looked beyond them to the quality of work being done and focused on improving it. This is, of course, a desirable lesson since it led them to focus on enhancing skill. Looking at quality also draws attention to the purpose of assessments: to provide the basis for making a decision, a fact that seems to have been forgotten by some to whom completing forms within the specified time had become the task itself rather than a means to an end.

This quote from Munro is a powerful reminder for social work (care) organisations that any processes that prevent rather than enable direct work with service users are counterproductive to all those involved in practice.

❖ REFLECTIVE ACTIVITY

- To what extent does managerialism harm services and is it possible to have a responsive form of managerialism in the workplace to meet conflicting demands?
- Consider this quote by Froggett (2002: 70) from Harlow et al. (2013: 542):

  The marketisation of relationships in health and welfare promotes efficiency among providers by subjecting them to bracing competition, and increased choice for users who are expected to exercise responsible and rational discretion on their own behalf. The assumption is that needs are transparent and obvious to the consumer, requiring no interpretation by professionals, and that welfare is merely a commodity.

- Thinking of organisations you work in or know, to what extent is Froggett's assumption correct? Can you provide examples that counter Froggett's view?

Leadership and management perspectives

Lawler and Bilson (2010) offer a preferred 'reflective pluralist' framework for organisations' leadership and management that guides employers and decision makers away from managerialism and 'rational objective' approaches. It recognises the complex nature of messy social work situations and that actions and solutions need innovative creative thinking that is nurtured by pluralism. The strength in organisations, for example when adapting to change, is provided by inclusive management practices recognising the diversity and resources in the workforce, rather than adherence to a rational, hierarchical, target-driven culture (see Table 5.1).

Table 5.1 Comparison of leadership and management perspectives

	Reflective pluralist	Rational objectivist
Epistemology/ontology	Pluralist/relativistic, observer dependent	Realist, observer independent
Management	Situated, locally variable	Transferable, independent of context
Views of change	Unpredictable, conflictual, emergent	Predictable, planned, managerially determined
Orientation	Social, emotional, reflective	Rational, linear, bureaucratic
Ethical position	Constructivist, feminist, compassionate concern	Utilitarian

Source: Lawler and Bilson (2010: 20)

There is some recent evidence that government and employers in social work are moving away from 'rational objectivist' managerialist positions, to be more reflective and innovative, for example the standards for employers of social work in England (LGA 2014) and the Knowledge and Skills Statements (KSS) for practice leaders and supervisors (DfE 2015) in child and family social work. See Appendix 5.1 for both sets of standards.

The employer standards (LGA 2014) set out clear expectations that social workers should have a well-led, enabling professional environment to improve service-user outcomes. It was a wide-ranging stakeholder consultation which agreed that resourced workforce planning, safe caseloads, and effective supervision are a right for social workers and key pillars for an effective and resilient workforce.

The KSS for practice supervisors and leaders (DfE 2015) is a seminal document for child care social work as it sets out clear expectations and roles for workforce management. It proposes that leadership is part of management, and that management at the front line or in senior positions is not a remote activity from practitioners when building an 'excellent' workforce. It sets clear standards of leadership for senior operational managers, i.e. practice leaders, ensuring they engage practitioners and children and families at the front line, and promotes strategy to ensure that practice is supported by informed decision making in an organisational culture that is accountable and effective.

This reflects that effective performance management should be set in a culture of purpose and emotional intelligence (Howe 2008) to govern and shape excellent practice. It is reflectively pluralist in the Lawler and Bilson (2010) concept, in that management is situated within the workforce – it is an internal change agent; it recognises the emotions in practice and seeks to construct knowledge and support which deals with the reality of practice and working in an organisation. These KSS (DfE 2015) for supervisors and managers could, if used creatively, be an antidote to managerialism.

KSS (DfE 2015) reflects a growing perception (Hunt 2010) that 'top-down' management structures in many areas of the economy and public service do not promote agility to meet service-user need. Moreover, the Innovation Fund (Innovation Unit 2016) is a social enterprise originally set up by central government (DfE) to situate local organisations at the 'front line' of practice to construct 'reflective pluralist' (Lawler and Bilson 2010) solutions to complex problems. They believe that '[p]ublic services

are critical to everyone's well-being, but often they don't mee[...]
skills, tools and planning create services and systems that help pe[...]
The radical co-construction of services with users builds caring ca[...]
and seeks innovative leadership often to prevent harm and disad[...]
early intervention in old age or with mental health issues. Indee[...]
'We work with ambitious people who lead, deliver and use publ[...]
we develop radically different, better, lower cost solutions to comp[...]

It will be interesting to discover if the social justice narr[...]
(Ferguson and Woodward 2009) can be rediscovered and maintained by revised leadership management paradigms from initiatives like the Innovation Fund (2016) and KSS (DfE 2015), with practitioners empowered to lead rather than be passive supervised subjects within larger organisations. McPherson (2011: 49) shows original insight when he concludes: 'Management isn't about controlling people, it isn't about knowing things and it isn't about doing things. It is about asking good questions, freeing people up to get on with it.'

This brings us to the concept of leadership, which is synonymous with management but should not be for managers alone − this is one of the many myths of leadership (Yukl 2010; Yukl and Lepsinger 2004; Achua and Lussier 2013). Leadership should be for the *many not the few* within social work and social care organisations, as noted by the Innovation Fund (2016) and DfE (2015), and can often include 'managing up' by practitioners in their settings. Leaders can be disturbance handlers and resource allocators in organisations, picking up these traditional hierarchical management decision-making roles (Mintzberg 1973). This concept of 'distributed leadership' (Yukl 2010) can be a liberating 'micro power' organisational concept, enabling more autonomous practice, closer to service users, with leading from the 'front line' of care in distributed leadership improving experiences of care and co-producing services, especially under the Care Act 2014 which seeks to integrate social care and health services (Cullen 2013; SCIE 2015). As noted above, hierarchical and/or narrowly accountable leadership models are often seen as bad for organisations (Schyns and Schilling 2013). Being destructive and inward looking, with the effect of preventing stability and creativity within practice, results in supervision being balanced to accountability alone. Hafford-Letchfield and Lawler (2010: 7) sum up the positive argument for the importance of organisational leadership when they conclude:

> Senior leaders have a big role to play in facilitating the rebalancing of power in which all transactions harness people's competence, capability and capacity. Such distributed leadership styles build on people's real experiences and rely on local meaning making to shape their own work and processes.

In this case, distributed leadership could be a form of authentic leadership (Yukl 2010) having purpose and meaning stemming from a pluralistic practitioner value base (Lawler and Bilson 2010) with a sophisticated understanding of real-world issues (after Gardiner 2012). Authentic leadership is underpinned by a positive organisational culture that allows employees to have self-belief when dealing with contemporary change and challenge (Bevan and Fairman 2014), i.e. leading from the edge! This is a form of 'strengths-based' management which, along with coaching and mentoring, maintains and grows the positive core of the workforce. However, Lawler (2007: 138) importantly

ts a note of caution about leadership initiatives in social work when he says: 'The
ent emphasis on leadership might be seen as a further attempt to encourage greater
ontributions from individual social workers rather than as a humanising or liberal
influence in current social work organisation.' Therefore, there are concerns (BASW
2015; Jones 2014) that leadership needs to allow practitioners choice and control, with
organisations having faith in professional judgement and providing a positive appreciative
culture for practitioners away from a blame-based deficit model.

Another leadership and management concept that is emerging in social work and
social care organisations is effective followership (Hafford-Letchfield et al. 2015). This
can be defined as a person '[w]ho is high on critical thinking and involvement ... are
not risk adverse nor do they shy away from conflict' (Achua and Lussier 2013: 238).
They respect their leader, for example line manager, and the complexity of their
professional practice, but offer constructive criticism to service the best interests of the
organisation. In short, they are the self-sustaining positive core of the workforce that
organisations need to identify and grow in response to pressure and change. But it is a
requirement for effective followers to have 'the ability to independently assess what is
required of them and the others to participate in the process of developing and
implementing ideas about how to get there' (Hafford-Letchfield et al. 2015: 151).

❖ REFLECTIVE ACTIVITY

- How can organisations support managers to be more efficient 'tightrope walkers' (Aronson and Smith 2011)? Refer to the standards for
  employers of social work in England (LGA 2014) and the Knowledge and
  Skills Statements (KSS) for practice leaders and supervisors (DfE 2015).
  See Appendix 5.1.
- Are you a follower? How could theories of followership promote
  distributed leadership?

Importance of reflective practice and supervision

The importance of reflective practice is enshrined within social work and other helping
professions and is underpinned and enabled by effective service-user-focused supervision
(Baim and Morrison 2011; Hawkins and Shohet 2006; Morrison 2006, 2010; Wonnacott
2011). However, Chapman and Field (2007: 23) highlight that organisational and
strategic pressures have led to a three-tier formulation of practice depth, with reflective
practice being harmed by conveyer-belt practice and pragmatic practice.

1 **Conveyer-belt practice.** Superficial practice, responsive to efficiency drivers; the
   system is seen in terms of casework and targets. Work is policy driven and compliant.
2 **Pragmatic practice.** More depth. Some engagement with service users but focus is
   on organisational efficiency drivers. Supervision is about case management.

3   **Reflective practice.** Deep practice. Critically reflective, quality decision making and interventions, assessing needs while safeguarding, mobilising resources and support in casework, access to critically reflective supervision.

Morrison (2006: 30) notes that reflective practice is impaired when the four functions of supervision (Figure 5.3) are imbalanced. Effective supervision needs to be balanced between the four stakeholders in supervision: supervisor, supervisee, agency and, significantly, the service user.

Morrison (2006) proposes that practitioners need to reflect for two important reasons. First to access their memory bank, locating practice in relation to their research and knowledge base. The worker needs to be encouraged in supervision to have a *'competing hypothesis'* within a *'dialectic mind-set'* (Reder and Duncan 1999: 100), a crucial questioning ingredient of critical thinking which enables the practitioner to justify their actions and recognise their assumptions (Rutter and Brown 2015). Second, social work, as all heath and care work, is an emotional task. Functional case-based supervision, ticking boxes in a managerial audit, impairs the manager's and practitioner's ability to place emotions in context and plan for the future.

These overly managerial functions of supervision can be a source of harm for workers if they are 'the tail that constantly wags the dog' in supervision. There is a danger that the latter unchecked could reduce the time for the enabling reflective supervision being provided by practice supervisors to their staff within their KSS

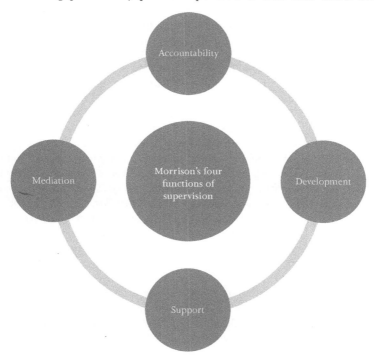

Figure 5.3 Morrison's (2006) four functions of supervision

(DfE 2015) from 2016. The growing need for accountability and the language of audit (Munro 2011, 2012) is still an issue in supervision (Lawler 2015). Izod and Lawson (2015: 208) conclude from their experience of supervision that the language of the 'technical' conveyer belt or pragmatic practitioner (after Chapman and Field 2007) becomes '[a] trap of certainty, evidence of knowing, rather than something that enables nuance and the capacity to change or develop one's ideas'.

The learning organisation

Learning is valued as a central component to organisational growth and development (Senge 1990), but the definition of a learning organisation is illusive (Kerka 1995; Porath et al. 2012). However, Kerka (1995: 3) pulls together some concepts which have commonality in most thinking about productive practices within organisations to promote learning. These are:

- providing continuous learning opportunities
- using learning to reach their goals
- linking individual performance with organisational performance
- fostering inquiry and dialogue, making it safe for people to share openly and take risks
- embracing creative tension as a source of energy and renewal
- being continuously aware of and interacting with their environment.

Learning should be part of everything that an organisation does, its heartbeat at the centre of the organisational system (Senge 1990). An effective learning organisation should be human, staff focused and have the ability to support its staff to be 'mindful' and think creatively, allowing mistakes to be learnt from, in contrast to any blame culture (Jones 2014).Therefore, social care and social work organisations should be 'risk enabled', allowing staff to work with service users on growing safety and protection within families and communities rather than a narrow managerial perspective (Carr 2011; WASOS 2011). This could be defined in contemporary learning organisations as relationship-based, value-led practice promoting social justice and empowerment.

In this case, vehicles for organisational learning in social work and safeguarding in health and social care, such as Serious Case Reviews (SCRs), should promote more learning than blame and be constructive in their developmental practice feedback (Rawlings et al. 2014). Sadly, there is mounting evidence in child protection at least (Jones 2014; Warner 2014) that SCRs can be dominated by fear of media reaction and agencies' 'reputation management', creating a shame and blame culture for individual social workers (Rawlings et al. 2014).

However, one recent significant SCR (Coventry LSCB 2013), with its subsequent 'Do it for Daniel Campaign' in 2013, provided a key element of organisational reflexivity, honestly admitting collective responsibility but also wishing to create a debate. Chief executive of Coventry City Council Martin Reeves (Guardian Social Care Network 2014) commented:

I'd like this to spark a debate around social care funding. With changes to Ofsted rules meaning more councils will continue to require improvement plans, we need to address – especially in a climate of drastic funding reductions – how the government can support those councils to make the improvements. Just inspecting councils and highlighting failures isn't going to save children. What will save them is learning from those issues and supporting councils to put them right.

In this context, a self-critical approach to how knowledge was generated about safeguarding and multi-agency working developed in Coventry, creating significant learning *and unlearning* about practice (after Wang and Ahmed 2003), radically reviewing the effectiveness of local child protection systems *and, importantly,* the nature of the support needed for practitioners. This led to the subsequent promotion of creative child-focused service planning within an open, informed local and national discourse about children's safeguarding, thereby facilitating a progressive learning organisation and culture. This was in contrast to previous aspects of managerialism within organisations, as seen above, which often concentrated on workplace processes rather than culture (Coventry LSCB 2013; *Guardian* Social Care Network 2014; Jones 2014).

Considering the importance of an effective learning organisation to organisational well-being and effective practice (Senge 1990; Kerka 1995; Wang and Ahmed 2003), some potentially key approaches (below) could sustain learning organisations, promoting a positive culture and creating connections and reflexivity between managers and practitioners to build practice creativity within the current climate of financial constraints.

- The promotion of a 'social learning culture' within teams (Rutter and Brown 2015: 69) to '*capture, codify but also share implicit knowledge*'. Reducing silo thinking, especially in multi-disciplinary teams developing a commonality of practice and critical thinking with service users.
- This would be a springboard for organisations to create 'communities of practice' (Wenger 2000) to sustain and drive continuous professional development and practitioner voices in service provision.
- The adoption of appreciative inquiry (AI) as a practice development approach, as noted by Hawkins and Shohet (2006). AI as outlined by Srivastva and Cooperrider (1987) is a strengths-based tool that asks questions about workers' potential and ability within an organisation. Its aim is to grow an ecology of strengths in the workforce by dialogue. It seeks to reduce a dysfunctional organisational focus on deficit planning and concentrate on what can be done and build on it. WASOS (2011: 30) also indicate that AI is a productive method for organisational learning with children and families practitioners co-constructing a positive workplace culture with employers. They conclude: 'In the child protection context building a culture of appreciative inquiry around front-line practice acts' as an 'antidote to the anxiety-driven defensiveness and the obsession with researching failure that bedevils this field'.
- The use of informed evidence-based practice (EBP) as a platform for discretion and relationship-based practice in professional decision making (Trevithick 2014) to reduce practitioner compliance and defensiveness about practice stemming from the current social work blame culture (Jones 2014). Recently, EBP can be evaluated

as having fallen foul of managerialism (Rogowski 2011; Trevithick 2014) and target setting (Munro 2011), with practitioners selecting narrow and uncritical evidence bases that meet the timescale speed or assessment form, rather than the complexity of the practice situation.

- The importance of action learning for managers (Brockbank and McGill 2003; Pedler 2011; Zuber-Skerritt 2002). Enabling managers to learn and develop from group discussions of their experiences, for example reflecting with others, networking and collectively owning organisational problems and their subsequent solutions. It builds confidence in management and supports an inquisitive positive learning culture in organisations about the 'powerful questions' that arise in the workplace. It is therefore effective with the 'wicked problems' (Grint 2010) that social work and other public sector leaders face today, i.e. uncertain problems of increasing complexity that need more active reflective collaboration to resolve. A typical action learning cycle is shown in Figure 5.4.

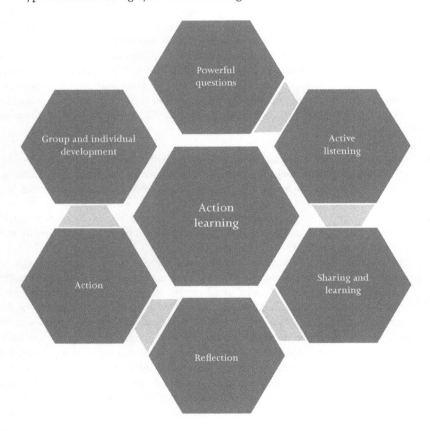

Figure 5.4 Action learning cycle

❖ REFLECTIVE ACTIVITY

- Taking Kerkas' (1995) assessment of the key requirements of a learning organisation (below), to what extent does the organisation you work in, or an organisation you know, function as a learning organisation? Reflect back on the key approaches discussed above.
  - Providing continuous learning opportunities.
  - Using learning to reach their goals.
  - Linking individual performance with organisational performance.
  - Fostering inquiry and dialogue, making it safe for people to share openly and take risks.
  - Embracing creative tension as a source of energy and renewal.
- Being continuously aware of and interact with their environment.

Conclusion

This chapter has examined contemporary organisational systems and the current challenges and dilemmas of promoting social justice within social work (care) practice in England. Concepts of co-creating services (Innovation Unit 2016) with organisations, practitioners and service users working together offers positive approaches, with innovation being informed by the values of humanism and relationship-based practice (Ruch 2005) between managers, practitioners and service users. However, exploring the 'shadow side' of organisations, i.e. a covert culture within organisations, indicates that even caring organisations can function to benefit themselves rather than service users or practitioners, especially in a climate of tight financial limitations. However, the development of standards, for example DfE (2015) and LGA (2014), and new conceptual frameworks for practice, for example Bevan and Fairman (2014), should be a progressive development in any organisation's culture.

More positively, 'reflective pluralism' (after Lawler and Bilson 2010), with its distribution of problems (and solution finding) throughout the workforce, is a valid alternative organisational concept to the more 'brittle', less flexible 'rational objective' approaches of process and predictability seen in managerialism. Being focused on timescale and outcomes to the detriment of direct work with service users is an endemic organisational problem in English social work as noted by Munro (2011) and Hardy (2015a). It is very possible that professional judgement and service outcomes could be enhanced by a 'reflective pluralist' approach emphasising practice relationships first and managerial and organisational-led matters second.

The latter is promoted by investment in a learning organisation, i.e. an organisation that is protective of the welfare of its workforce, generating knowledge and skills to promote the well-being of service users. Developing an active social learning culture, community of practice and appreciative inquiry are key building blocks in an effective learning organisation. Indeed, without an overt commitment to social justice as a heuristic guiding principle the speed, acceleration and performance management of managerialism could halt any progress that could be made by recent government initiatives in England (DfE 2015; LGA 2014) to improve social work (and care) learning organisations.

Finally, the 'wicked problems' (Grint 2010) in England for social work and social care should not fundamentally be any worse than in any other part of the United Kingdom. However, it is possible that organisations in other parts of the country tackle these problems in a different way. The *Guardian* (Hardy 2015b) survey of 2000 Scottish social care staff in 2015 found that, despite the real and substantial pressures facing the sector, the good majority (78 per cent) of people working in social care services in Scotland were happy in their jobs.

References

Achua, C. F. and Lussier, R. N. (2013) *Effective Leadership*. Stamford, CA: South-Western.

Aldrich, H. (1999) *Organizations Evolving*. London: Sage.

Aronson, J. and Smith, K. (2011) Identity work and critical social service management: Balancing on a tightrope? *British Journal of Social Work*, 41(3), 432–48.

Ayre, P. and Preston-Shoot, M. (eds) (2010) *Children's Services at the Crossroads: A Critical Evaluation of Contemporary Policy for Practice*. Lyme Regis: Russell House Publishing.

Baim, C. and Morrison, T. (2011) *Attachment-Based Practice with Adults: A New Practice Model and Interactive Resource for Assessment, Intervention and Supervision*. London: Pavilion.

BASW (British Association of Social Work) (2012) *The State of Social Work 2012: What Social Workers Think about the State of their Profession in 2012*. Birmingham: BASW.

BASW (2015) *Review of the Professional Capabilities Framework*. www.basw.co.uk/pcf/pcfreview2015.pdf (accessed 02/02/16).

BASW (2016) *The Professional Capabilities Framework for Social Work*. www.basw.co.uk/pcf/ (accessed 04/02/16).

Baum, J. A. and Rowley, T. J. (2002) Companion to organizations: An introduction. *The Blackwell Companion to Organizations*. Oxford: Blackwell.

Beckett, C. and Maynard, A. (2013) *Values and Ethics in Social Work: An Introduction*. London: Sage.

Bevan, H. and Fairman, S. (2014) *The New Era of Thinking and Practice in Change and Transformation: A Call to Action for Leaders of Health and Care*. United Kingdom NHS Improving Quality. Leeds: UK Government White Paper.

Broadhurst, K., Wastell, D., White, S., Hall, C., Peckover, S., Thompson, K., Pithouse, A. and Davey, D. (2010) Performing 'initial assessment': identifying the latent conditions for error at the front-door of local authority children's services. *British Journal of Social Work*, 40(2), 352–70.

Brockbank, A. and McGill, I. (2003) *The Action Learning Handbook: Powerful Techniques for Education, Professional Development and Training*. London: Routledge.

Carr, S. (2011) Enabling risk and ensuring safety: Self-directed support and personal budgets. *Journal of Adult Protection*, 13(3), 122–36.

Casey, L. (2015a) *Report of an Inspection of Rotherham Metropolitan Borough Council*. London: Stationery Office.

Casey, L. (2015b) *Reflections on Child Sexual Exploitation.* http://dera.ioe.ac.uk/23762/1/ Louise_Casey_report_into_CSE_template_format__4_.pdf (accessed 09/02/16).

Chapman, M. and Field, J. (2007) Strengthening our engagement with families and understanding practice depth. *Social Work Now*, 23, December 2007.

Coventry Local Safeguarding Children Board. (2013) Daniel Pelka SCR (Serious Case Review). www.coventry.gov.uk/lscb (accessed 12/12/15).

Cullen, A. F. (2013) 'Leaders in our own lives': Suggested indications for social work leadership from a study of social work practice in a palliative care setting. *British Journal of Social Work*, 43(8), 1527–44.

Dalrymple, J. and Burke, B. (2006) *Anti-Oppressive Practice: Social Care and the Law.* Maidenhead: McGraw-Hill Education (UK).

DfE (Department for Education) (2015) *The Knowledge and Skills Statements for Practice Leaders and Supervisors.* London: DfE.

DfE (Department for Education) and DOH (Department of Health) (2013) *Office of the Chief Social Worker: New Appointees Start.* www.gov.uk/government/news/office-of-the-chief-social-worker-new-appointees-start (accessed 12/12/15).

Do it for Daniel Campaign (2013) Example: www.coventrytelegraph.net/news/coventry-news/job-ad-campaign-urges-social-7726889 (accessed 01/11/15).

Dunleavy, P. and Hood, C. (1994) From old public administration to new public management. *Public Money and Management*, 14(3), 9–16.

Egan, G. (1993) The shadow side. *Management Today*, 21(8).

Evans, E. (2012) Organisational rules and discretion in adult social work. *British Journal of Social Work*, 43(4), 739–58.

Featherstone, B., White, S., Morris, K. and White, S. (2014) *Re-imagining Child Protection: Towards Humane Social Work with Families.* Bristol: Policy Press.

Ferguson, I. and Woodward, R. (2009) *Radical Social Work in Practice: Making a Difference.* Bristol: Policy Press.

Forrester, D., Westlake, D., McGann, M., Thurnham, A., Shefer, G., Glynn, G. and Killian, M. (2013) *Reclaiming Social Work? An Evaluation of Systemic Units as an Approach to Delivering Children's Services.* Bedford: University of Bedfordshire.

Francis, R. (2013) *The Mid Staffordshire NHS Foundation Trust Public Inquiry – Chaired by Robert Francis QC. Report of the Mid Staffordshire NHS Foundation Trust Public Inquiry. Executive summary.* London: The Stationery Office.

French, W. L. and Bell, C. H. (1999) *Organisation Development.* Upper Saddle River, NJ: Prentice Hall.

Gardiner, R. A. (2012) Leadership, authenticity, and the Arendtian world. *The Word Hoard*, 1(1), 8.

Gardner, A. (2014) *Personalisation in Social Work.* London: Learning Matters.

Goodman, S. and Trowler, I. (eds) (2011) *Social Work Reclaimed.* London: Jessica Kingsley Publishers.

Grint, K. (2010) *Wicked Problems and Clumsy Solutions: The Role of Leadership.* Basingstoke: Palgrave Macmillan.

Guardian Social Care Network (2014) 'Do it for Daniel': the story behind Coventry's social work recruitment campaign. www.theguardian.com/social-care-network/2014/sep/22/do-it-for-daniel-coventry-social-work-recruitment (accessed 01/11/15).

Hafford-Letchfield, T. and Lawler, J. (2010) Reshaping leadership and management: The emperor's new clothes. *Social Work and Social Sciences Review*, 14(1), 5–8.

Hafford-Letchfield, T., Lambley, S., Spolander, G. and Cocker, C. (2015) *Inclusive Leadership in Social Work and Social Care.* Bristol: Policy Press.

Hardy, R. (2015a) Targets take priority over time with service users, social work survey finds. *Guardian* Society Social Care Network. www.theguardian.com/social-care-network/2015/may/06/targets-take-priority-over-time-with-service-users-social-work-survey-finds (accessed 08/02/16).

Hardy, R. (2015b) *Guardian* Social Care Network Survey: Social care staff in Scotland are happy despite the pressures. www.theguardian.com/social-care-network/2015/oct/28/social-care-staff-in-scotland-are-happy-despite-the-pressures (accessed 08/02/16).

Harlow, E. (2003) New managerialism, social service departments and social work practice today. *Practice*, 15(2), 29–44.

Harlow, E., Berg, E., Barry, J. and Chandler, J. (2013) Neoliberalism, managerialism and the reconfiguring of social work in Sweden and the United Kingdom. *Organization*, 20(4), 534–50.

Harris, J. (2003) 'Businessology' and social work. *Social Work and Society*, 1(1).

Harvey, D. (2005) *A Brief History of Neoliberalism*. Oxford: Oxford University Press.

Hawkins, P. and Shohet, R. (2006) *Supervision in the Helping Professions*. Maidenhead: McGraw-Hill Education (UK).

HCPC (Health and Social Care Professions Council) (2016) *Revised Standards of Conduct, Performance and Ethics*. London: HCPC.

Hood, C. (1991) A public management for all seasons? *Public Administration*, 69(1), 3–19.

Howe, D. (2008) *The Emotionally Intelligent Social Worker*. Basingstoke: Palgrave Macmillan.

Howe, D. (2014) *The Complete Social Worker*. Basingstoke: Palgrave Macmillan.

Hughes, M. and Wearing, M. (2013) *Organisations and Management in Social Work*. London: Sage.

Hunt, J. (2010) In social care, leadership is not always top-down. *Guardian* Society. www.theguardian.com/social-care-careers/good-leadership (accessed 02/02/12).

Ince, D. and Griffiths, A. (2011) A chronicling system for children's social work: Learning from the ICS failure. *British Journal of Social Work*. http://computing-reports.open.ac.uk/2010/TR2010-02.pdf (accessed 08/02/16).

Innovation Unit (2016) *The Leading Innovation Partner for Public Services* www.innovationunit.org/our-mission (accessed 26/01/16).

Izod, K. and Lawson, C. (2015) Reflections from practice: Supervision, knowledge and the elusive quality of credibility. *Practice*, 27(4), 277–89.

Jay, A. (2014) *Independent Inquiry into Child Sexual Exploitation in Rotherham: 1997–2013*. Rotherham Metropolitan Borough Council.

Jones, R. (2014) *The Story of Baby P: Setting the Record Straight*. Bristol: Policy Press.

Kerka, S. (1995) *The Learning Organization. Myths and Realities*. ERIC Digest 166.

Kirkpatrick, I., Ackroyd, S. and Walker, R. M. (2005) *The New Managerialism and Public Sector Professionals*. Basingstoke: Palgrave.

Laming, H. (2003) *The Victoria Climbié Inquiry*. London: HMSO.

Lawler, J. (2007) Leadership in social work: A case of caveat emptor? *British Journal of Social Work*, 37(1), 123–41.

Lawler, J. (2015) Motivation and meaning: The role of supervision. *Practice*, 27(4), 265–75.

Lawler, J. and Bilson, A. (2010) *Social Work Management and Leadership: Managing Complexity with Creativity*. London: Routledge.

Lawson, J., Lewis, S. and Williams, C. (2014) *Making Safeguarding Personal 2013–14*. London: Local Government Association.

LGA (Local Government Association) (2014) *The Standards for Employers of Social Work in England*. London: LGA.

McPherson, B. (2011) *Equipping Managers for an Uncertain Future: Developing Your Managers on a Tight Budget*. Lyme Regis: Russell House Publishing.

Melrose, M. and Pearce, J. (eds) (2013) *Critical Perspectives on Child Sexual Exploitation and Related Trafficking*. Basingstoke: Palgrave Macmillan.

Mencap (Mentally Handicapped Children and Adults) (2012) *Stuck at Home: The Impact of Day Service Cuts on People with a Learning Disability*. London: Mencap.

Mintzberg, H. (1973) *The Nature of Managerial Work*. New York: Harper Collins.

Morrison, T. (2006) *Staff Supervision in Social Care: Making a Real Difference for Staff and Service Users*. Hove: Pavilion.

Morrison, T. (2010) The strategic leadership of complex practice: Opportunities and challenges. *Child Abuse Review*, 19(5), 312–29.

Munro, E. (2011) *The Munro Review of Child Protection. Pt. 1. A Systems Analysis*. London: Department for Education.

Munro, E. (2012) *Progress Report: Moving Towards a Child Centred System*. London: Department for Education.

Munro, E. R. and Stone, J. (2014) *The Impact of More Flexible Assessment Practices in Response to the Munro Review of Child Protection: A Rapid Response Follow-Up*. London: Department for Education.

Needham, C. (2014) Personalization: From day centres to community hubs? *Critical Social Policy*, 34(1), 90–108.

Pedler, M. (2011) *Action Learning in Practice*. Farnham, Surrey: Gower Publishing.

Pollitt, C. (1993) *Managerialism and the Public Services: Cuts or Cultural Change in the 1990s?* Oxford: Blackwell Business.

Porath, C., Spreitzer, G., Gibson, C. and Garnett, F. G. (2012) Thriving at work: Toward its measurement, construct validation, and theoretical refinement. *Journal of Organizational Behavior*, 33(2), 250–75.

Practice Governance Group (2011) *Scottish Government. Practice Governance Framework: Responsibility and Accountability in Social Work Practice*. www.gov.scot/Resource/Doc/347682/0115812.pdf (accessed 12/12/15).

Rawlings, A., Paliokosta, P., Maisey, D., Johnson, J., Capstick, J. and Jones. R. (2014) *A Study to Investigate the Barriers to Learning from Serious Case Reviews and Identify Ways of Overcoming these Barriers*. DFE- RR340 www.safeguardingchildrenea.co.uk/wp-content/uploads/2014/08/A-study-to-investigate-barriers-to-learning-from-serious-case-reviews.pdf (accessed 12/12/15).

Reder, P. and Duncan, S. (1999) *Lost Innocents. A Follow-up Study of Fatal Child Abuse*. London: Routledge.

Rix, J. (2011) How Hackney reclaimed child protection social work. *Guardian* Society www.theguardian.com/society/2011/nov/08/reclaiming-social-work-hackney-breakaway-success (accessed 01/01/16).

Rogowski, S. (2010) *Social Work: The Rise and Fall of a Profession*. Bristol: Policy Press.

Rogowski, S. (2011) Social work with children and families: Challenges and possibilities in the neo-liberal world. *British Journal of Social Work*, 42(5), 921–40.

Rogowski, S. (2013) *Critical Social Work with Children and Families: Theory, Context and Practice*. Bristol: Policy Press.

Ruch, G. (2005) Relationship-based practice and reflective practice: Holistic approaches to contemporary child care social work. *Child and Family Social Work*, 10(2), 111–23.

Rutter, L. and Brown, K. (2015) *Critical Thinking and Professional Judgement in Social Work*. London: Learning Matters.

Schyns, B. and Schilling, J. (2013) How bad are the effects of bad leaders? A meta-analysis of destructive leadership and its outcomes. *The Leadership Quarterly*, 24(1), 138–58.

SCIE (Social Care Institute for Excellence) (2015) *Leading the Care Act. Report from SCIE Roundtable held on 5 March 2015.* SCIE Report 72.

Senge, P. M. (1990) *The Fifth Discipline: The Art and Practice of the Learning Organization.* Broadway, NY: Publishing Group.

Simmons, L. (2007) *Social Care Governance Workbook.* Social Care Institute for Excellence (SCIE) Social Care Governance Support Team.

Srivastva, S. and Cooperrider, D. L. (1987) Appreciative Inquiry into Organizational Life. *Research in organizational change and development,* 1. Bingley: JAI Press.

Thorlby, R., Smith, J., Dayan, M. and Williams, S. (2014) *The Francis Report: One Year On.* London: Nuffield Trust.

Trevithick, P. (2014) Humanising managerialism: Reclaiming emotional reasoning, intuition, the relationship, and knowledge and skills in social work. *Journal of Social Work Practice,* 28(3), 287–311.

VCF (Victoria Climbié Foundation) (2014) *Voices from the Front Line: Supporting Social Workers to Deliver Quality Services to Children.* http://vcf-uk.org/vcf-calls-for-urgent-action-in-new-research-voices-from-the-front-line/ (accessed 12/10/15).

Virilio, P. (2012a) *The Great Accelerator.* Cambridge: Polity.

Virilio, P. (2012b) *The Administration of Fear.* New York: MIT Press.

Wang, C. L. and Ahmed, P. K. (2003) Organisational learning: A critical review. *The Learning Organization,* 10(1), 8–17.

Warner, J. (2014) 'Heads must roll'? Emotional politics, the press and the Death of Baby P. *British Journal of Social Work,* 44(6), 1637–53.

WASOS (West Australian Government Signs of Safety Framework) (2011) *The Signs of Safety Child Protection Practice Framework* www.dcp.wa.gov.au/Resources/Documents/Policies%20and%20Frameworks/SignsOfSafetyFramework2011.pdf (accessed 09/02/16).

Wenger, E. (2000) Communities of practice and social learning systems. *Organization,* 7(2), 225–46.

White, S., Hall, C. and Peckover, S. (2009) The descriptive tyranny of the common assessment framework: Technologies of categorization and professional practice in child welfare. *British Journal of Social Work,* 39(7), 1197–217.

Wonnacott, J. (2011) *Mastering Social Work Supervision.* London: Jessica Kingsley Publishers.

Yukl, Y. (2010) *Leadership in Organisations,* Global Edition. Harlow: Pearson.

Yukl, G. and Lepsinger, R. (2004) *Flexible Leadership: Creating Value by Balancing Multiple Challenges and Choices* (Vol. 223). Oxford: John Wiley & Sons.

Zuber-Skerritt, O. (2002) The concept of action learning. *The Learning Organization,* 9(3), 114–24.

Acknowledgements

Figures 5.1, 5.2 and 5.4 are available from Google Images (2016) https://images.google.com/ (accessed 09/02/16). Table 5.1 is with the permission of the authors.

Appendix 5.1

The Knowledge and Skills Statements (KSS) for Practice Supervisors and Leaders (DfE 2015) in Children and Family Social Work in England.

The Practice Supervisor will be able to do the following:

1   **Promote and govern excellent practice**

Establish and maintain a highly valued position of influence within the organisation, and be recognised for extensive knowledge and skill in the profession of child and family social work. Help shape and influence an environment which enables excellent practice by setting high standards and motivating others to do the same. Demonstrate optimistic behaviour, and build positive relationships with children and families and other professionals. Lead by example, showing integrity, creativity, resilience and clarity of purpose. Be visible and accessible to all staff, children and families.

Be accountable for ensuring the highest professional standards and professional conduct. Design and implement measures to assure the quality of practice and the effective throughput of work. Interrogate decisions, ensuring they are underpinned by theory and the best evidence and that they will contribute to the goals of the family and their social work plan, whilst ensuring that the safety of children remains the highest priority. Closely monitor the wellbeing of children in public care, ensuring that they grow up in homes in which they are happy and thriving, holding high ambitions for their futures.

2   **Developing excellent practitioners**

Recognise, respect and value the expertise of practitioners and provide a practice framework, underpinned by theory and the best evidence, within which they can work effectively. Explain and champion the framework to practitioners, other professionals, children and families and set an expectation that this framework will be applied to practice. Facilitate use of the best evidence to devise effective interventions, which are most likely to support family welfare and reduce risk to children. Secure excellent practice through an analytical understanding of different patterns of family functioning, matched with service responses which are most likely to effect change for families, as well as support children in public care and young people leaving care.

Recognise the strengths and development needs of practitioners, and use practice observation, reflection and feedback mechanisms, including the views of children and families, to develop practice. Develop a culture of learning and improvement, where staff are sufficiently stretched and mentored to meet their aspirations. Gauge different learning styles and recognise when the role of the Practice Supervisor is to teach and when it would be more effective to draw on practitioners' own knowledge. Invest available resources into staff and service development, drawing on the expertise of children and families.

AQ

3 **Shaping and influencing the practice system**

Provide a safe, calm and well-ordered environment for all staff, ensuring that processes are fit for purpose and efficient. Create an ethos within which staff are motivated and supported to be ambitious on behalf of children and families. Use resources, including those that lie within families and communities, to the best effect. Facilitate constant reflective thinking about the welfare of families and the safety of children. Build and develop influential and respectful partnerships between practitioners and partner agencies. Pay attention to different structures, pressures, priorities and levers for influencing and shaping the thinking of others.

Share practice knowledge and expertise and influence the wider organisation and national system to function to the best effect. Offer constructive advice and creative, strengths-based solutions to difficulties.

4 **Effective use of power and authority**

Apply a proportionate and ethical approach to the exercise of authority, which develops and maintains relationships with families and professionals and ensures the protection of children. Maximise opportunities for children and families to make informed choices. Secure an up to date, working knowledge of relevant legislation and case law. Exercise statutory powers where social work assessment shows that families require help and support and children are at risk of significant harm, ensuring that actions are proportionate to risk. Support practitioners to always communicate clearly, honestly and respectfully the purpose and content of the social work plan.

Recognise the patterns of relationships between professionals, identifying where these are likely to compromise the welfare of families and the safety of children, taking immediate and corrective action. Invite challenge and debate and be accessible to children, families and professionals. Ensure the professional network identifies the logic by which children and families are functioning and use this as a basis for effective engagement. Take into account diversity, the experience of discrimination and the impact of poverty.

5 **Confident analysis and decision-making**

Create a culture of focused thinking which consistently explores a wide range of contexts (including family and professional stories, the chronology of critical events, social and economic circumstances). Generate multiple hypotheses which make sense of the complexity in which children and families are living. Help practitioners to make decisions based on observations and analyses, taking account of the wishes and feelings of children and families. Ensure that practitioners are ambitious for children and families and that the long-term and life-long consequences of decisions are fully considered at all stages of planning and review, and in consultation with children and families. Build relevant relationships with children and families and professionals to test current hypotheses and dominant perspectives. Ensure that children and young people's expectations are met where possible and any disappointment sensitively acknowledged and sufficiently addressed.

Establish recording processes, provide the full analysis underpinning decisions, making sure the rationale for why and how decisions have been made is comprehensive and well expressed.

6 **Purposeful and effective social work**

Ensure practitioners adopt an approach to practice which is proportionate to identified risk and need. Use supervision processes to challenge the balance of authoritative intervention and collaborative engagement to determine how current practice is achieving the best long-term outcomes for children and families. Use focused questioning with practitioners to clarify the direction of work, and identify whether practitioners need to adopt a more reflective and curious approach, or respond with greater pace and assertion. Ensure that family narratives are sought and listened to, that all relevant family members, including fathers, are engaged in shaping plans and supported to carry these out, and that practice empowers families to make positive changes.

Ensure methods and tools used are based on the best evidence, that progress is frequently reviewed and that the social work plan is adjusted accordingly. Reflect upon and review the welfare and support needs of children and families and be alert to evidence of actual or likely significant harm ensuring that identified risks are managed and new risks identified, assessed and addressed.

Implement effective strategies for ensuring throughput of work. Frequently review the requirement for continued involvement so that cases are closed in a timely manner and that families have an appropriate and long-term support plan where that is required, and ensure that no child or family is left unnoticed in the system.

7 **Emotionally intelligent practice supervision**

Recognise how different relationships evoke different emotional responses, which impact upon the effectiveness of social work practice and provide responsive, high quality individual supervision. Use mechanisms such as peer supervision and group case consultation to help identify bias, shift thinking and the approach to case work in order to generate better outcomes for children and families. Recognise and articulate the dilemmas and challenges faced by practitioners and use this expertise and experience to guide, assist and support the provision of services.

Identify emotional barriers affecting practice and recognise when to step in and proactively support individuals. Promote reflective thinking to drive more effective discussions so that reasoned and timely decision-making can take place. Demonstrate a high level of resilience within pressured environments, be attuned to the effect of high emotion and stress and respond in calm, measured and pragmatic ways.

Reflect upon the confidence of practitioners and adapt management and leadership style according to the needs of individuals and the organisation. Protect practitioners from unnecessary bureaucratic or hierarchical pressures and have in place strategies to help manage the root causes of stress and anxiety. Continually energise and reaffirm commitment to support families and protect children.

8 **Performance management and improvement**

Explain to practitioners the full legal, regulatory, procedural and performance framework within which they operate and be accountable for their work within it. Provide opportunities for staff to give and receive constructive feedback on performance. Recognise and commend hard work and excellent practice and build social workers' confidence in their practice. Challenge complacency with a commitment to continued improvement and confidently hold poor practice to account.

Establish available capacity so that work is allocated appropriately across the staff group and ensure best use is made of resource, ability, interests and ambitions. Devise and implement systems which both demonstrate effective practice and trigger immediate corrective action where necessary. Produce and utilise data to understand current demand, historical patterns and likely future trends. Scrutinise system performance and devise and implement effective and timely improvement plans.

Strike a balance between employing a managerial, task-focussed approach and an enabling, reflective leadership style to achieve efficient day-to-day functioning. Develop a strategy for future improvements and contribute to similar within the wider organisational system. Draw on and share best practice within local and national contexts. Implement communication channels with children, young people, families and other professionals inviting feedback and ideas for improvement. Respond thoughtfully and proactively to complaints and mistakes, creating learning opportunities for self, staff and the organisation.

The Practice Leader will be able to do the following:

1   **Lead and govern excellent practice**
Be a highly visible and highly valued figure, occupying a position of significant influence at a local and national level, and be known for exceptional knowledge and skill in the profession of child and family social work. Hold accountability for child and family social work practice and its impact on the lives of children and families locally.

Provide clarity of organisational purpose and the values underpinning that, focusing on providing a world-class service for children and families. Demonstrate optimistic behaviour, and positive relationships and attitudes towards children and families, other professionals and partner agencies, politicians and the public. Drive change and constant progress so that children and families get the very best help and support. Secure an up to date, working knowledge of relevant legislation and case law. Show the strongest commitment to children in public care by ensuring they grow up in homes in which they can thrive and, having left care, receive all the support to which they are entitled.

Lead by example with integrity, creativity, resilience, and clarity of purpose. Sustain wide, current knowledge and understanding of child and family social work practice and broader child protection and welfare systems, locally, nationally and globally.

2   **Creating a context for excellent practice**
Engage staff, children and families and the wider partnership in constructive thinking about the future. Create a shared strategic vision which inspires, motivates and encapsulates the organisational commitment to supporting families, protecting children and providing safe and stable childhoods for children in public care.

Champion this vision and drive strategic leadership throughout the organisation, so that it is applied to everyday practice.

Focus on best outcomes for children and families and ensure that the vision, purpose and plan for the organisation is welcomed and owned by all. Continuously evaluate how best to keep the vision a reality, and what needs to change to build upon existing strengths.

Create a culture in which excellent practice is expected and celebrated, critical incidents handled with grace and discipline, and public commitment to protecting children and supporting families frequent and authentic.

3   **Designing a system to support effective practice**
Design with political and financial astuteness, and within a clear set of principles, a practice system which enables excellent child and family social work practice to flourish. Ably translate local and national policy into the organisational context, without compromising high quality professional practice. Prioritise budgets in order to meet demand and ensure quality of service provision. Confidently illustrate the relationship between efficiency, children's outcomes and financial flexibility so that services can respond to changing need and risk.

Provide a safe, calm and well-ordered environment for all staff, ensuring that process is well considered, fit for purpose and efficient. Create sufficient capacity for practitioners to build relationships with children and families and undertake effective direct work with families which enhances family wellbeing and reduces risks. Use resources, including those that lie within families and communities, to best effect and have mechanisms in place to ensure constant reflective thinking about the welfare of families and the safety of children. Build influential and productive relationships across the organisation and the wider local partnership, across regions and nationwide, to secure the very best support to families and the protection of children.

Establish communication channels which report on the welfare of children and families, and the safety of those at risk. Be alert to anxiety and pressures within the organisation, even at the earliest stages. Secure high quality legal, financial and human resource services for the organisation and ensure communication technology is fit for purpose. Challenge orthodoxies in the best interests of achieving excellence for children and families, and model entrepreneurial and innovative approaches to practice and leadership.

4   **Developing excellent practitioners**
Critically appraise theory, the best evidence and rationale for different practice approaches. Select robust methodologies to form an overarching practice framework. Identify the skills needed to practise within the complexity of children's and families' lives, and in particular the population being served by the organisation. Secure the resources and support needed to implement the practice framework and shape, in partnership with others, the current and future quality of practice through effective training and sustained professional development for all staff and throughout a practice career. Recognise and utilise the resource that children, families and communities can bring to the development of staff and services.

Recognise the value of excellent social workers remaining in frontline practice. Provide sufficient organisational, professional and personal support to ensure the wellbeing of practitioners so that they can provide excellent social work services to children and families. Identify and develop people with emerging leadership talent, and support retention through the provision of challenging, interesting and motivating opportunities.

5 **Support effective decision-making**
Build a culture where managed risk is accepted and understood as being inherent in every decision that is made. Encourage practitioners to make decisions and take subsequent actions in this context making sure they know they have the backing of the organisation to act reasonably and in a child's best interests. Actively demonstrate trust in the workforce and develop a culture which promotes learning, reflection and the acceptance of accountability.

Publicly acknowledge the enormity of separating a child from their parents. Participate and add rigour to decision-making about children coming into public care, returning home or to the wider family, or moving to new permanent families. Ensure that all long-term consequences of current decisions are properly explored and understood.

Make sound and complex decisions in high pressured, fast paced conditions, striking a balance between speed and depth of thought. Draw on the best evidence to help inform thinking and decision-making.

6 **Quality assurance and improvement**
Set and uphold high quality practice standards, instilling a strong sense of accountability in staff for the impact of their work on the lives of children and families. Establish rigorous and fair processes for managing the performance of staff, including accurate measures of practice through direct observation. Secure an in-depth, comprehensive and current understanding of the realities of practice across the organisation and know how to address early signs of difficulties. Recognise and commend hard work and excellent practice which builds social workers' confidence in their practice. Meet complacency with a commitment to continued improvement and confidently hold poor practice to account.

Learn from local, national and international review, inspection and research and lead local and national debate. Ensure local children, families and communities play an active role in assessing the quality of services received and developing ideas for service and staff development. Pay close attention to the organisation's local and national reputation, taking steps to manage its public profile successfully. Establish the organisation as a credible and respectable public service, proudly promoting the achievements of staff, children and families.

Accessible at www.gov.uk/government/uploads/system/uploads/attach ment_data/file/448491/Consultation-document-knowledge-and-skills-practice-supervisors-and-practice-leaders.pdf

Appendix 5.2

Standards for the Employers of Social Workers in England (LGA 2014). This applies to adult and children and families social work.

1   **Clear Social Work Accountability Framework**:
    Employers should have in place a clear social work accountability framework informed by knowledge of good social work practice and the experience and expertise of service users, carers and practitioners.

2   **Effective Workforce Planning**:
    Employers should use effective workforce planning systems to make sure that the right number of social workers, with the right level of skills and experience, are available to meet current and future service demands.

3   **Safe Workloads and Case Allocation**:
    Employers should ensure social workers have safe and manageable workloads.

4   **Managing Risks and Resources**:
    Employers should ensure that social workers can do their jobs safely and have the practical tools and resources they need to practice effectively. Assess risks and take action to minimise and prevent them.

5   **Effective and Appropriate Supervision**:
    Employers should ensure that social workers have regular and appropriate social work supervision.

6   **Continuing Professional Development**:
    Employers should provide opportunities for effective continuing professional development, as well as access to research and-relevant knowledge.

7   **Professional Registration**:
    Employers should ensure social workers can maintain their professional registration.

8   **Effective Partnerships**:
    Employers should establish effective partnerships with higher education institutions and other organisations to support the delivery of social work education and continuing professional development.

Accessible at www.local.gov.uk/workforce/-/journal_content/56/10180/3511605/ARTICLE

Chapter 6
Critical practice: 'Touching something lightly many times'

Some thoughts on language and reparation in relation to mental health and social justice

Linda Kemp

Chapter outline

This chapter introduces:

- language as a medium for expressing experience
- the relationship between professional and service user in relation to mental health
- a critical theory of health care.

In this way, the psychiatrist can work economically with three kinds of black space at once. An economy is a system of apparently willing but actually involuntary exchanges. A family, for example, is a really a shopfront, a glass plate open to the street. Passers-by might mistake it for a boucherie, splashed as the customer/butcher are with blood.

Bhanu Kapil, Schizophrene (2011: 42)

In this chapter we examine the contention that the shaping function of language can limit or expand the articulation and agency of both service users and health care workers. In the book you are reading now the discussion of health and social care is taking place through the medium of language. You are reading these words and it is through these words and your own words that you think about health and social care and how what you are reading relates to your own experiences. Language is the medium which facilitates understanding and generates possibilities of creating new knowledge. This chapter will take a critical look at the role language plays in circumscribing lived experience and how this relates to your understanding of yourself as a professional working in health and social care, as well as everyone's experiences of receiving care. Drawing broadly on the insights of critical theory as applied to health care (Morgan et al. 2016: 71–75), the poetic hybrid writing of Bhanu Kapil and Simone Weil's philosophical writing, this chapter takes a critical lens to health and social care through examining practices relating to mental health care. The aim is to foreground ways in which a critical approach to language can contribute to an amelioration of the relationships between people accessing health and social care services and those working within those services.

Drawing inspiration from the sphere of mental health activism I take as my starting point the assertion of survivor/user-led critical mental health that the 'Recovery' model of mental health care (Repper and Perkins 2003) 'continues an onslaught of neoliberalism in mental health, in which people are to be made individually responsible for difficulties which would be better thought of as originating in society' (Gadsby 2015). Jonathan Gadsby discusses the manifestation of this neoliberalisation of mental health care in the form of the Mental Health Recovery Star, a tool designed in 2007 by Triangle Consulting Social Enterprise to provide outcome measures for progression in mental health recovery. The ten 'points' of the star comprise 'managing mental health', 'self-care', 'living skills', 'social networks', 'work', 'relationships', 'addictive behaviour', 'responsibilities', 'identity and self-esteem', and 'trust and hope'. Simply through reading these labels it will be clear to the reader that grave difficulties are encountered when attempting measurement in any of these areas, not to mention further difficulties in appending values to the subjective evaluation – whoever completes it, in any capacity – of fundamental areas of life and then extending these 'measurements' into an interpretation of effectiveness in the form of whether the desirable targets have been met. It is quite possible to imagine a scenario where the desirable target for the mental health service provider is the throughput of service users who are 'recovered' sufficiently to be discharged from the service, and where the service itself retains a metric to demonstrate its own effectiveness. Here 'recovery' becomes a project which can be delivered through meeting established targets, a process which in turn also commoditises service users. The transactional basis of the Recovery Star positions actions and other people as means for personal benefit: value is ascribed to transactions which bring about 'progress' (towards prescribed targets) for the service users. It is a short step from this to the assumption that actions, 'transactions', which do not 'progress' the service user towards these targets are negligible transactions, even where those transactions may be actions and social relations which the service user deems desirable and do indeed contribute, perhaps significantly, to their health and wellbeing. The immeasurable and the unmeasured become waste, or excess, and the service user non-compliant or deviant. Conversely, one might argue that the Recovery Star serves as a guide for conversation, a tool to assist the carers' or mental health professionals' conversation with their service users, perhaps of particular benefit during instances where encouragement is required to foster conversations characterised by deep listening and empathy. However, without these skills being in place one might question the agility with which the Recovery-Star-based conversations might be directed.

The purpose of the above gloss of this particular tool as symptomatic of problematic ethics underpinning the measurement of outcomes for people experiencing mental distress is to gesture towards a survivor/user-led counter-argument that foregrounds the neoliberal agenda subtending the Recovery Star. The Recovery in the Bin survivors group have designed and presented the UnRecovery Star (Recovery in the Bin, 2015). UnRecovery is an emergent term, originating in survivor-activist circles, designed as a political critique of the aforementioned neoliberalisation of mental health care generally and the co-option of 'Recovery' by the State specifically (Recovery in the Bin, 2015). The ten 'points' of the UnRecovery Star are 'unstable housing', 'sexism', 'loss of welfare state', 'loss of rights', 'economic inequality', 'homophobia/transphobia', 'racism', 'discrimination', 'trauma/iatrogenic trauma' and 'poverty'. The labels on the points of this star are clearly very different from those on the Recovery Star. Jonathan Gadsby (2015) notes of this distinction:

> Their attack is a political one: far from opening the frames of reference from narrow medical illness to more holistic personal wellbeing, the Recovery Star continues an onslaught of neoliberalism in mental health, in which people are to be made individually responsible for difficulties which would be better thought of as originating in society. Through this lens, the holism of the Recovery Star becomes a complete colonisation of a person with a set of ideas that appear to be liberating but in fact absolve the powerful from the need to acknowledge and address inequalities of all kinds. For example, widening the conversation to include work and financial skills might seem welcome because loss of role, loss of meaningful activity and financial worries are very significant drivers of distress. However, in so doing, we may be failing to notice with the service-user that they live in an unjust society in which finding one's way and having access to decent housing, meaningful roles, security, having protected rights and simply being allowed to be different seem to be increasingly the domain of the privileged.

Moreover, the service user's ability to overcome these social inequalities are negligible, more likely to emerge from chance of circumstance than design. Laying these limitations at the feet of the service user places an implied responsibility upon the service user which the health care worker themselves would likely be unable to overcome in similar circumstances. Whilst the language of the labels appended to the points of the Recovery Star, the words 'managing mental health', 'self-care', 'living skills', 'social networks', 'work', 'relationships', 'addictive behaviour', 'responsibilities', 'identity and self-esteem', and 'trust and hope', appear perhaps as reasonable approximations of discrete areas of an individual's life, the carving out of subsets in this way emphasises a normative behavioural standard. The words themselves, the language against which the measuring of outcomes will take place, are, arguably, not in and of themselves value-laden. The value is imposed in their context, their application as devices against which behaviours will be scored. Switching these labels to the words deployed in the UnRecovery Star uncovers the self-reliance and self-culpability implicit in the original star. Survivor-led critiques, such as the re-appropriation of the Recovery Star, illustrate the power of discursive formations. The totalising effect of outcome measures denies the service user their own agency over their own lives.

Here we might usefully turn to the work of the French philosopher Michel Foucault and his notion of 'discursive formations' which, broadly, posits 'discourses' as the controlling systems for the production of knowledge. Foucault's works examine a range of different discourse formations with *Madness and Civilization* (1961), in particular, examining how Western society came to define what it considers to be 'madness' and the idea of incarceration as a 'solution' to this perceived 'problem'. Foucault's style of writing forms part of his project of deconstructing metanarratives; refusing definition often seems to support a multiplicity which defies more conventional interpretive gestures towards power. Eliding the attribution of a direct meaning to the term 'discursive formations', Foucault comes close to defining his use of the word 'discourse' through illustrating his understanding thus: 'the edges of a book are neither clear nor rigorously delineated. No book exists by itself ... it is a point in a network' (Foucault 1998: 304). This is followed by two further elaborations in the same interview: 'The description of discourse asks a different question: How is it that this statement appeared, rather than some other in its place?' (Foucault 1998: 307) and,

> What permits the individualization of a discourse and gives it an independent existence is the system of points of choice which it offers from a field of given objects, from a determinate enunciative scale; and from a series of concepts defined in their content and use. Therefore, it would be inadequate to look for the general foundations of a discourse ... a single discourse can give rise to several different options.
>
> (Foucault 1998: 320)

Without defining his terms, an action which would invite limitations, Foucault indicates a fluidity with which assumptions about the fixity of discourse may be overturned. Previously 'closed' discourses are opened up to an ongoing investigation that *never* reaches a final point of closure because to do so would make the discourse static and therefore a form of stasis. Foucault's 'discursive formation' is an ongoing activity, both in terms of the active involvement of the person reviewing how any discourse has been formed, and the inscribed activity of documents/discourses as they relate to other documents/discourses through history. Accepting this Foucauldian proposition has significant implications for the practice of health and social care, broadly, and mental health care specifically. Where a discourse such as that inscribed into the Recovery Star forecloses its own outcomes, outcomes which are implicitly value-laden and ultimately judgemental – implicating the service user in their own 'failure' to achieve the outcomes imposed from *without* their own discursive understanding of themselves – an unravelling of the Recovery Star itself as a system of discourse, those neoliberal values of self-reliance and independence as separate from the society in which the individual lives, exposes the Recovery Star as a coercive tool which further estranges the service user from a healthful belonging to society. Integration into society on terms other than those identified by the service user effectively contributes to the further fragmentation of society. This itself is symptomatic of mental health care in the contemporary moment, typified as it is by communicative fragmentation, the substitution of one set of values inscribed into the language of health 'care' as against the self-articulations of the service user who, with the required resources, identifies and articulates in their own words the terms (desires) with which they seek to reintegrate into society. If this seems to overemphasise the importance of language and the willingness of individuals to articulate, with words, their own values, we might revisit the UnRecovery Star to contemplate how highly any given individual rates themselves against the ten social oppressors articulated therein. Faced with these outcomes, might one not be further empowered through defining one's own values rather than being faced with a demand to measure oneself against structural forces one is more or less powerless, at least on an individual level, to alter? The totalising of closed discourse formations such as the Recovery Star at best side-step and at worst eradicate the human capacity for creativity, the force which enables the individual to shape their own life rather than the alternative, which is to have life shaped by another.

Staying with the notion of individual capacity for creativity and the agency to shape one's own life we will now look at some alternative takes on how this agency might manifest. Writing in the context of understanding the effects and affects of trauma, Sandra Bloom 'make[s] the case that artistic performance, in all its variations, is a primary integrating mechanism in an organism highly susceptible to the protective, but ultimately destructive mechanism we call *dissociation*' (Bloom 2010: 199). Disassociation, as the word itself suggests, is linked to fragmentation and loss of integration. Bloom's argument posits evolutionary purposes for the development of artistic practices, recognising that artistic creativity performs a communicative function enabling integration of the individual (back) into their society. Belonging to the wider society, symptomatic of the essential social nature of the human animal, is core to the integration of the individual whose individuality depends upon a healthful belonging (communicative function within) to the social group. Bloom's attention to the loss of language function which accompanies trauma points towards the communicative schism and the reparative work art is capable of performing (Bloom 2010: 204). Bloom's model here is one of integration, reintegration, based on a social model where rather than an individual isolated from the social culture in which s/he lives, s/he (re)integrates within the cultural terms of that society, which here I place in opposition to the theorised society posited in the Recovery Star. Taking this further, Griselda Pollock argues that,

> We are accustomed to think about trauma with the model of cure. Bad things happen to individuals. We should try to get over them. Time will heal. They are in the past. We must move on and let go. Or, if the event is historical, we build a monument, set up a memorial day, make a movie and leave our burden to them. The problem is that trauma, as we now understand the wounding of the psyche by

an extreme event or by accumulated suffering, is not like that. When we borrow trauma as a term for personally affecting psychological shocks or as a metaphor for historical events that exceed existing representational resources, we also confront a problem that will not sort itself out by itself.

(Pollock 2013: 1)

Pollock's argument foregrounds an essential social-ness and the social function of the 'symptomologies such as the compulsion to repeat and acting out' (Pollock 2013: 1). Pollock queries the assumption of a cure model as a useful framework for considerations of trauma, cure implying a resolution taking the form of relief from symptoms. One cannot be 'cured' or 'recover' from trauma but one can be relieved from or learn to manage its effects and affects. Such concern with the specificities of trauma drills down through the generalisations demarked through the terms 'health and social care' with its catch-all embrace, through to the immediate concern with 'mental health' of this chapter, to a concern with a specific – and yet still generalised – symptomatic of dissociative 'ill health' and in particular one marked by the loss of language. The accounts written by Bloom and Pollock above participate in their own fields of discursive formations, speaking within, to and beyond their particular disciplinary bases. Their value to health and social care as both academic discipline with its institutionalised forms of educational pedagogies and the institutionalised forms of practising health and social care jobs, careers and professional roles effecting and affecting the lives of other human beings, lies in their advocacy of a politicised holism. Both Bloom and Pollock argue for dynamism, a continual becoming, rather than representation which, like a star, is fixed, remote, and awarded for 'good' (conforming) behaviour.

On the subject of representation this seems an opportune moment to reflect on the status of textbooks, including this one, and their propensity to be read as textbooks. Once again language betrays the difficulty. Commonplace definitions of the word 'textbook' would have it defined as 'a manual of instruction', 'a work recognised as an authority', approaches which endow the textbook with an authoritative status (OED Online 2015). Textbooks, read without caution, can also be taken as representative of something far greater than their contents profess.

Discussing trauma and its relation to art, Sandra Bloom posits that:

in individual pathology no one else agrees with the view of reality shared by that individual. Instead, the person is called delusional, mad, or at the least eccentric. There is a borderline between these two realities, however. Children, artists, prophets, visionaries spend time there.

(Bloom 2010: 202)

Allowing acknowledgement of more than one 'reality' steps beyond the usual call of the health and social care domain, a 'discursive formation' where it is commonly carried out as though an acceptable 'reality' is firmly defined. This reality can be found in those descriptors labelling each point of the Recovery Star. The shaping function of language can limit or expand the articulation and agency of both service users and health care workers. The agency of language can be acutely witnessed when it appears in one of its most condensed forms, poetry. In poetry the compressed use of language foregrounds its intricacies, revealing otherwise hidden or forgotten meanings which are revealed through context. Words and language are revealed to be and do considerably more than simply represent.

The epigraph at the start of this chapter is taken from *Schizophrene* by the poet-writer Bhanu Kapil. In these few lines Kapil brings together multiple and distinct concepts which, combined, reveal each as more complex than normative assumptions permit. In this way the discourses associated with psychiatry as a medical model for understanding how the mind functions or more often with its disfunction, is analogous with an economy, a discourse usually associated with financial transactions and, in Kapil's gloss, also the *dysfunctional*, because 'involuntary', nature of these transactions. Mention of 'a family', in this context meaning any family system, can then be interpreted through this lens of enforced emotional and mental entanglements. Furthermore, these exchanges are merely a (shop) 'front', the shopping speaking back to the transactions of economic exchange, situating the family as a network of economic exchanges, and one vulnerable to the destruction implied by the breakability of the 'glass plate' and its location in a public place, inviting any passer-by to look in, observe, perhaps shatter the glass window. Completing this passage with reference to 'boucherie' (butcher's) finalises the impression of slaughter, the bloody mess of family life as the enforced economic unit of the family thrashes against one another, distorting and disturbing one another as the involuntary performance, demanded by the shop window of a consumer-driven, socially-sanctioned family life, is enforced through economic blood ties. The conjoining of 'customer/butcher' lets no one escape: the reader, too – us, ourselves – is complicit in this economy of distorted desires. This depiction of the 'family' estranges our understanding of 'the family' as it is constituted in familiar terms where the family is a source of belonging and, by extension, comfort. The refrain 'family and friends' occurs so often in health care literature as the recourse to which service users are urged to turn for support, it forms a discursive framework which reinforces a normative standard of the family in particular as a source of support and thus eliding the prospect of the family as a source of damage, as depicted in Kapil's image.

Difficulties between language and notions of healing are addressed through Kapil's foregrounding of a fissure between the two, not least in the title of her book. The third section of *Schizophrene* carries the title 'A Healing Narrative' and offers eight fragments of text. The entire book comprises fragments of text. Kapil writes, 'Sometimes I think it was not an image at all but a way of conveying information' (Kapil 2011: 40). Kapil also writes, 'I cannot make the map of healing and so this is the map of what happened in a particular country on a particular day' (Kapil 2011: 48). In these statements, and the book itself as a practice, Kapil rejects the representative inherent in the image (metaphor is declined) and rejects the possibility of constructing an authoritative description of steps to be taken for healing to occur (the 'map'). In their place she posits the image as transmitting information, an active process rather than statically representative, and healing as rooted in the particular rather than the general.

The fissure of the book's title manifests as an account of immigration and trauma. In a book which declares a concern with healing it is notable that encounters with health care, as the reader of this textbook might recognise it, are encounters of absence:

What digs into the head?

(Kapil 2011: 7)

I went to the Institute of Community Health Sciences in London, to interview Kamaldeep Bhui. Getting as far as his door.

I pressed my forehead to the door, which was cross-hatched. I could see his radio, his books, his clutter.

(Kapil 2011: 17)

Digging into the head is the role of the psychiatrist. The implication of the scene beyond the cross-hatched door is that the health worker Kapil seeks to interview is absent. She is unable to ask her questions. There is a gap, which she leans into with her forehead, an area of the body traditionally associated with foresight. The action of leaning into, touching, the door, the threshold into the space where healing happens or is understood, signifies a search for healing and an intuitive reaching towards an 'other' in order to facilitate this healing. The communication of touch is important in this book, where the fissure Kapil describes as schizophrenia 'is rhythmic, touching something lightly many times' (Kapil 2011: 61). In the 'Quick Notes' which close *Schizophrene*, Kapil writes of 'making a book that barely says anything, I hoped to offer: this quality of touch' (Kapil 2011: 71). The 'touch' of Kapil's book is the touch of her writing, her language, which by, in her own terms, 'barely saying anything' ensures a lightness, the opposite of instrumentalist, coercive language.

The family scene appears once again in Kapil's book. Here it is quoted in its entirety:

The schizophrenic's work is to make the house schizophrenic: an illuminated yet blackened construction at the centre of the field. All of the lights are on and the curtains are not drawn, exposing the occupants in the rituals of their illnesses. There is the butcher with his hatchet, compulsively chopping the meat. There is the butcher's wife, washing the table then setting the meat down upon it. There are the butcher's children sitting down to eat. When the meal is done, they remove their clothing as a family and put it in a bucket to soak. Even this far from the centre of the regional metropolis, their nudity comes as a shock.

(Kapil 2011: 54)

'Exposing the occupants in the rituals of their illness' the poet reveals, through exposure, stripping back and laying bare, unthinking conformity to prescribed social roles as a definition of illness. The 'work' of the schizophrenic here is at once symbolic and real, s/he reveals, through schism, through detaching from the 'shared reality' described by Bloom (2010: 202) to share a visionary experience of the family unit (dis)functioning upon a tableau scene, 'illuminated' by the emphasis placed upon it by a society which reveres one particular social construct of relations over and above others, 'yet blackened' too by the enforcement of this 'construction' – the placing of it 'at the centre of the field', as the centrepiece of life and by implication de-centring, devaluing, alternatives. The brutality returns, as in the original appearance of this family (the epigraph to this chapter), through butchery. Here family life is a form of butchery. Butchers hack pieces of meat, animal carcasses, to be consumed by humans. The animal nature of humans is made evident through the butchery, killing to survive, but here the distinction between who and what is being killed is blurred, the boundaries between 'family' and 'murder' are drawn closer together, an association which is recognisable within Western culture through the archetypes found in stories handed down through generations in forms such as fairytales, Shakespeare and classical Greek plays. In Kapil's book this 'visionary' insight reveals the proximity of family behaviour to the behaviour of (packs of) animals, 'their nudity' serving as a final reminder of their meat/animal status. Disguising this insight through the lens of 'the schizophrenic' facilitates Kapil's 'visionary' insight; however, the insight is really the exposure or reframing offered through her deft, clear usage of language, ordering her words in the most powerful arrangement to conjure an arresting scene.

In *The Iliad or The Poem of Force* the writer and visionary Simone Weil writes of the effects of violence on both the perpetrator and the victim. Weil begins with a definition of force:

> To define force – it is that x that turns anybody who is subjected to it into a thing. Exercised to the limit, it turns man into a thing in the most literal sense: it makes a corpse out of him. Somebody was here, and the next minute there is nobody here at all.
>
> (Weil 2005: 183)

'That x' is a violence which dehumanises. In Kapil's *Schizophrene* butchery becomes the line which distinguishes the human from the animal. Weil goes on to say,

> An extraordinary entity this – a thing that has a soul. And as for the soul, what an extraordinary house it finds itself in! Who can say what it costs it, moment by moment, to accommodate itself to this residence, how much writhing and bending, folding and pleating are required of it? It was not made to live inside a thing; if it does so, under pressure of necessity, there is not a single element of its nature to which violence is not done.
>
> (Weil 2005: 185)

Here Weil is revealing the harm of violence at an individual level, the private harm which is here figured as the contortions of a soul. In Kapil's writing that private harm extends to the harms revealed in the destructiveness of the family as an institution where conformity to prescribed social roles is enforced and policed by one another and by the onlookers who watch through that glass-plated shop window. Force within relationships instrumentalises relationships, turning people into things. In fact Weil is writing about Homer's poem *The Iliad* towards the start of the Second World War and her writing about force concerns the instrumentalisation of human life as it unfolded under Hitlerism and the Nazi regime. In this way Weil links public concerns, the widest social sphere, with the private troubles witnessed in her description of the contortions of the soul attempting to survive in the contorted body. The soul, the individual level, is contorted if society, the body, is instrumentalised, becomes a thing. In our context of thinking about what it means to become a professional working in one of the health and social care professions we need to think about how the discursive formation between the public sphere, society, and the apparently private concerns of an individual's health and wellbeing are circumscribed within the day-to-day language of practice. Any professional or paraprofessional working in health and social care fields holds a position of power and responsibility in relation to those in their care and this power and responsibility includes the potential for force. The language of the Recovery Star collapses public and private discourse formations, shifting public concerns such as the workforce, marketplace and inequalities in access to housing onto the individual. Force in the form of coercion is exerted when these public concerns are treated as private and operationalised in the form of the Recovery Star's measurement scale. In this way the Recovery Star represents an instrumentalisation of the concept of 'recovery' and what is understood by the term 'mental health'. People in receipt of these instrumentalised forms of 'care' risk harm in the form of dehumanisation. In this chapter the insights of Bhanu Kapil's *Schizophrene* and Simone Weil's *The Iliad or The Poem of Force* help to illuminate the role of language in creating discourse formations which shape our understandings of the world around us and how the coercive the force of instrumentalised forms of language can become causes of harm.

References

Bloom, S. L. (2010) Bridging the black hole of trauma: The evolutionary significance of the arts. *Psychotherapy and Politics International*, 8(3), 198–212.

Foucault, M. (1961) *Madness and Civilization: A History of Insanity in the Age of Reason*. New York: Pantheon Books.

Foucault, M. (1998) *Aesthetics: Essential Works of Foucault 1954–1984, volume 2*, edited by James D. Faubion. London: Penguin.

Gadsby, J. (2015) The Recovery Star meets the Unrecovery Star. *Critical Mental Health Nurses' Network*. http://criticalmhnursing.org/2015/10/19/the-recovery-star-meets-the-unrecovery-star/ (accessed 18 February 2016).

Kapil, B. (2011) *Schizophrene*. New York: Nightboat Books.

Morgan, A., Felton, A., Fulford, B., Kalathil, J. and Stacey, G. (2016) *Values and Ethics in Mental Health: An Exploration for Practice*. London: Palgrave.

OED Online (2015) 'Text-book, n.' *OED Online*. Oxford University Press, December 2015 (accessed 18 February 2016).

Pollock, G. (2013) *After-Affects/After-Image: Trauma and Aesthetic Transformation in the Virtual Feminist Museum*. New York/Manchester: Manchester University Press.

Recovery in the Bin (2015) 18 key principles. www.studymore.org.uk/binrec.htm (accessed 18 February 2016).

Repper, J. and Perkins, R. (2003) *Social Inclusion and Recovery: A Model for Mental Health Practice*. Edinburgh/London: Baillière Tindall.

Weil, S. (2005) The Iliad or The Poem of Force. In *Simone Weil: An Anthology*. London: Penguin, pp.182–215.

Chapter 7
Globalised practice

Adam Barnard

Chapter outline

This chapter introduces:

- definitions of globalisation
- the processes of globalisation
- the intersectionality of globalisation
- the challenge of McDonaldisation and McReflection
- the impact on health and social care services and communities.

Introduction

The current process of globalisation is defined and examined to explore how it is having an impact on communities and social care services. The chapter explores globalisation's defining features such as flows, barriers, stretched social relations, interpenetration of cultures and the emergence of global infrastructures. Ritzer defines globalisation as 'an accelerating set of processes involving flows that encompass ever-greater numbers of the world's spaces and that lead to increasing integration and interconnectivity among those spaces' (Ritzer 2004). Global networks and flows operate differently for different groups of people and communities. Debates around class, 'race', gender, age, sexuality and disability, so often central to social care, have been subsumed or marginalised in the mainstream of globalisation (Adam 2002). Sassen (1998) argues than in global cities (such as London, Tokyo, New York) most of the daily servicing jobs are carried out by women, immigrants and people from minority ethnic groups (often the same person). Health and social care provision is often delivered by a similar person where the intersection and intertextuality of social difference is experienced in the provision and reception of 'care'.

Dominelli (2007) explores the opportunities and constraints that the dynamics of globalisation present for human development in a range of different countries and situations. Arguing that globalisation is currently a system of organising social relations along neo-liberal lines, Dominelli examines practical examples of how people respond to significant social changes in their communities. Globalisation has collapsed the boundaries of time, space and place in ways that have exacerbated inequalities, at the same time giving rise to unparalleled riches for some and the illusion of equality for all. The chapter concludes by examining the impact of globalisation on communities and the possibilities of the political dimensions of social work in a UK context.

Globalisation

Children as young as two recognise the golden arches of McDonald's. Starbucks, Disney, Nike and Adidas have become global brands that are instantly recognisable and have permeated every high street and home. The Nike 'swooshstika' is reportedly the most requested tattoo in North America (Klein 2004). Political events from around the world are reported immediately such as 9/11 or the Asian tsunami. We mostly use Microsoft on computers and have shopped in a Wal-Mart store. The argument is that a process of globalisation has led to distinct changes in our everyday life. Drugs, crime, sex, war, protest, terrorism, disease, people, ideas, images, news, information, entertainment, pollution, goods and money all travel the globe (Held 2004). Ritzer (2010) suggests globalisation is increasingly omnipresent and is the most important change in human history. Consequently health and social care theory and practice has increasingly needed to become aware of, and respond to, the challenges of globalisation.

In terms of culture (Hopper 2007), society (Barnett et al. 2005), politics (Bayart 2007) and economics (Held and Kaya 2006; Kaplinsky 2005), rapid and dramatic changes have taken place due to globalisation. Wikipedia – a good example of this process – suggests Globalisation (or Globalization) – depending on which globalised term you use – refers to increasing global connectivity, integration and interdependence in the economic, social, technological, cultural, political and ecological spheres.

What does this suggest to us about the contemporary world? How are we to understand this process? What impact does this have on health and social care? What does this mean for globalised communities? What challenges and opportunities does it raise for social care and helping professions in the twenty-first century?

What's going on?

There is no question that the world is currently undergoing significant and profound acceleration in the process of globalisation, but globalisation itself is not new. For example, trade has existed for millennia between areas such as the Roman Empire, Arabia and China. The movement of peoples has a long, rich and troubled history. Knowledge, science, technology and culture have always been global throughout history. New forms of communication have emerged from the spoken, written to printed word, along with numerical systems or new technologies of communication such as the Victorian telegraph. However, many commentators would suggest we are now witnessing a qualitatively different set of processes.

Globalisation, although not new, has achieved unprecedented heights in the last half of the twentieth century and has accelerated further in the early twenty-first century. That dramatic growth has led to much work in many different fields on the topic of globalisation and many efforts to define it. Held (2004) suggests globalisation involves four dimensions. The first dimension is social relations so stretched that cultural, economic and political networks are connected across the world. For example, different and dispersed communities are part of global 'diasporas' of peoples stretched beyond any nation or locality. Communities are constituted across territorial boundaries. Families can keep touch with relatives in Pakistan, India, China, Australia and Africa. Gilroy explores black peoples' experience in the 'black Atlantic' (Gilroy 1992) and the Jewish diaspora suggests that this aspect of globalisation is nothing new. Health and social care theory and practice increasingly needs to recognise the significance of stretched social relations. For example, family members involved in receiving health and social care services may be in different countries, with different expectations and cultural understandings of health and social care. Diverse and heterogeneous cultural needs must be addressed by health and social care services. European enlargement has meant that health services are seeing increased use by migrant populations. Social care services are benefiting from older relatives moving to the UK to care for a new generation of children born to migrant communities.

The second dimension of globalisation is an intensification of flows of interaction so that instant communication is available to many (if you have access to the mass media, TV, internet or telephone). Ritzer (2010) insightfully notes the differentiation among different types of flows, such as interconnected, multi-directional, conflicting, and reverse flows. Trade and commerce, entertainment, news and media, sport, art and culture are all experienced rapidly and in a far greater volume than before. Information on health and social care is communicated instantly, so far-flung, localised events take on a global significance such as the 'swine flu' epidemic of 2009. The relative success of web-based National Health Service information has been well received by most users. It is also helpful to note Ritzer's (2010) suggestion that globalisation can be seen to 'hop' unevenly rather than flow smoothly.

The third dimension is the increasing interpenetration of distant cultures and events as societies come face to face with each other. For example, Bollywood films, the diversity of food available, the global recognition of brands such as Coke, Disney, Microsoft and McDonald's suggests this interpenetration of culture. 9/11 shows how we are influenced and affected by geographically distant and remote events. Health and social care services, theory and practice, have needed to respond positively to transcultural understanding and action in the design and delivery of services.

Finally, the fourth dimension is the emergence of global infrastructures to support and drive these changes. The internet is often identified as a key emerging infrastructure that supports stretched social relations, intensified communication and brings people and places closer together, although in an uneven and divided way (Drori 2006). The emergence of 'health tourism' where people travel to, and access, health and social care services from global providers has been a recent development. So how might we summarise these changes and these processes?

Towards a definition

Ritzer defines globalisation as 'an accelerating set of processes involving flows that encompass ever-greater numbers of the world's spaces and that lead to increasing integration and interconnectivity among those spaces' (Ritzer 2004). Ritzer (2010) argues globalisation is not just money, but virtually everything else that knows no (or at least fewer) limits in the global age. Giddens (2002) refers to these processes as a 'runaway world' and Marshal McLuhan and Bruce Powers (McLuhan and Powers 1989) speak of the 'global village'.

Woodward (2003: 171) suggests globalisation is a:

> social, cultural, political and economic phenomenon, which is subject to many different interpretations, ranging from those who see its impact as minimal and nothing new, to globalists or globalizers who argue that it is a recent and very significant phenomenon which has transformed life across the world. Some read this as a positive experience whilst others see it as having disastrous effects on local communities and those outside the western, especially US, mainstream. Most commentators agree that it has had some transforming impact.

Ritzer (2010: 3) argues:

> globalization is a transplanetary *process* or set of *processes* involving increasing liquidity and the growing multidirectional *flows* of people, objects, places and information as well as the *structures* they encounter and create that are *barriers* to, or *expedite*, those flows

Ritzer (2010) eruditely suggests globalisation can bring with it greater integration (especially when things flow easily), but it can also serve to reduce the level of integration (when structures are erected that successfully block flows). He provides a multidimensional and contemporary examination of globalisation.

Globalisation transforms our everyday lives, from minor considerations of what to have for dinner to major world-changing events. It involves social, economic, political, cultural and environmental processes and is characterised by conflict (such as terrorism and war) as well as consensus (such as communication and entertainment). It is also characterised by a weakening of boundaries of nation states (Woodward 2003: 137). Ritzer (2010) usefully captures this process as the increasing liquidity at the core of today's global world and a conceptual apparatus of 'flows' and 'barriers'. Events in one country are no longer isolated, such as the fall of the Berlin Wall, pollution or natural disasters. All have far-reaching effects that are transnational and global. Health and social care is not immune from these transformations and a globalised system of services and service users has emerged in response to these processes.

Another area that demands attention with globalisation is that it is divided between winners and losers. 'Positive globalisers' see everyone benefiting from the expansion of globalisation, whilst 'negative globalisers' see losers missing out on the benefits and suffering increased exploitation. Globalisation allegedly presents opportunities of greater democracy and participation such as through the internet but this technology remains dominated by the wealthy areas of the world. There is rapid transmission of information, easy access for individuals and communities and new opportunities for ideas, markets, democracy and choice. However, speed is of more importance to rich nations and it is this very speed that leads us into a rapid and manic sense of consciousness where we often fail to reflect on the consequences of the impulse of the immediate, or the consequences of our actions. Health and social care is caught in trying to respond positively and appropriately to these impulses. Ideas can be censured, choice is restricted to global brands and products, and democracy can be blocked, stifled or monitored. Globalisation has allowed easier movement of people across the globe but migration is often blocked for many refugees and migrants. Migration is often economically driven; exploitation remains and deepens. Health and social care services have been reconstituted in terms of who accesses services and who provides these services. Any economic benefits of globalisation need to be extended across all countries to challenge the health divides between the global rich and poor nations. Economic benefits need to be translated into health benefits. Adverse effects of globalisation on population-level health influences (e.g. on tobacco marketing and cross-border transmission of infectious disease) must be minimised, and globalisation's change of infrastructures needs to recognise health provision (Woodward et al. 2001). Changes and reduction in health and social care services have often been motivated by a perceived need to reduce social provision, with a view to becoming more competitive within the global economy (Deacon 2000).

Milestones in global health have had a wide-ranging and profound impact on communities – for example, in the US, vaccines and the eradication of smallpox, automotive safety, environmental health, infectious disease control, cancer, cardiovascular disease, safer and healthier foods, advances in material and child health, oral health and addictions (Lueddeke 2016: 13). In the UK, the sanitary revolution of the introduction of clean water and sewage disposal were the most significant milestones. These milestones have impacted on the physical state of individuals rather than the emotions, personal well-being and mental disorders of individuals (Lueddeke 2016: 13). There is still a significant amount of work to be done on these aspects of health and social care so professionals can make the overall well-being of individuals and communities their first concern and have a more significant impact on the social determinants of health.

The challenges of mental health, the gender gap, finances, world health and policy reforms present a challenging picture for globalised health and social care.

Globalisation and communities

Let us consider just a few examples of money, communication, 'sameness' (homogeneity) and consumption with special emphasis on their impact on community (the discussion that follows draws heavily on the work of Appadurai (1996) and his sense of global 'scapes'). Vast sums of money circulate around the world through government treasuries, banks, brokerage houses and so on. However, most of this flow of money is largely invisible to us, although it can have a profound effect on us. The focus throughout this chapter is the impact of globalisation on health and social care and communities, so how do global flows of money affect them? In many ways, of course, but one of the most important effects occurs when global traders in money decide that a currency of a given nation is overvalued. The result is a decline in the value of that currency with devastating effects on whole societies (for example, several East Asian countries in 1997; Argentina in 2002), as well as most communities within them. Buying power declines as local currencies are devalued. Jobs are lost and increasing numbers find themselves out of work and short of money. The community suffers in various ways without any control over the process. Globally, the poor are at risk from globalisation. Ritzer (2010) helpfully makes a distinction between the 'lightness' of the 'northern' tourist who can move easily and the heaviness of the 'southern' vagabond who is likely to move because they are compelled to do so (for example, forced to migrate to escape poverty [and to find work], by war, because of discrimination, and the like). Health and social care needs an awareness of the flows and barriers to globalisation and the movements of people.

Let us also consider communication. Some commentators have suggested the world has become 'flat' (Friedman 2005) due to the horizontal and less hierarchical forms of communication available, and it is the case that a far wider range of people are capable of communicating their views and getting out their messages. We can become aware of Chinese struggles for democracy, the living conditions for Iraqi people or popular protest in South America. This can have a salutary effect on communities which are able to get their views out and to have them reaffirmed by others scattered throughout the world. That said, the reverse is the case because those who seek to destroy a community can use the same media to organise and carry out their destructive activities. Terrorism, crime, drugs have all benefited from globalisation. This suggests that the world has not become anything approaching flat (Friedman 2005) as there are still great inequalities, barriers to equal participation and dangers in all sorts of things, including the internet.

A major issue in globalisation, as discussed by Ritzer (2004, 2005) is the degree to which it is related to growing homogeneity (becoming the same or 'sameness') or sustained heterogeneity (being diverse and different). This has great implications for communities since the latter would imply the continued survival and vitality of diverse and distinct communities whilst the former would involve a loss of distinctiveness among communities that would increasingly grow to look more and more alike.

'McDonaldisation' is the process by which the principles of the fast food restaurant are affecting more and more sectors of society and more and more societies around the world (Ritzer 2004). It is the latter, of course, that makes this a globalising process. The idea that more sectors of society and more societies around the globe are being affected by, and are adopting, the same principles (for example, efficiency) means that McDonaldisation tends to be associated with increasing homogenisation. At a most basic level many communities around the world look increasingly alike because so many of them have one, or more, McDonald's restaurants (there are over 30,000 of them, most outside the US), to say nothing of many of its clones in the fast food business (for example, Burger King, KFC, etc.). McDonaldisation can have a significant impact on health and social care issues. For example, the rise of obesity and particularly childhood obesity, partly due to increased consumption of fast food, is becoming a major area of concern for health care providers. Fast food has also decreased the social and community involvement of mealtimes. More generally, more and more organisations operate on basically the same principles so we can talk about things like 'McUniversities', 'McDoctors', 'McPharmacies' and 'McChurches'. Ritzer (2004) ably discusses the McDonaldisation of life and death, where health and social care services such as in vitro fertilisation are becoming more common place and the use of euthanasia clinics as well as a sanitised and efficient process of funerals has brought McDonald's principles to the end of life.

From our discussion on reflection there is a pressure for the processes and principles of McDonalisation to be brought into reflective practice. Calculation, prediction, control and the replacement of human labour with non-human technology is framing much contemporary reflection. A reflective app is seen as the promise of reflective practice. Reflection demands a global awareness so reflection can be located in the wider set of force fields of a globalised world.

As powerful as the process of McDonaldisation may be, it is a long way to get to homogeneous communities, from wiping out community diversity. Much remains different about communities from one area of a given nation to another, to say nothing of one part of the world to another. Furthermore, McDonaldisation produces enemies and that leads to counter-reactions that lead to more, rather than, less diversity. Individuals, groups, communities and even large, global organisations such as Slow Food based in Italy have mounted significant opposition to McDonald's and McDonaldisation. Slow Food is particularly important in this regard for its defence of distinctive cities ('Slow Cities'), local communities, and traditional food and other products. For example, in his defence of locally produced food, José Bové, a modest agricultural farmer, has become an international icon of resistance to global capitalism (Bové and Dufour 2005). The recent global debate on the provision of health care has seen the value of localised provision and the health and social care failing of the USA.

However, there is a deeper kind of homogeneity in the sense that more people become ever more deeply enmeshed in consumer culture. This means that consumption becomes increasingly important to them, perhaps becoming the centre of their lives. We can enjoy sun-dried Italian tomatoes, drinking American Coke on Ikea settees whilst watching Big Brother. There is a threat to heterogeneity when local, diverse products and practices are eroded by a global consumer culture. Would you rather have cheap standardised shoes made in sweat-shop conditions in a distant country by child labour or a bespoke pair of handmade shoes by a local artisan? If the global economy had not made the former so cheap, we might all prefer the latter. These threats to heterogeneity and diversity include communities that grow to be increasingly oriented to satisfying and expediting consumption and which all start to resemble each other. A similar position can be raised in health and social care. The homogeneity of provision has led to a standardised and monolithic provision of services whilst heterogeneity has emerged as a transcultural need and from service-user groups.

Those who want to sustain communities and their diversity will want to oppose much of what is described above. Heterogeneity at many levels is what makes life and communities interesting and rewarding. Threats to that heterogeneity are regarded by many as leading to less interesting and meaningful lives. More importantly, control shifts from inside the community to external powers that then have the capacity to alter or even destroy that community (as Wal-Mart or Tesco has famously done on a number of occasions). Even more tangibly, these organisations are essentially in the business of making money and very often they do so by exploiting communities and their people, as well as by taking profits to another community, perhaps even to another nation (Klein 2004). All of this can leave a community greatly impoverished, economically, politically and culturally. In terms of health and social care, the control of Big Pharm has seen the provision of certain types of service and the neglect of others. The World Health Organization (WHO) established the Commission on Social Determinants of Health (CSDH) in 2005, on the premise that action on social determinants of health is the fairest and most effective way to improve health for all people and reduce inequalities brought about by globalisation.

However, we must not forget that globalisation is not a one-way street but a unidimensional process. Just as many things flow into any given community, many things flow out, as well. Ritzer (2010) is particularly enlightening in his discussion of the various aspects of flows. Importantly, globalisation can have many positive effects on many things, including communities. Many communities have been greatly enhanced by the entrance of global businesses, the global media, global sports teams and the like. In assessing the impact of globalisation we need to look at both a community's gains and losses. Positive commentators have suggested it is not clear that anything needs to be done about globalisation in general, but it is clear that communities need to seek out that which enhances them and to block the entrance of that which threatens them and their integrity, or to limit their impact if they cannot be blocked.

The future of health and social care professions

What of the future? It seems clear that globalisation is here to stay and the future will bring an acceleration of it and its effects on everything, including communities and health and social care services. There will certainly continue to be many positives associated with this process, but it is also the case that the negatives will continue as well. The thrust of this discussion leads us to worry that the negatives will come to outweigh the positives. After all, the great power and a disproportionate share of the wealth are on the side of the forces that support McDonaldisation, consumerism and homogeneity. In confrontations with most communities, they have the upper hand (although there are certainly instances where the community 'David' has slain the corporate 'Goliath'). Thus, it is hard to envision a bright future for communities, at least as we have traditionally thought of them. A highly McDonaldised community, one in which much of what transpires is centrally conceived, controlled, and lacking in distinctive content, is a long way from what we have thought of (perhaps over-romantically) as community. We will need to rethink what we may mean by community, but this is far less of a problem than being forced to abandon communities to the larger forces that seek to eviscerate them and to profit from denuding them of what makes them unique and special.

Similarly, the rise in the movement of people is a positive force of migration for more diverse communities such as European enlargement, but also presents a bleaker picture of an increase in trafficking, dispossessed populations and the growth of excluded diasporas.

There can be distinctly advantageous bi-products to globalisation: the sharing of customs, traditions, ways of life, increased variety and richness in culture, entertainment, sport and the arts, and the breaking down of territorial boundaries and insular mentalities. It can give us a vibrant, diverse, dynamic and independent culture that draws from a multitude of sources. On the other hand, globalisation can give us a homogenised culture. Cities appear the same with uniform chain stores, global brands and supermarkets. We relax watching Disney films or the insipid Endemol format of Big Brother. It can give us a lifeless, alike, static, consumer culture imposed from corporate sources. This suggests we are in a contemporary era of globalisation, understood as a positive and negative process that has substantial and significant impact on communities and health and social care wherever they may be.

For health and social care, and the helping services, both positive and negative globalisation presents a huge range of challenges. For example, child protection issues are now global concerns with trafficking, exploitation, sex tourism and abuse increasingly coordinated across national boundaries. Adult care services need to account for and be mindful of global dimensions to care such as respecting and valuing diversity of peoples and culture, and respecting links to geographically distant communities. However, few commentators have focused on how globalisation has impacted on health and social care practice. Dominelli and Hoogvelt (1996) demonstrate the significance of globalisation on the process of intervention and the labour process in health and social care. As a result of global market forces, needs-led assessments and relationship building have given way to budget-led assessments, increased managerial control over practitioners and bureaucratised procedures for handling consumer complaints. These changes seek to reorient health and social care away from its commitment to holistic provisions and social justice towards technocratic competencies of homogenised and bureaucratic responses. Globalisation adds to the pressure for health and social care to abandon its historic mission to promote equality and social justice. It can also accelerate the breakdown of communities and lead to aggravated social problems amongst marginalised and excluded groups.

The challenge to the globalised health and social care worker is to retain the humanity, holism, justice and the opportunities that globalisation can bring, whilst protecting communities from exploitation and inequalities. Beckett and Maynard (2005) suggest that helping professions, generally, deal with people who in one way or other are marked as different and are, to various degrees, excluded from mainstream society. The challenge for health and social care and helping professions is to operate in a way which as far as possible challenges and reduces that exclusion, rather than in a way that confirms and legitimises it. The danger of the McDonaldisation of health and social care in a 'globalised' world is a challenge ever more important and central to health and social care and helping professions.

❖ MOMENTS OF REFLECTION

- Consider the times when you have thought about the global process of health and social care (for example, health and social care services on holiday, holiday tourism, the health and social care of friends and family not in this country). What issues does this raise? What would be the most effective way of dealing with them?
- Would you be happy with an American-style health and social care provision? (For example, most American health care is provided by private insurance companies.)
- Watch Michael Moore's *Sicko*.
- Think about the impact globalisation has on your life, the life of your community, and the services that you and your community use. Would you see this as positive or negative?

References

Adam, B. (2002) The gendered time politics of globalization: Of shadowlands and elusive justice. *Feminist Review*, 70, 3–29.

Appadurai, A. (1996) *Modernity at Large: Cultural Dimensions of Globalization*. Minneapolis: University of Minnesota Press.

Barnett, A., Held, D. and Henderson, C. (2005) *Debating Globalization*. Cambridge: Polity Press, in association with openDemocracy.

Bayart, F. (2007) *Governance of the World*. Cambridge: Polity Press.

Beckett, C. and Maynard, A. (2005) *Values and Ethics in Social Work: An Introduction*. London: Sage.

Bové, J. and Dufour, F. (2005) *Food for the Future: Agriculture for a Global Age*. Cambridge: Polity Press.

Deacon, B. (2000) Eastern European welfare states: The impact of the politics of globalization. *Journal of European Social Policy*, 10(2), 146–61.

Dominelli, L. (2007) (ed.) *Revitalising Communities in a Globalising World*. London: Ashgate.

Dominelli, L. and Hoogvelt, A. (1996) Globalization and the technocratization of social work. *Critical Social Policy*, 16(47), 45–62.

Drori, G. (2006) *Global E-Litism: Digital Inequality, Social Inequality, and Transnationality*. New York: Worth.

Friedman, T. (2005) *The World is Flat: A Brief History of the Twenty-First Century*. New York: Farrar, Straus and Giroux.

Giddens, A. (2002) (2nd edn) *Runaway World: The Reith Lectures*. London: Profile Books.

Gilroy, P. (1992) *The Black Atlantic: Modernity and Double Consciousness*. London: Verso.

Held, D. (2004) (2nd edn) *A Globalising World? Culture, Economics, Politics*. London: Open University Press.

Held, D. and Kaya, A. (2006) *Global Inequality: A Comprehensive Introduction*. Cambridge: Polity Press.

Hopper, P. (2007) *Understanding Cultural Globalization.* Cambridge: Polity Press.

Kaplinsky, R. (2005) *Globalization, Poverty and Inequality: Between a Rock and a Hard Place.* Cambridge: Polity Press.

Klein, N. (2004) *No Logo: No Space, No Jobs, No Choice: Taking Aim at the Brand Bullies.* London: Flamingo.

Lueddeke, G. R. (2016) *Global Population Health and Well-Being in the 21st Century: Toward New Paradigms, Policy and Practice.* New York: Singer.

McLuhan, M. and Powers, B. R. (1989) *The Global Village: Transformations in World Life and Media in the 21st century.* Oxford: Oxford University Press.

Ritzer, G. (2004) *The McDonaldization of Society.* Revised New Century Edition. Thousand Oaks, CA: Pine Forge Press.

Ritzer, G. (2005) *Enchanting a Disenchanted World: Revolutionizing the Means of Consumption.* Thousand Oaks, CA: Pine Forge Press.

Ritzer, G. (2010) *Globalization: A Basic Text.* Chichester: Wiley-Blackwell.

Sassen, S. (1998) *Globalization and the Discontents: Essays on the New Mobilities of People and Money.* New York: The New Press.

Woodward, D., Drager, N., Beaglehole, R. and Lipson, D. (2001) Globalization and health: A framework for analysis and action. *Bulletin of the World Health Organization,* 79(9), 875–81.

Woodward, K. (2003) *Social Sciences: The Big Issues.* Buckingham: Open University Press.

Chapter 8
Reflections on conditionality

Issues of social policy for the emerging professional

Chris Towers

Chapter outline

This chapter introduces:

- the nature of conditionality
- role-play methods
- reflective practice.

Introduction

This chapter is a reflective engagement on conditionality, one of the most consistently important themes in my teaching of social policy over many years. Students have enjoyed talking of or debating if or to what extent the receipt of welfare benefits should be dependent upon what the claimant does in return for his or her monies or services. This chapter will reflect not only on the nature of conditionality but on the issuers of morality, asking whether we should judge some of the most poor or vulnerable people, withdraw services if they are not behaving 'well' or impose sanctions. Should such individuals, despite such backgrounds, show responsibility or should we meet need regardless? These questions are matters of rights and entitlement; in short, social justice. The chapter will also reflect on how these issues are likely to concern a would-be practitioner, such as a 'young' housing officer working with issues of anti-social behaviour in social housing or a housing support officer considering the behaviour of someone abusing alcohol in supported housing. Such a practitioner may be embarking on employment in one of the many diverse fields of health and social care. I will refer to some issues explored in the classroom, in particular how teaching methods, with particular emphasis on role play, have facilitated exploration of conditionality and allowed for reflection by students. I will refer to the fictional character 'Colin', a middle-aged man who makes various claims for benefits and services. Students of health and social care have witnessed live and pre-recorded role plays as the lead character, played by myself, has acted out situations with practitioners from job centre staff to health service personnel, played by colleagues in the department. I have sought to enact reflective learning in the classroom and bridge any gaps between theories and practice so that students can assimilate new knowledge. These have been examples of enactment where teachers enact what they know in the classroom, transferring it to students in ways that make sense to them, so that they can ask themselves questions surrounding how the ideas and theories translate into practice (Lyons 2010). This is a process whereby in the 'doing', social phenomena is brought into focus (Weick 1995), with individuals constantly involved in the self-formation or indeed social construction of issues, dealing with tensions between autonomy and constraint. My teaching and role play dealt with matters of enactment, 'showing' tensions between social actors and acting them out before the students.

Conditionality, morality, rights and responsibilities

These enactments have brought issues like conditionality to students and allowed for some reflective learning based on what they have seen and heard as well as read, to introduce ideas that could be made tangible through their own experiences. Conditionality welfare relates, or can relate, to trying to impose behaviour change on an individual by linking their receipt of a service to how they may behave (Classen and Clegg 2007). In such an instance the person fails to engage in a relationship of reciprocity (Watts et al. 2014), where he or she recognises they have responsibility as well as rights. This does not always accord with how service users may think or act. Dunn (2010) found that benefit claimants rejected the notion of reciprocity, held by the benefits office, that they had responsibilities as well as rights. This did not mean, however, that they did not want to 'work', they did, but on their terms. They undertook voluntary work and in doing so exerted some autonomy and control of their own options and choices. It may also be that in doing so they are also reflecting a sense of entitlement, a notion that has grown with the development of the welfare state in the UK in which welfare entitlement became seen as something of a given (Bosanquet 2012). The idea is that individuals have entitlement to welfare rather than it being something that has to be earned or whereby entitlement is conditional upon certain behaviours or belonging to a defined category of claimant. It may be important perhaps to consider that people do hold values, such as the importance of participation and contribution to society or some notion of 'fairness', albeit a highly contested and contestable notion, but would rather make choices that seem meaningful to them. Students in my classes, teaching social policy to learners of health and social care, have engaged with these issues of morality. Of course, in saying this one must recognise that morality is both situated and contextual (Caruana 2004), with sociologists seeing morality as something that regulates and structures behaviours whereas psychologists will see it as something individuals may grow towards or aspire to as part of their psychological development. Indeed it can be argued that morality is bound and situated in socio-cultural and socio-structural conditions present at the time (Edelstein and Nunner-Winkler 2005), in relative rather than absolute terms, and understanding social actors means 'knowing' something of those conditions. Students have constantly made judgements on the welfare claims of a fictional case study, 'Colin'. Many have said that he 'should' work for his welfare and that he has no right to simply claim without 'doing' anything to justify it. They have employed their own moral frameworks without necessarily acknowledging how morality is situated and contextual.

The issue of rights (the right to, say, free health care) can couple with issues of morality, such as questions of 'proper conduct' from patients of the National Health Service when they physically abuse NHS staff. There are, moreover, other manifestations or expressions of conditionality such as 'conditions of category' and 'conditions of circumstances' (Classen and Clegg 2007) and these may relate, to use the same example, to patients not being 'old enough' or 'young enough' to qualify for a certain health care. In the first instance, one gets help according to membership of a group; in the second instance one may fail to meet requirements or circumstances, such as failing a means test. Students have considered how 'deserving' the claimant is or how much they have a genuine rather than fraudulent claim. These are early reflections of would-be practitioners and the responses from students have revealed diverse moral compasses as well as different levels of knowledge and awareness around issues of entitlement. Role plays around a claim for personal independence payments, a benefit paid according to if, or the extent to which, a claimant is defined as having care and/or mobility needs, evoked strong passions. Students revealed conflicting reflections on the rights and wrongs and on issues of responsibility and morality. They engaged on the moral level and it was for this reason passionate, revealing their inner worlds, their sense of 'deserving and undeserving', 'right and wrong'.

Morality, social construction and historical perspectives

Social policies are not simply responses to social problems or issues but they can certainly be, to some extent, viewed through such a lens. Social problems can, of course, be in part social constructions, or there is at least some element of social construction in the way issues are defined or thought of (Dorey 2005). These are not neutral or unbiased constructions, and it can be argued that all constructions are value based and therefore not neutral. Social groups, each with different levels of entitlement, can also be considered less or more worthy or deserving of this support. Groups can be named and thus defined in certain, quite restrictive, ways. Watts et al. (2014) say that the principle of conditionality has roots in laws made in centuries past, such as the Vagrancy Act of 1824 which outlawed begging with the condition that if the destitute did not refrain from it they would be 'asked' to go to a 'free place of shelter' where they could receive some assistance. One could argue that the workhouse system, with the poorest receiving welfare in institutions in return for 'work', was enshrined with the principle of conditionality. Whilst the Poor Laws and workhouse system came to an end in post-Second World War Britain, one can argue that the principle on which they centred, the principle of less eligibility (Rainwater 2009) that only the poorest shall receive support, survives today in the workings of the modern welfare state. There are other discourses and conflicting ways of seeing, for one could argue that the Second World War, and in particular the aftermath, brought with it a shift away from conditional welfare to more universal systems designed to meet need. The post-war Labour government introduced a raft of reforms which bolstered a sense of citizens' economic security (Bochel et al. 2005). It was also hoped that in doing so there would be a greater sense of social inclusion. People had or were given a sense of rights, social rights and a chance to feel part of society. This era has sometimes been dubbed the 'golden age' (Esping-Anderson 1994): a time of reconstruction not only of the economic base but of the moral and political one, when the focus was on social justice, solidarity and a sense of universalism.

It was a time when Britain saw the development of state services, universal benefits that could cover the good majority of citizens. That said it does not mean that they did not believe in some sort of social contract; they had, through National Insurance, an obligation to make weekly contributions through work, in exchange for these benefits. Students on the health and social care degree are encouraged to look back at historical events such as the formation of the welfare state and be critically reflective, identifying that conditionality on some level may have and is present, or can be present, even within systems of welfare that would appear universal. But however one looks at these events it has been argued that the post-war consensus around universal benefits was starting to break in the later part of the 1970s with a new emphasis on selective approaches to welfare (Bochel et al. 2005).

The pace of change towards a more conditional welfare has perhaps quickened since the 1970s. Criticism of universalism took a 'new' turn with the election of the New Labour government in the late 1990s. It was Labour who developed the concept of the 'third way' and a balance between rights and responsibilities (Dwyer 2004). This focus started with reference to claimants and welfare providers forming contracts with each other, but became increasingly moral in tone and put the emphasis very firmly on economic cost-cutting rather than the rights of citizens (Dwyer 2004). Watts et al.

(2014) argue that there has been a kind of creeping conditionality over decades, with migrants, disabled people, young offenders and others targeted for specific conditionality measures. The sanctions imposed on welfare recipients became stronger and more apparent in October 2012 when welfare reforms meant that one could effectively lose benefits, for up to three years in the worst-case scenario, if one did not comply with the requirements to look for paid work.

Different perspectives: supporting arguments for conditionality

Whilst tracing the roots of conditionality and observing them across time and place is important for students, so also is a critical awareness of arguments both for and against the concept of conditional welfare. Issues of conditionality can be linked to issues of social justice in many diverse ways. British prime minister David Cameron stated that merely getting people back into paid employment is a form of social justice (Dunn 2010) as well as displaying a form of compassion in the way there is a desire to assist claimants. This would be 'justice' for claimants but perhaps also justice for the 'taxpayer'. Dunn (2010) makes reference to ex-Labour minister John Hutton (2006) and his comment that it was 'unfair' to ask what he regarded as 'hard-working families' to pay for those out of work. It was not fair, he said, that they should shoulder the burden for people who did not show responsibility in their approach to looking for work. So for Hutton, social justice is linked to issues of fairness, rights and responsibilities and conditional welfare supports such a drive for justice, not so much for the claimant but for the wider taxpayer. These ideas link to notions of what matters to people, what they value, and it may be argued that 'responsibility' and 'conditionality' are held as important values or ideas along with ideas around people being accountable for themselves but also accountable to the wider community. It can be argued, however, that the notion of 'public interest' is highly contestable and that there is no firm definition of what this means (Morrison and Svennevig 2002). Students in my role plays worked with notions of public interests and responsibility towards others. Some of the students on the health and social care degree have commented that for them work and conditionality are linked and that it is important that claimants form some kind of contract with the state whereby they promise to make effort to look for work. In saying so they are making sense of that notion of reciprocity referred to earlier. This link between work and conditionality is emphasised by Dwyer (2004), when referring to White (2000), who argues that conditionality is important in that

> access to welfare benefits is one side of the contract between the citizen and community which has as its reverse side various responsibilities that the individual citizen is obliged to meet: as a condition of eligibility for welfare benefits the state may legitimately enforce these responsibilities, which centrally include the responsibility to work.
>
> (White 2000: 57)

There are arguments for conditionality with the notion of reciprocity related to ideas of citizenship. Conditionality as seen from this perspective promotes societal well-being and in addition to this it is making the best possible use of resources available (Watts et al. 2014). Sanctions may cause distress and indeed hardship in the short term but in the long term such conditions could be seen as liberating, freeing people up from poverty. Conditionality from this perspective frees people from dependency whilst at the same time reduces costs to the state.

Arguments against conditionality

Whatever the cost or benefit to the state from conditional policies there is the argument that rights come with citizenship. Dwyer (2004) refers to Marshall's theory of citizenship (1992), stating that for Marshall universal and unconditional welfare should be a distinguishing feature of citizenship. Health and social care students will do well to reflect on the implicit assumptions around the idea of citizenship as a means to access or entitlement for it is quite possible that students may simply argue that welfare should depend on the claimant making 'moral' or 'correct' decisions in order to access benefits rather than ones that are defined by something like citizenship. Watts et al. (2014) argue that there is the unsaid or perhaps sometimes stated argument that these are just behavioural issues. We impose conditions with the assumption that finding work is something that the individual has great control over. This accords with my experience of teaching health and social care students where some students are more aware of the potential behavioural issues, such as the lack of willingness to work, and less aware of the wider and more complex issues in the labour market, such as weak demand for labour (Shildrick et al. 2012), which make work harder to attain. Explanations for unemployment will quite obviously incorporate structural understandings of unemployment and more nuanced understandings that integrate agency and structure. Students will need to show more depth of understanding and recognise the different contexts in which unemployment occurs, to reflect on these different contexts, to consider wider issues that affect viability to work in order to understand different perspectives on conditionality. Maybe this expresses a wider goal for the reflective practitioner, to reflect on how each context and the life of each claimant brings together new knowledge and new insights into the relationship between behavioural and wider explanations of not just unemployment but homelessness, poverty and other social issues or problems.

They may also need to reflect not only on the behaviours of claimants but also on their lives and emotional and physical states, for it is also argued that individuals with complex needs may sometimes not even understand the consequences of their actions or indeed inactions (DrugScope and Homeless Link 2013). Conditionality may in such cases mean very little and a contract between the benefits agency and the claimant may exist in a very different form whereby there could be confusion over where rights and responsibilities begin and end.

Issues of mental capacity also come into play in such a discussion for if conditionality requires the person to make calculations over courses of action and weigh up whether to go for this or that job, bearing in mind the conditions, then that person surely must have capacity of mind. Ashley (2014) questions how far some service users are able to do that. Looking at issues of autonomy, responsibility, social welfare and entitlement she suggests that in order to make decisions and be autonomous the person must be able to enact good decisions. Speaking within the realm of mental health she says that in order for one to make decisions in one's 'best interests' we need more than legally defined decision-making capacity. If a person can show, retain, weigh up information they need more than that, they need to critically reflect, they need motivational skills and they need some self-esteem. In short, they need support, needing some enforcement perhaps, to motivate, but equally some support. It is noted that the Department of Work and Pensions (DWP) can appoint someone to give assistance to a claimant of state benefits who is struggling to manage their monies because they have problems with issues of either mental capacity and/or physical disability (Durham County Council 2015).

These are issues for deep reflection by students of health and social care, asking them to consider wider issues of vulnerability and risk in relation to matters of conditionality. Even if a practitioner embraces the idea of conditional welfare they still need to address important issues concerning the actual capacity of vulnerable service users to make decisions over what job to apply for when they lack the ability to even comprehend the choices they appear to have. One could also reflect on issues of social justice but not from the point of view, argued earlier, that 'justice' is done for wider society if the workless show responsibility as well as claiming rights but from another angle. This is the idea of providing universal support in order to simply provide justice to the poor and the needy. Fitzpatrick (2005) makes reference to how social policies that aim to meet the basic needs of a wider population, of all its citizens, invite a greater sense of participation and a sense of social justice, responding to a commonality of needs and reducing social inequalities in the first place. The author also argues that ethnic minorities can also benefit from universalism rather than selective or conditional welfare. Black men, he argues, are disproportionately represented amongst the unemployed and so conditional welfare is particularly harsh on such disadvantaged people. He goes on to say that the New Labour government of 1997–2010 and its move towards punitive workfare carried within it a set of individualising and pathologising assumptions about the unemployed – ideas that missed out recognising underlying causes of their situations and instead focused on behavioural aspects only. There is perhaps a need to develop a critical reflective practice that has an understanding of disadvantages and inequalities but more critically is able to 'see' these disadvantages within their own specific contexts. A housing officer is thus able to 'know' how disadvantaged individuals experience homeless legislation that focuses on 'intentionality' as a key issue for the homeless person accessing or perhaps not accessing housing. They are able to 'see' how someone unemployed may come to 'know' a Department of Employment work scheme for the workless within the context of both the Guidelines of the Department of Work and Pensions and the employment narrative of a particular individual.

Whilst there are philosophical arguments against conditionality one can also argue that there are issues around the effectiveness of ascribing conditions to the continued receipt of welfare. I have focused so far purely on the issue of conditionality as applied to unemployment benefits, but it also exists within the housing sphere for, as Dwyer (2004) points out, the 1996 Housing Act, delivered by the then Conservative government, brought conditional or behavioural aspects into housing, saying that the right to stay in social housing was dependent upon certain kinds of behaviour. That government brought in probationary tenancy periods of twelve months, with the right to stay beyond that period linked to issues of anti-social behaviour, and landlords were also found to make it easier for them to evict tenants as a result of poor behaviour. Jones et al. (2007) point to various studies that have taken place to ascertain if the idea of making welfare conditional appears successful, of if it appears to motivate. They point to the work of Hoffman et al. (2010) who investigated the impact of enforcement action on individuals and families living in social housing as a way of responding to anti-social behaviour. There was a monitoring of tenant behaviour to see if the withdrawal of support or the threat of such withdrawal reduced their levels of anti-social behaviour. The research found that these sanctions compounded the existing social disadvantages faced by vulnerable individuals. They also increased the risk of social exclusion and homelessness. The authors suggest that other approaches, not focusing on conditionality, are more likely to lead to greater success in tackling anti-social behaviour, countering a trend towards more punitive actions and encouraging more sustainable outcomes for families, communities and landlords.

These alternative approaches recognise that those engaging in such behaviour can be both victims as well as perpetrators of such actions (Nixon and Parr 2006). They also share one common feature – they experience issues of social exclusion, facing what have been described as 'severe and multiple difficulties' (Dillane et al. 2001: 41). Hoffman et al. (2001) refer to the work of the Home Affairs Select Committee, informed by working practitioners in the field, who suggest a so-called 'twin-track' strategy of enforcement and support. This may involve helping such families with parenting advice or with anger management. Reflective practitioners will take an interest in approaches that may or may not have conditionality at their centre and will reflect on the relative measures and outcomes of such approaches. They will also need to view particular contexts and circumstances in which various approaches are adopted, be critical in their reflection and aware of how different approaches may influence their work.

Working with conditionality

Students of health and social care have been encouraged to examine all policies and identify where and how conditional welfare impacts upon service users. I actively encourage them to think the issues through from the point of view of both the service user and those assessing a claim. They are aware, through reflection, of the tensions and conflicting priorities, of how issues of social justice can be interpreted in different ways and how matters of 'need' may conflict with ideas around the 'deserving' and 'undeserving'. Displays of such awareness are evidence of more holistic assessments, thinking through the wider issues around policies and practice. They may struggle to think in this way but they may not struggle with particular issues. Many practitioners for example may struggle with conditionality; they certainly can struggle with the way public service workers are constrained by prevailing orthodoxy and they can reflect on these struggles. Colley (2012) documents how, in an age of austerity since the banking crisis in 2008 in the UK, the language and practice of managerialism has stifled workers; with an emphasis on targets, the ethos of client-centred professional practice has suffered. Clarke and Newman (1997) cited in Colley (2012) have noted how managerialism and its imposition have generated deep-running conflicts between different sets of values with ideas of person-centred or client-centred values in opposition to ideas relating to auditing and accounting for the work of agencies' services.

Valuing reflection

Reflection is important for emerging professionals and certainly when they are working with service users who may be subject to conditional welfare. Of course, one needs to understand what reflection and reflective practice actually is. Farrell (2012) reflects on the understanding of educationalist and philosopher John Dewey and his reference to reflective thinking as that which practices reflective rather than what he calls 'routine thinking'. He questioned any thinking that was routine or just in line with authority. Of course, students as practitioners may have to work with the so-called 'routine thinking'. Malthouse et al. (2014) argue that professionals do not always have much autonomy or control in professional practices. Drawing on Giddens and structuration theory, it is said that social life is an interplay between agency and structure but in this interplay the person can be relatively powerless. White et al. (2006) argue that critical reflection aids the practitioner in opening up new perspectives on the lives and choices of service users and opens up the idea that there are power dynamics involved which can, if not reflected upon, leave service users powerless and open to less possibilities. This critical reflection allows for the exposure of dominant assumptions.

It is vital that students learn how to be reflective practitioners for whilst they may not have a say in how these policies and indeed social groups are constructed, they will have to work with them to the best of their ability and show commitment towards supporting service users whilst possibly having to sanction them or impose a condition upon them for their continued receipt of welfare. There have been attempts to value reflection within social work and health and social care settings. Heel et al. (2006) argue that it is an essential part of good practice to reflect, although there are voices against it or cautioning the use of it, stating that it lacks theoretical grounding (Vandenberge and Huberman 2006). Jude and Regan (2010) suggest that reflective work is when practitioners take the time to reflect on their own work, their values as well as their actions. It is about 'standing back' and taking time to reflect on their actions, to think of how they are relating to others in a wider context. It allows or affords the practitioner time to reflect on different ways of working and alternative perspectives of ways of doing things. The same authors reflect from their experience of working reflectively in social work settings. Their research project found that the practitioners were encouraged to try new ways of working, new ways of thinking and learning. They, like myself, used role plays and various techniques to encourage such reflection.

Conclusions

Students and emerging professionals can learn so much from reflection, reflecting on some key issues in practice in a world of more and more conditional welfare. I have learned through teaching students that they have reflected on their learning through role play. Practitioners will have to learn to discover the surprising nuances in people's lives before imposing any potential sanctions or rules of conditionality. They will have to work within the system rather than act outside of it but they can still try to help service users negotiate their way through a complex system and difficult choices. They can then practice in a way that takes different issues into account and reflects not only on their own policy making and their own constraints but the constraints service users have to work with each day.

References

Ashley, V. L. (2014) *Great Expectations: Autonomy, Responsibility and Social Welfare Entitlement.* Thesis submitted for the Degree of Doctor of Philosophy, University of Essex, April 2014.

Bochel, H., Bochel, C., Page, R. and Sykes, R. (2005) *Social Policy: Issues and Developments.* London: Prentice Hall.

Bosanquet, N. (2012) From welfare state to entitlement programmes. Futures 44, 666–70. http://ac.els-cdn.com/S0016328712001061/1-s2.0-S0016328712001061-main.pdf?_tid=17ad356a-9a74-11e5-b6f1-00000aacb35d&acdnat=144922 (accessed 4 December 2015).

Caruana, R. J. (2004) Morality in consumption – towards a multi-disciplinary perspective. University of Nottingham. No. 24-2004 ICCSR Research Paper Series, ISSN 1479-5124.

Clarke, J. And Newman, J. (1997) *The Managerial State. Power, Politics and Ideology in the Remaking Of Social Welfare.* London: Sage. Quoted in Colley, H. (2012) Not learning in the workplace: Austerity and the shattering of illusions in public service work. *Journal of Workplace Learning*, 24(5).

Classen, J. and Clegg, D. (2007) Levels and levers of conditionality. Measuring change within welfare states. In Watts, B., Fitzpatrick, S., Bramley, G. and Watkins, D. (2014) *Welfare Sanctions and Conditionality in the UK.* York: Joseph Rowntree Foundation.

Colley, H. (2012) Not learning in the workplace: Austerity and the shattering of illusions in public service work. *Journal of Workplace Learning*, 24(5).

Dillane, J., Hill, M., Bannister, J. and Scott, S. (2001) Evaluation of the Dundee Families Project, University of Glasgow. In Hoffman, S., Mackie, P. K. and Pritchard, J. (2010) Anti-social behaviour law and policy in the United Kingdom: Assessing the impact of enforcement action in the management of social housing. *International Journal of Law in the Built Environment*, 2(1), 26–44.

Dorey, P. (2005) *Policy Making in Britain: An Introduction.* London: Sage.

DrugScope and Homeless Link (2013) Joint submission of the Work and Pensions Select Committee, inquiry into role of the JobCentre Plus. London: Drugscope and Homeless Link. Quoted in Watts, B., Fitzpatrick, S., Bramley, G. and Watkins, D. (2014) *Welfare Sanctions and Conditionality in the UK.* York: Joseph Rowntree Foundation.

Dunn, A. (2010) Welfare conditionality, inequality and unemployed people with alternative values. *Social Policy and Society*, 9(4), 461–73.

Durham County Council (2015) Fact Sheet: Mental Capacity. www.durham.gov.uk/media/6427/Factsheet-Mental- capacity/pdf/FactsheetMentalCapacity.pdf (accessed 4 December 2015)

Dwyer, P. J. (2004) Creeping conditionality in the UK. From welfare to rights to conditional welfare entitlements? *The Canadian Journal of Sociology*, 29(2), 365–87.

Edelstein, W. and Nunner-Winkler, G. (2005) *Morality and Context.* Amsterdam: North-Holland.

Esping-Anderson, G. (1994) After the golden-age. The future of the welfare state in the new global order. Occasional Paper no. 7, World Summit for Social Development. United Nations Research Institute for Social Development.

Farrell, T. S. (2012) Reflecting on reflective practice: Revising Dewey and Schön. *TESoL Journal*, 3(1), 7–16. http://onlinelibrary.wiley.com/doi/10.1002/tesj.10/full (accessed 20 October 2015).

Fitzpatrick, T. (2005) Alternative approaches to social policy. In Bochel, H., Bochel, C., Page, R. and Sykes, R. (2005) *Social Policy: Issues and Developments*. London: Prentice Hall.

Heel, D., Sparrow, J. and Ashford, R. (2006) Workplace interactions that facilitate or impede reflective practice. *Journal of Health Management*, 8, 1–10. Quoted in Jude, J. and Regan, S. (2010) *Practitioner Led Research, Integrated Working. An Exploration of Reflective Practice within a Social Care Team. Social Policy: Issues and Developments*. London: Prentice Hall.

Hoffman, S., Mackie, P. K. and Pritchard, J. (2010) Anti-social behaviour law and policy in the United Kingdom: Assessing the impact of enforcement action in the management of social housing. *International Journal of Law in the Built Environment*, 2(1), 26–44.

Hutton, J. (2006) Welfare reform: 10 years on, 10 years ahead, Speech, 18 December available at www.dwp.gov/aboutus/200618-12-06asp (accessed 11 June 2008). Quoted in Dunn, A. (2010) Welfare conditionality, inequality and unemployed people with alternative values. *Social Policy and Society*, 9(4), 461–73.

Jones, N., Vargas, R. and Villar, E. (2007) *Conditional Cash Transfers in Peru: Tackling the Multi-Dimensionality of Childhood Poverty and Vulnerability*. New York, NY: UNICEF. Quoted in Forde, I., Bell, R. and Marmot, G. (2011) Using conditionality as a solution to the problem of low uptake of essential services among disadvantaged communities: A social determinants view, *American Journal of Public Health*, August 101(8): 1365–69.

Jude, J. and Regan, S. (2010) *Practitioner Led Research, Integrated Working. An Exploration of Reflective Practice within a Social Care Team*. London: Children's Workforce Development Council.

Lyons, N. (2010) *Handbook of Reflection and Reflective Enquiry: Mapping a Way of Knowing for Professional Reflective Enquiry*. London: Springer.

Malthouse, R., Roffey-Barentsen, J. and Watts, M. (2014) Reflectivity, reflexivity and situated reflective practice. *Professional Development in Education*, 40(4).

Marshall, T. H. (1992) *Citizenship and Social Class*. Quoted in Dwyer, P. J. (2004) Creeping conditionality in the UK. From welfare to rights to conditional welfare entitlements? *The Canadian Journal of Sociology*, 29(2), 365–87.

Morrison, D. E. and Svennevig, M. (2002) *The Public Interest, the Media and Privacy*. London: BBC.

Nixon, J. and Parr, S. (2006) Antisocial behaviour: Voices from the front line. In Flint, J. (ed.), *Housing, Urban Governance and Anti-Social Behaviour: Perspectives, Policy and Practice*. Bristol: Policy Press. Quoted in Hoffman, S., Mackie, P. K. and Pritchard, J. (2010) Anti-social behaviour law and policy in the United Kingdom: Assessing the impact of enforcement action in the management of social housing. *International Journal of Law in the Built Environment*, 2(1), 26–44.

Rainwater, L. (2009) *Social Policy and Public Policy, Inequality and Justice*. New York and London: Transaction Publishers.

Shildrick, T., Macdonald, R., Furlong, A., Roden, J. and Crow, R. (2012) *Are 'Cultures of Worklessness' Passed Down from Generations?* York: Joseph Rowntree Foundation. Quoted in Watts, B., Fitzpatrick, S., Bramley, G. and Watkins, D. (2014) *Welfare Sanctions and Conditionality in the UK*. York: Joseph Rowntree Foundation.

Vandenberge, R. and Huberman, A. M. (2006) *Understanding and Preventing Teacher Burnout: A Sourcebook of International Research and Practice*. Cambridge:

Cambridge University Press. Quoted in Jude, J. and Regan, S. (2010) *Practitioner Led Research, Integrated Working. An Exploration of Reflective Practice within a Social Care Team*. London: Children's Workforce Development Council.

Watts, B., Fitzpatrick, S., Bramley, G. and Watkins, D. (2014) *Welfare Sanctions and Conditionality in the UK*. York: Joseph Rowntree Foundation.

Weick, K. E. (1995) *Sensemaking in Organizations*. Thousand Oaks, CA: Sage.

White, S. (2000) Review article: Social rights and social contract-political theory and the new welfare politics. *British Journal of Political Science*, 3, 507–32. Quoted in Dwyer, P. J. (2004) Creeping conditionality in the UK. From welfare to rights to conditional welfare entitlements? *The Canadian Journal of Sociology*, 29(2), 365–87.

White, S., Fook, J. and Gardner, F. (2006) *Critical Reflection in Health and Social Care*. Maidenhead: Open University Press.

Chapter 9
Professional supervision

Jane Challinor

Chapter outline

This chapter introduces:

- reflection and supervision
- supervision, coaching and mentoring – what's the difference?
- supervision during your studies
- supervision in the workplace
- criticisms of professional supervision.

Supervision plays a key role in professional education and practice and underpins the development of professional identity. However, what is meant by supervision may be different for different professions or organisations. At its heart is the process of reflection. In this chapter the role of reflection in learning and personal development is discussed and supervision itself – as a reflective process – is defined in the context of work and professional education, contrasting this with other developmental processes such as mentoring and coaching. We will also consider challenges facing supervision practice in the current climate and question whether supervision is a positive force for social justice or whether it is simply a subtle way of controlling the individual and society at large.

Supervision and reflective practice

When considering what it means to be a health and social care professional, a significant part of the role is that of the reflective practitioner. Whether it is reflecting on an intervention made with a service user, taking time to reflect on a new practice that has been introduced or a theory we have come across, or whether it is a more introspective action in which we consider our own feelings, behaviours and responses to a difficult situation, reflection is a process which is intrinsically bound up with learning, development and evidence-based practice.

In the field of professional education a deliberate act of reflection is normally applied to an experience or critical incident which has already occurred in practice, with the aim of enabling the professional to understand the significance of what has occurred, both for themselves and the service user, to relate the occurrence to theory and to formulate from this a plan of how to act in a similar future scenario. This is the foundation of much professional or clinical supervision as well as of professional practice education (Boud and Walker 1998; Moon 1999).

Reflection is usually described as a process of recounting a past event in order to learn from it:

> The way in which the word 'reflection' is commonly used suggests several understandings. First, that reflection seems to lie somewhere around the process of learning and the representation of that learning ... Second, to be of significance for study, we have to regard reflection as implying purpose (Dewey 1933; Hullfish and Smith 1961) ... The third understanding is that it involves complicated mental processing of issues for which there is no obvious solution (Dewey 1933; King and Kitchener 1994).
>
> (Moon 1999: 4)

> The common-sense view of reflection is that it is a mental process that is couched in a framework of process of purpose or outcome.
>
> (Moon 1999: 15)

There have been many other people writing about the reflective process and its importance in learning – notably David Kolb (1984), Graham Gibbs (1988) and Jenny Moon (1999, mentioned above). All seem to generally agree on the iterative and cyclical nature of learning – summed up in Figure 9.1.

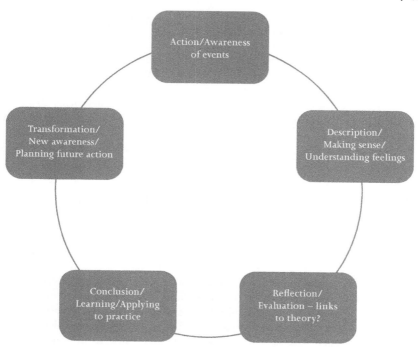

Figure 9.1 The iterative and cyclical nature of learning

David A. Kolb (with Roger Fry) created his famous model out of four elements: concrete experience, observation and reflection, the formation of abstract concepts and testing in new situations. He represented these in the famous experiential learning circle that involves (1) concrete experience followed by (2) observation and experience followed by (3) forming abstract concepts followed by (4) testing in new situations (after Kurt Lewin). It is a model that appears time and again.

Kolb and Fry (1975) argue that the learning cycle can begin at any one of the four points – and that it should really be approached as a continuous spiral. However, it is suggested that the learning process often begins with a person carrying out a particular action and then seeing the effect of the action in the situation. Following this, the second step is to understand these effects in the particular instance so that if the same action was taken in the same circumstances it would be possible to anticipate what would follow from the action. In this pattern the third step would be understanding the general principle under which the particular instance falls (Smith 2001, 2010).

So why do we need to develop reflective skills as professionals? Because the problems we meet day to day ('real-world problems') are 'messy and indeterminate, problematic situations' and cannot be 'solved' through step-by-step, rule-based problem-solving skills (Schön 1987, 1992, in Moon 1999: xx). Therefore, an ability to reflect 'in action' – as well as after the event – is essential:

The methods used in teaching and nursing [and social work], for example, involve review, interpretation and reconstruction of ideas and reflection is employed in these processes. Another reason is that practice in these professions is often based on rapid action and the proof of expertise in the subjects emerges from the actions (Argyris and Schön 1974; Schön 1983). Thus, for the teacher managing a class of difficult children, the teacher's action at any point matters more than their knowledge of the dictates of theory or even their own prior theorizing about their action. A similar situation exists for the nurse encountering a crisis. Action is what counts.

(Moon 1999: 55)

Reflection and professional development: coaching, mentoring and supervision

Supervision, coaching and mentoring are all forms of professional and personal support that are available to health and social care practitioners. They are distinct but related processes, which in their different ways support practitioners in their reflections.

Coaching and mentoring are terms that are sometimes used interchangeably, but a useful way of distinguishing them is that coaching can be defined as supporting a practitioner in the development of a skill or set of skills pertinent to their practice or role, whilst mentoring is often seen as a form of advice-giving from an older, or more experienced, colleague especially – but not exclusively – in relation to career development.

> Jeni is finding her workload overwhelming at times. She feels she just doesn't have enough time to answer emails, keep her files up to date, and complete the reports the manager needs from her on a regular basis. Her desk seems to be disappearing under a sea of paperwork. In a discussion with her line manager, she agrees to book some **coaching** sessions to focus on her time management. The coach, who is a member of the central training division, helps Jeni to set goals for herself and discusses various strategies that will help her to tackle her work more systematically – including having a wall planner and an electronic diary that flags up reminders when important tasks are due. Jeni also reviews her method of dealing with emails and comes up with some simple rules for herself that help her to keep on top of her inbox.

> Amin has been in his post as a junior finance officer in the NHS for four years and really loves his work. However, he notices that some colleagues who started the job some time after him have already moved up to the next grade, joined another team or even moved to another city to get a promotion. He has never thought of himself as particularly ambitious but he feels he is at least

as able as those colleagues – he just lacks confidence when it comes to interviews and job applications. One day he receives an email from HR which announces a staff **mentoring** scheme. After a brief chat with the HR officer for his team, he is assigned a mentor who is a senior manager with a different team in another part of the city. Amin meets with his mentor once every few weeks for about six months. He finds it helpful to hear the mentor describe her own career path from practitioner to manager and this gives him a clearer idea of what he wants to do next. The mentor looks with him at current job vacancies and encourages Amin to talk about his skills and experience and identify where these would meet the person specifications. The mentor encourages Amin to put in an application for a Team Leader post and offers to act as a referee.

Coaching has over many years developed a professional body of theory, skills and knowledge in its own right, starting within the sports coaching field and more recently transferring into other work environments. It is not uncommon nowadays to find performance coaches or business coaches employed in large organisations and even 'life coaches' now advertise their services, usually in a private or freelance capacity. Coaching is generally seen as a non-directive form of development which focuses on improving performance and developing individuals' skills.

A common model used in the coaching session is GROW:

Goal: What is the goal you want to achieve? What is the longer-term objective? What is the objective for this discussion?

Reality: What is the situation now? Who is involved? What is it costing? What is happening?

Options: What are the possible (not necessarily practicable) solutions? What could be done?

Will: What will be done? When? With whose support?

(Whitmore 2009)

Different versions of this model do exist (see also Downey 2003), but essentially they are focused on the development of options for future action. The Reality part of the model could also be thought of in terms of reflection. It is here that the client might describe and evaluate the situation they wish to change.

Here is Jeni again, discussing her time management issues with her coach (we already know that her goal is to become better organised):

'I just don't seem to be able to get on top of things. My desk is awash with paper, books, post-its, messages on scraps of paper – I can't seem to get a grip on things! I used to be much better organised – at uni I had a wall planner to help me manage my workloads and plan ahead for my assignments, but when I started this job I didn't ever seem to have time to set up a system before the work started piling in. My boss doesn't help – she is really busy and she just flies in every morning with a heap of things for me to sort out: I don't have any idea which is the most urgent or important, she just expects me to know ... I am really scared that she just thinks I am stupid or wildly inefficient and when my probation review comes up she is just not going to renew my contract!'

In following the GROW model, Jeni's coach might next help her to generate a number of possible options for future action. These might include taking a day to sort through and reorganise her desk, ordering a desktop filing system and wall planner, or – as mentioned above – setting up that reminder system on her electronic diary. She might also think about negotiating a regular catch-up session with her boss to discuss work priorities, as what seems to be emerging from the coaching session is a growing realisation that Jeni is not the only one who needs to be better organised! Jeni may also need help in becoming more assertive – learning how to say no, how to ask for help and how to negotiate deadlines.

Jeni will go on to discuss a range of options with her coach and then decide on which of these she has most 'will' or desire to carry out. She would then be encouraged to create a SMART (Doran 1981) action plan to help her realise her goal.

Supervision: three dimensions and seven eyes!

Clinical or professional supervision shares some characteristics with coaching, but its remit is usually wider than developing skills. In fact, there are often considered to be three main dimensions of supervision: **educational**, **supportive** and **managerial** (Proctor 1991).

The **educational** aspect may be about learning new skills or understanding theory or putting these into practice; it may also be about supporting the supervisee to undertake further research, to carry on with their studies or progress to a new level of practitioner.

Managerial supervision can have as its focus legislation, organisational procedures, normal processes or conventions pertaining to the professional role; there may also be an element here of the supervisor monitoring the performance of the supervisee.

Emotional support may also be needed in the supervision session – many aspects of work in the health and social care field can be upsetting and the supervisee – however experienced – may need simply to talk through their feelings or discuss how they have been affected by events, in order to be able to make sense of them and move on.

Supervision problem 1: when emotional support is needed

Sam is a student on a health and social care course who works as a volunteer befriender for a cancer charity. For several weeks, she has been visiting an elderly woman, Frema, who has terminal cancer. Sam's role includes popping in to make coffee and pick up shopping. She enjoys chatting with Frema who seems to find it a relief to have someone to talk to about her concerns. Over the Christmas break, whilst staying with her family back at home, Sam receives a message to say that Frema has died. When she returns to university, Sam is contacted by the lead volunteer from the charity to arrange a supervision session. Sam feels upset that she had missed seeing Frema before she died because of the university holidays. In supervision she is able to discuss her feelings with the lead volunteer and recognise that she had been able to bring Frema a lot of comfort during their chats. She also recognises that as a befriender she is inevitably going to be faced with the loss of many clients in the future and whilst she isn't going to stop caring about them, she has to balance her sadness with the memory of the happy times she spent with each of them.

Shohet and Hawkins' 2012 process model of supervision (sometimes called the seven-eyed supervisory model) is a useful one. First published in 1989, it looks at the processes that operate both within and outside the supervision session itself – in the relationship between supervisor and supervisee (the social worker, counsellor or nurse who has come for supervision, for example) and between the supervisee and their client.

At the most basic level, the supervisor is concerned with the well-being of the client under discussion (the first 'eye', or level 1) then the relationship between client and supervisee and what the supervisee did and said in their interactions with their client (levels 2 and 3). Next (level 4) they will be concerned about the internal processes – the thoughts and feelings – of the supervisee (this is the reflexive aspect of supervision referred to by White 2015). This is also about the supervisee's needs for emotional and developmental support.

Some elements of the supervision session will inevitably be concerned with the relationship between supervisor and supervisee (level 5). On a strictly procedural level, this may be about the contract between the parties – issues of confidentiality, clarifying the boundaries between operational management, performance appraisal and supervision. It may also be about the less obvious psychological relationship between the two – do they like working together? Do they differ in their approaches to issues? Are they politically or culturally opposed? These are aspects of the relationship that may have a bearing on its success or failure as a supportive and educational process as it is within this dimension that feelings of trust between supervisor and supervisee are established. To some extent, the relationship between supervisor and supervisee also reflects the relationship between supervisee and client. This is often referred to as the parallel process. At its simplest, this can be about the supervisor modelling appropriate behaviours which the supervisee then transfers into the relationships with their client.

A more complex aspect of the parallel process is where the supervisee unconsciously brings to supervision some aspect of their relationship with a client, perhaps even involuntarily adopting some of the clients' mannerisms and behaviours. With deeper reflection, supervisor and supervisee can use this process to understand the client's needs (McNeill and Worthen 1989).

The supervisor also needs to take care of their own thoughts and feelings (level 6) (this refers to the aspect of the *supervisor's* reflexivity), as they arise within the supervision session and also afterwards – through *their own* supervision. BASW's emphasis on supervision, for example, encompasses the idea that social work managers are appropriately trained in the skills of supervision and subject to appropriate governance arrangements (BASW/CoSW England 2012).

Finally, but importantly for the furtherance of social justice, Shohet and Hawkins (2012) recognise that the supervisory relationship sits within a wider context (level 7) – that of the organisation or system to which the supervisor and supervisee belong (the local authority, the hospital, etc.) with its rules, procedures and codes of ethics – and beyond that to society at large. The supervision session therefore needs to take account of the social context of the client – their immediate family, community, societal and political pressures to which they are subject – as well as focusing on any immediate problem that they are facing and which might be the focus of the therapy session, care plan or needs assessment that has been carried out.

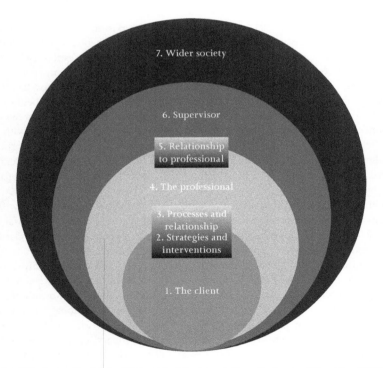

Figure 9.2 The Seven-Eyed Supervision Model adapted from Shohet and Hawkins (2012)

Supervision for your final-year dissertation

During your studies at university you may have supervision in relation to a final-year dissertation. This is somewhat different from what we mean by professional supervision but the process can be very similar. Although in this instance the main focus will be educational (discussing the findings from your literature search, refining your research methods, improving your written expression), there can also be managerial aspects related to procedures or university regulations (understanding the system used for referencing your sources, understanding the assessment criteria or the format required for submission of your final dissertation) and even some emotional support, as the process of working on such a large piece of writing can be very stressful!

When you are allocated a supervisor for your final-year dissertation, think of this as your first experience of professional supervision. You may be asked to sign a learning agreement or to maintain a reflective log of your supervision sessions, or arrangements may be more informal. Nonetheless, approaching these sessions with a professional attitude will help you to get the most from them and will also prepare you for the experience of professional supervision when you start work in the health and social care field.

Making the most of supervision

- Ask your supervisor to let you know what s/he expects of you and what the process is if things don't work out as expected.
- Understand that *you* are responsible for your own work – not your supervisor. Decisions about research topics, dissertation title, workload planning and presentation are *yours*. Your supervisor can advise and guide but not tell you what to do.
- Make sure you know how long your appointments will last, how often they will take place and what is the final deadline for supervision meetings to be completed.
- Make appointments (and if need be, cancel them) well in advance so both you and your supervisor can prepare.
- Be clear about what you want from each supervision session: come with questions to discuss; bring copies of your work to look at if necessary.
- Keep your own notes of what has been discussed, and after each session make a brief plan of what you need to do next in order to address any issues raised.
- Be prepared to be honest about your feelings so that you can get the advice and support you need but conduct yourself in a professional manner. You may feel angry, upset, frustrated or disappointed, but you need to manage your feelings appropriately and take responsibility for them.

Managerial, reflective and reflexive supervision in social work

Supervision has a long and somewhat chequered history in the field of social work. In the early days, supervision of professional staff borrowed much from psychoanalytical approaches that were developing in the 1930s. The focus of the supervisory relationship was on support for the worker to reflect on their caseload (Wonnacott 2012).

In the 1980s, a far more managerialist approach developed within social work generally, with an emphasis on targets and auditing practice. Even recent research into social work supervision has found that the boundary between management and supervision can still be very unclear and that far from being a supportive and developmental process which aims to be emancipatory (that is, supporting the supervisee to act autonomously), it can be far too concerned with meeting objectives, staying within rules and policies and generally avoiding risk to the organisation (Noble and Irwin 2009).

According to White (2015: 252), 'social workers in England have been pressured towards becoming unreflective people processors'. However, after a number of high-profile public enquiries which have profoundly questioned the role of supervision in social work practice, the thinking behind supervision has turned full circle and the relationship is now far more likely to be one in which the worker is supported to exercise their professional judgement, using skills of critical thinking (Wonnacott 2012).

The British Association of Social Workers currently has very specific policies about the format of supervision:

> All social work practitioners have the right to receive formal, one to one, professional supervision in relation to practice and personal development from registered and appropriately experienced social workers. This includes those working in integrated structures, multi-disciplinary teams and specialist roles.
>
> (BASW 2011)

The definition of supervision from BASW goes some way towards setting out very clear guidelines about the purpose and conduct of supervision.

Definition of social work supervision

The BASW definition of supervision below includes the definition and description of supervision in the Skills for Care and Children's Workforce Development Council (CWDC) guidance on supervision and the definition of professional supervision in the Scottish Association of Social Work Manifesto. Supervision is a regular, planned, accountable process, which must provide a supportive environment for reflecting on practice and making well-informed decisions using professional judgement and discretion. Supervision should enable social workers to:

- be accountable for their practice and ensure quality of service for people who use services
- uphold professional standards
- build purposeful professional relationships and communicate effectively
- make sound professional judgements based on good practice
- manage risk and protection alongside their duty to respect rights and address need
- reflect on, analyse and evaluate their practice
- manage the emotional impact of their work

- share, debrief and identify any further required resources to address responses to stressful situations
- challenge constructively in the interests of client, worker and agency
- develop the knowledge, skills and values required for their own role, professional development and as part of an integrated, multi-professional or multi-agency team or service
- contribute to research and use knowledge and experience to explore new ways of working
- identify and manage stress factors that may impinge on the worker, service user or agency
- ensure peer and management review of professional decisions and to encourage mutual learning and development
- communicate with their line manager on organisational issues
- manage realistic workloads and caseloads.

(BASW 2011: 7)

This definition is interesting in that it supports the idea of supervision having a number of functions:

- **Educational** ('develop knowledge, skills and values ... contribute to research ... encourage mutual learning and development').
- **Supportive** ('manage the emotional impact of their work ... manage realistic workloads ... identify and manage stress factors').
- **Managerial** ('be accountable for their practice ... uphold professional standards ... manage risks').

BASW also talks about the relationship between supervision and reflection ('reflect on, analyse and evaluate ... practice') as part of the process of professional development.

In supporting this return to reflective models of supervision, White (2015) introduces the idea of *reflexivity* – where practitioners are allowed to 'locate themselves in the picture, to appreciate the influences on their knowledge and values and how all of this impacts on their practice'. This fits well with Shohet and Hawkins' (2012) seven-eyed supervisory model, discussed above, which firmly locates the supervisee in the picture and makes a legitimate space for this kind of reflexivity alongside the managerial and educational dimensions of supervision.

The wider role of supervision: Facilitating social justice

The focus of supervision can range far beyond the client, the supervisee and the organisation in which they work to look at society in general and the power structures within it. In this aspect of supervision, the supervisor may encourage their supervisee to think about the wider environment in which their client exists, to think about working cross-culturally, recognising diversity and employing anti-discriminatory practices: 'Examples of social justice action include advocating for financial relief and suitable housing or challenging views that stereotype or subjugate people according to cultural identities such as ethnicity, race, gender or class (Cooper, 2002)' (Hair 2015: 350).

It is also essential that the supervisor models this approach in the relationship they establish with their supervisee by explicitly exploring how issues of race, culture, religion, ethnicity, disability, gender and sexual orientation might impact their relationship, as well as that between the supervisee and their client (Wonnacott 2012).

Another dimension of supervision that is taking on increasing significance is the protection of vulnerable service users. Whilst this is implicit in all types of supervision, this has become even more critical in clinical settings such as nursing, particularly following on from scandals such as Winterbourne View, Mid Staffordshire NHS Trust and Bristol Royal Infirmary.

❖ REFLECTIVE ACTIVITY

Read the example below and think about how as a supervisor you might support Kieran to look at the issues presented by Laila from the perspective of promoting social justice.

Supervision problem 2: A 'messy' problem in the classroom

- Kieran is experiencing problems with a particular child in his class. A new girl, Laila, who speaks fairly basic English but has difficulty with written work, frequently misbehaves in class, running around or nudging other children whilst they are working and laughing loudly. Recently a number of small items have gone missing in the classroom and one Friday afternoon, Kieran notices what he feels sure is one of these items, a board marker, sticking out of Laila's pocket. Some of the other children have started to exclude Laila and call her names. At times arguments are overflowing from play time into the classroom, making it very difficult for Kieran to continue with lessons. It has been suggested that Kieran should spend extra time with the new girl to bring her English up to standard as quickly as possible. He has also tried to work with the family on some of the behavioural and learning issues, but Laila's mother speaks no English and the meetings have to be arranged so that Laila's brother, who is in the class above, can act as translator.

Reflective commentary

No clear answers ...

At present Kieran is looking at the problem from the point of view of behaviour management and the learning needs of the whole class. But there are other issues here: Laila is clearly a recent immigrant to the UK. How could the diversity she brings to the class be celebrated? Other pupils are acting towards Laila in a discriminatory way (calling her names) – how could Kieran challenge **their** behaviour, to promote greater acceptance? And what about the wider needs of Laila's family? Is there some way the school could be better at supporting them rather than relying on another child to interpret in meetings that are potentially quite sensitive? Is stealing a **cause** of the problems here or is it a symptom of Laila feeling excluded and bored?

The supervisee's experience

Most supervision happens after the event – with the counsellor, nurse, social worker, etc. reflecting on a busy week or month of working with a range of clients. In some organisations, however, supervision is immediate – even happening at the same time as the intervention with the client is taking place.

This extract from an online article about working for ChildLine as a volunteer counsellor highlights the importance of supervision in supporting the counsellor:

Every week my shift at ChildLine begins with a briefing to get us all up to date with anything we need to know and every shift ends with a debrief where a *supervisor* can check out how you are feeling about the calls and online contacts you have taken. There are three-and-a-half hours on each shift so it's important that you talk about what you have done and how you feel about it ... The ChildLine staff really value our contributions and they want to keep us safe.

Over the course of the past six months I have clocked-up more than 75 hours in the counselling room. I've also spent nearly fifteen hours taking part in workshops on suicide, self-harming, eating disorders and sexual abuse.

The training never stops. You are so aware that ChildLine is always striving to make their counsellors ever more equipped and the service more effective.

What kind of things do children contact you about?

[One] of the first calls I received was from an eleven-year-old who was being bullied at school. This was the first time she had called ChildLine. She knew about ChildLine because we had visited her school. She had been punched by another girl and her mobile phone had been stolen.

She was extremely upset, about the bullying and about how she was going to be able to tell her dad that she had lost her phone. We talked about how she felt about being bullied, how bullying was never the fault of the person being bullied and how she might talk to her dad about what had been happening. We talked about what might happen if she told the one teacher in the school she liked what had been happening inside and outside school. She said she felt better and that she was going to call ChildLine back to let us know how she got on.

The following week I took a call from a fifteen-year-old. It was the first time she had called ChildLine. Someone had mentioned it to her on a social networking site. She had been self-harming, she was desperately ill from anorexia, and soon into the call she confided in me that she was contemplating taking her life.

As with any calls that pose an immediate danger to a young person I stuck my hand up and received the support and guidance of a supervisor for the rest of the call.

(This is Devon 2010)

Criticism of professional supervision

For some, supervision can give rise to concerns about power relationships – in particular the way the supervision session becomes a 'confessional' and is used to extend control over the population through the process Foucault referred to as Governmentality – the exercise of moral regulation and discipline (Gilbert 2001). From this perspective, the managerial aspect of supervision is predominant, making it too much concerned with ensuring that practice follows rules and regulations. Through the disciplining or regulating of the supervisee, the norms or rules are transmitted to the service user – in an attempt to control particular sections of society.

However, Gilbert goes further in suggesting that even the supportive aspects can be intrusive and a subtle way of enforcing self-regulation, through the creation of a relationship which is likened to the religious idea of the confessional. Gilbert quotes Foucault in the following description of the status of the confessional in modern society:

> The obligation to confess is now relayed through so many points, is deeply ingrained in us, that we no longer perceive it as an effect of a power that constrains us: on the contrary, it seems to us that truth, lodged in our most secret nature, 'demands' only to surface.
>
> (Foucault 1981: 60, quoted in Gilbert 2001)

Far from being a space for developing reflective practice, the supervision session is here seen as a dialogue between penitent and confessor. The supervisee is assumed to be at fault or in need of fixing and is persuaded to disclose intimate feelings or beliefs in the hope of receiving 'redemption'.

Chapter summary

Ideas of reflective practice and professional or clinical supervision are deeply embedded in health and social care professions, from initial training through to professional standards of continuous professional development. Supervision, mentoring and coaching can support individual practitioners in their personal development but also offer a means of regulating professional practice.

Supervision is generally seen as having three main components – support for the individual on an emotional level; help with their educational development or further professional training; and a managerial dimension which ensures that professionals are practicing in accordance with policy and procedure laid down by organisations and regulatory bodies.

Models of supervision describes a complex relationship. Supervisors need to develop skills of self-awareness or reflexivity whilst also ensuring that the process focuses on the empowerment of the individual supervisee (and their client) thus furthering the cause of social justice. An uncritical acceptance of supervision's role in developing reflective practice precludes a consideration of its sometimes not-so-subtle role in regulating the actions of the individual. Balancing the various dimensions of supervision requires skill and supervisors therefore need to be appropriately trained – and supervised!

References

BASW (2011) *UK Supervision Policy* [online]. Available at http://cdn.basw.co.uk/upload/basw_73346-6.pdf (accessed 21/06/2015).

BASW/CoSW England (2012) *Research on Supervision in Social Work, with Particular Reference to Supervision Practice in Multi-Disciplinary Teams* [online]. Available at http://cdn.basw.co.uk/upload/basw_13955-1.pdf (accessed 25/10/2015).

Boud, D. and Walker, D. (1998) Promoting reflection in professional courses: The challenge of context. *Studies in Higher Education*, 23(2), 191–206.

Doran, G. T. (1981) There's a S.M.A.R.T. way to write management's goals and objectives. *Management Review (AMA FORUM)*, 70(11), 35–36.

Downey, M. (2003) *Effective Coaching: Lessons from the Coach's Coach*. London: Texere.

Gibbs, G. (1988) *Learning by Doing: A Guide to Teaching and Learning Methods*. Oxford: Further Education Unit, Oxford Polytechnic.

Gilbert, T. (2001) Reflective practice and clinical supervision: Meticulous rituals of the confessional. *Journal of Advanced Nursing*, 36(2), 199–205.

Hair, H. J. (2015) Supervision conversations about social justice and social work practice. *Journal of Social Work*, 15(4), 349–70.

Kolb, D. A. (1984) *Experiential Learning*. Englewood Cliffs, NJ: Prentice Hall.

Kolb, D. and Fry, R. (1975) Towards a theory of applied experiential learning. In C. L. Copper (ed.), *Theories of Group Processes*. London: John Wiley, pp. 33–58.

McNeill, B. W. and Worthen, V. (1989) The parallel process in psychotherapy supervision. *Professional Psychology: Research and Practice*, 20(5), 329–33.

Moon, J. E. (1999) *Reflection in Learning and Professional Practice*. Oxford: Routledge.

Noble, C. and Irwin, J. (2009) Social work supervision: An exploration of the current challenges in a rapidly changing social, economic and political environment. *Journal of Social Work*, July 2009, 9(3), 345–58.

Proctor, B. (1991) Supervision: A co-operative exercise in accountability. In Marken, M. and Payne, M. (eds), *Supervision in Practice*. Leicester: National Youth Bureau and Council for Education and Training in Youth and Community Work, pp. 21–23.

Shohet, R. and Hawkins, P. (2012) (4th edn) *Supervision in the Helping Professions*. Maidenhead: McGraw Hill.

Smith, M. K. (2001, 2010) David A. Kolb on experiential learning. *The Encyclopedia of Informal Education* [online]. Available at http://infed.org/mobi/david-a-kolb-on-experiential-learning/ (accessed 21/06/2015).

This is Devon (2010) Making a difference to children on the edge. *Western Morning News* [online]. Available at www.westernmorningnews.co.uk/Making-difference-children-edge/story-11655801-detail/story.html#ixzz3diDEfBgq (accessed 21/06/2015).

White, V. (2015) Reclaiming reflective supervision. *Practice*, 27(4), 251–64.

Whitmore, J. (2009 [1992]) Coaching for performance: GROWing human potential and purpose: The principles and practice of coaching and leadership. In *People Skills for Professionals* (4th edn). Boston: Nicholas Brealey.

Wonnacott, J. (2012) *Mastering Social Work Supervision* [electronic resource]. London: Jessica Kingsley.

Chapter 10
Reflective writing for professional practice

Siân Trafford

Chapter outline

This chapter introduces:

- reflective writing
- activities to support reflective writing
- reflective writing as a valuable tool for professional practice.

To understand the term 'reflective writing', we first need to consider the meaning of reflection. Moon (1999a: 3) maintains that finding a definition is problematic, and refers to a 'chaotic catalogue of meanings' yielding numerous understandings of the term. While its most typical meaning evokes a faithfully reproduced image in a mirror, or indeed any shiny surface, albeit back to front (Bolton 2005), a more helpful definition in this context is 'serious thought or consideration ... expressed in writing or speech' (Stevenson and Waite 2011). This latter definition, with its connotations of being actively involved in the process of reflecting, begins to shed light on how reflection can be applied in an academic or professional context to facilitate thinking and clarify ideas. Moon (2004) explains that the process of reflection involves shaping and modelling our knowledge, thoughts and feelings, an echo of Dewey's (2010 [1910]) observation that reflection crucially involves organising seemingly disconnected facts and elements to identify links and patterns. This, in turn, allows the reflector to view their actions and experiences from different perspectives and consider their own feelings and motivations, as well as those of any other protagonists involved.

❖ ACTIVITY 1

Consider a time when you felt nervous – perhaps your first week back at study. What were you thinking and how did it make you feel? Examine why you were thinking and feeling these things. What were your perceptions about the people around you? Did you think they seemed confident and self-assured and that you were the only one feeling out of your depth?

While reflection is now regarded as an important skill for practitioners, Moon (2004) maintains that the concept of reflective practice is relatively new, having entered the mainstream as a result of Schön's work. Schön (1983) explains that, for several decades, professionals have been encountering increasingly complex 'problems' and dealing with emerging value conflicts: for example, the current call for person-centred practice while also delivering increased efficiency demanded by ever-shrinking budgets. These factors require a different approach from the old, relatively inflexible application of knowledge and theory. The professional practitioner has to consider the individual situation and the array of approaches available to him or her and select the most appropriate or, indeed, tailor an approach using a combination of strategies and interventions. For this reason, the development of reflection is now acknowledged to be a vital skill for practitioners in many professions and is therefore taught as an integral part of many undergraduate courses (Moon 2004; Hargreaves and Page 2013). Although there are many ways to reflect – in a one-to-one situation, in a group setting, writing, undertaking creative activities (Knott and Scragg 2007) – writing is certainly an accessible and effective way to develop an understanding of reflection, to articulate and analyse one's thoughts and feelings and to deepen learning (Moon 2004; Bolton 2005; Cottrell 2003). A learning journal can be a useful way to capture details of events, and thoughts and feelings about those events. It can be kept entirely private, or it can be shared with others, whether fellow students or colleagues, to discuss experiences and share strategies for tackling problems (Cottrell 2003). Cottrell also argues that a learning journal can help students to chart progress, and even develop their writing because it is a private space where they can experiment with writing styles to find their own 'voice'.

> ### ❖ ACTIVITY 2
>
> Devise and keep a learning journal for a week. Useful sections could include:
>
> | Description | What I thought/felt | What was good/bad (Evaluation) | Why was it good/bad? (Analysis) | Could I have done something different? | How will I improve it for next time? |
> | --- | --- | --- | --- | --- | --- |

Reflection is inextricably related to learning, whether in an educational or a professional setting. Moon (2004: 186) tells us that 'we reflect in order to learn something, or we learn as a result of reflecting'. She explains that when we record our reflections by writing them down, we are tracing the thought processes we followed in a given situation, or in order to arrive at a particular solution or decision. Cottrell (2003), too, in advocating the use of a learning journal, maintains that writing things down helps to clarify thoughts and feelings and to devise solutions to problems or dilemmas. However, reflection is not only helpful when a situation has not gone as smoothly as anticipated, or when there have been negative consequences: it can be equally useful to reflect on successful outcomes. Hargreaves and Page (2013) argue that it can prove invaluable when considering everyday practice because it can lead to new insights which will support personal development and improve skills.

Writing reflectively about a particular episode or period allows us to examine it in detail, and to immerse ourselves in the thoughts, feelings and actions that were prevalent at the time. This focus allows us to recall a surprising amount of detail and to question our behaviour and thinking processes at the time. Bolton (2005) maintains that reflective writing creates both distance (because we are externalising it and also committing it to paper) and also closer contact, because it facilitates connection with thoughts, feelings and experiences. However, it can be daunting to sit down with a blank sheet of paper to begin writing, which is why it is helpful to break the experience down into the sections of a learning journal. Another effective way to overcome this is to employ Peter Elbow's (1998) 'freewriting' technique. This entails sitting down with a piece of paper and a pen or pencil, and just writing *without stopping* about any given thought or topic without worrying about punctuation, structure, spelling or even coherence. The exercise can last for two, five, ten minutes or even longer. The important point is that the writer does not stop, even if they simply keep repeating a word or phrase because they cannot think of anything else to write. Freewriting is designed to remove the paralysing fears about writing such as worries about spelling mistakes, writing the right thing or making sense, so it can even be useful as a warm-up exercise before an extended piece of writing, such as an assignment, or even an exam. It can also lead to 'I didn't know I thought/knew/remembered that until I wrote it' moments (Bolton 2005: 47), which are particularly valuable for reflective writing.

❖ ACTIVITY 3

Practise freewriting for five to ten minutes about a recent incident where you behaved uncharacteristically. Did the freewriting lead to any insights into your behaviour?

To be effective, however, reflective writing needs to go further than merely describing an episode: the writer needs to analyse, challenge, perhaps evaluate, what has occurred, or even to consider the perspectives of others (Moon 2004). The writer needs to consider their behaviour in that particular situation and to seek reasons for their reactions. To facilitate this, many different models of reflection (or experiential learning) have evolved, such as Schön (1983), Kolb (1984, see Moon 1999a), Gibbs (1988, see Hargreaves and Page 2013) and Cowan (1998). Boud and Walker (1998), however, state that caution needs to be exercised when using reflective models. They advise that the models should be viewed as 'scaffolding' to help the student in the process of reflection rather than rigid 'recipes' for reflection (Boud and Walker 1998). This 'scaffolding' takes the form of a series of stages, and many models are represented as a cycle:

● experiencing the event
● reflecting on and reviewing the experience by observing the circumstances, thoughts and feelings that were current at the time
● developing insights about what happened, and why, and devising strategies to produce a more effective outcome when in a similar situation – learning from the experience
● testing those plans – trying out what has been learned.

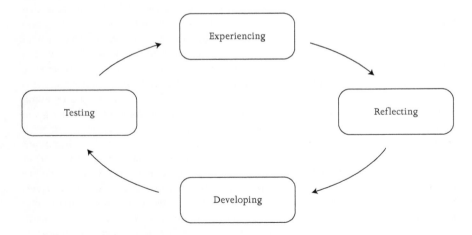

Figure 10.1 Kolb's reflective cycle

Here it is worth noting that Cowan's model is represented as a loose spiral (Cowan 1998: 38), which more accurately illustrates the progression generated by reflection. This will be more clearly illustrated later. Cowan also incorporates elements of both Kolb and Schön. Whereas Kolb's model generally includes only one mode of reflection, Schön differentiates between *reflection-in-action* and *reflection-on-action*. The former involves adapting to a situation as it unfolds (thinking on your feet), while the latter involves the Kolbian idea of reviewing a situation that has already taken place. Cowan adds a further period of reflection – *reflection-for-action* – to be carried out *before* the experience. This allows individuals the opportunity to consider any prior knowledge, experience or learning which might prove valuable for the task to be undertaken (Cowan 1998). Examples of these three modes of reflection at work can be seen in professional practice. For example, a social worker needs to gather as much information as possible about a service user before an initial visit (reflection for action). During the visit, it might be discovered that the service user is not eligible for a certain benefit, or a particular intervention is not appropriate, so an alternative strategy needs to be considered and explored (reflection in action). After the visit, a formal review constitutes reflection-on-action (Knott and Scragg 2007). During this process, the strategies and interventions are discussed to determine whether they have been successful in achieving the anticipated outcomes, and to identify corrections or improvements for subsequent action. It is this continual examination and evaluation of situations, assumptions, attitudes and even emotions which contributes to the development of professional practice.

❖ ACTIVITY 4

Consider examples of reflection for-, in- and on- action from your own experience or practice and record them in writing.

- Think of a time when you prepared thoroughly, or not thoroughly enough, for a visit (reflection for action).
- Think of a time when you had to adapt your approach during a visit (reflection in action).
- Think of a time when you analysed your performance following a visit (reflection on action), perhaps questioning your particular approach or considering how another approach might have affected the outcome. Did this reflection lead to a different way of approaching a subsequent similar situation?

Reflection, then, is a valuable tool which allows an individual, whether student or professional, to make sense of situations they encounter, sometimes involving complex problems. The additional act of using writing to reflect allows learning to occur as it captures the prevailing thoughts and feelings and allows the writer not only to organise and examine them, but also to process them (Moon 1999a). This is an invaluable skill for many professionals, not just those working in, say, education or health and social care, as the ability to reflect on an incident and consider how different outcomes may be achieved if one or more aspect is altered allows for professional development and, therefore, more effective professional practice.

❖ CASE STUDY

Sarah was anxious about the practice interview which was being recorded as part of her course and which would be shown to the whole class for peer review.

Outcome

However, at the end of the process she was pleased that her colleagues had praised her warm, approachable manner and the fact that she had been very well informed when explaining the services available to the client. They also suggested that she needed to involve the client a little more in the discussion. Sarah reflected on why she had been so nervous about undertaking the interview and receiving the feedback, and also on why she failed to involve the client, and how she was going to address that.

Sarah's possible reflections:

- I was nervous about how I was going to look 'on camera'.
- I was worried I wouldn't be able to recall all the necessary information.
- I was worried that I might appear silly or self-conscious or poorly prepared.
- I was worried about what my peers might say in feedback.
- I failed to involve the client because I was anxious to convey all the information I had prepared.
- Next time, I will ask the client about their desired outcomes and I will also ask the client at regular intervals whether they have any questions or comments they would like to make.

Although this is a very rudimentary form of reflection, it demonstrates that Sarah is considering the thoughts and feelings she was experiencing before the event, and is also considering not only what led her to neglect to involve her client in the interview, but also the steps she can take to overcome this in the future. These are the first steps towards professional development: making changes so that the outcomes of a given situation are improved on a subsequent occasion. This relates to Cowan's spiral of reflection as it depicts a breaking out of the closed loop of reflection described by Kolb and Gibbs. This 'breaking out' is a visual representation of the learning and progression that results from reflection, thus indicating continual development.

It would also seem to suggest that reflection is therefore an aid to developing self-awareness. Knott and Scragg (2007) and Hargreaves and Page (2013) explain that conscious reflection first helps an individual to become aware of their own feelings and what causes them, which then leads to noticing the feelings and reactions of others, thus developing empathy and emotional intelligence. For example, Sarah could go on to ask herself how her client might have felt during and after the interview. Possible feelings might have included frustration, even anger, at not being invited to ask questions or express their opinion; feelings of low self-esteem because they may have inferred that the professional did not consider their opinions worth listening to; feelings of powerlessness and lack of control because they may have been excluded from the decision-making process.

❖ ACTIVITY 5

Case study

A home care worker is clearly in a hurry and rather short-tempered with an elderly service user. Consider what might have caused the home care worker to behave in this unprofessional manner. Consider, too, how the service user might feel. How could the situation have been improved?

Commentary

The home care worker may already feel under pressure because of the short amount of time they are allowed with each service user. Additionally, they may be running late due to heavy traffic; perhaps they had difficulty finding a parking space which further shortened the time; perhaps, too, personal problems were preoccupying him/her.

The elderly service user may have felt intimidated and undervalued or worthless. They might have felt confused if the usual routine could not be followed, perhaps causing them to be slower than usual, which might have caused the home care worker to become even more delayed, and possibly more irritable.

Possible solutions

The home care worker could have explained the situation to the elderly service user and negotiated which tasks to complete. This might even have created a more trusting and open working relationship.

Reflection, then, can lead to new insights about events and problems, helping practitioners to make sense of complex situations (Moon 2004; Schön 1983; Hargreaves and Page 2013). It enables them to consider not only how their own emotions and personal circumstances might have influenced the events that occurred, but also how their actions might have impacted on the others involved. Their growing emotional intelligence will also enable them to consider how the other participants (service users, clients, patients, young offenders) might have been feeling before they approached the encounter, and also which emotions might have been aroused by the actions of the practitioner during the encounter. Since social workers and health and social care professionals almost inevitably work in situations which involve a range of heightened emotions – fear, anxiety, anger, frustration – self-awareness, empathy and emotional intelligence are vital skills to master, and reflection provides a way to do this.

Along with developing these skills, reflection provides a route to 'deep learning' because it allows, even encourages, the learner (the reflector) to challenge and to change what they already know, believe or practise (Moon 1999b). Deep learning, as the name suggests, leads to a deeper understanding of a subject or, in this case, of a situation, because the individual has engaged fully with the learning process to find meaning and to 'own' the knowledge (Moon 1999b: 26). Reflecting on events provides the space and time to consider what happened; what might have been influencing the practitioner's thoughts, feelings and actions; what might have been influencing the other participants' thoughts, feelings and actions; the impact the interaction of these variables might have had on the situation; whether a change in any one of these variables would have greatly altered the outcomes for better or for worse; and, if so, how to ensure that an improved outcome is achieved next time. Moon (1999b: 26) refers to this process as 'cognitive housekeeping' because it requires the learner to sort and reorganise thoughts, feelings and ideas, as they seek to make sense of, or find an explanation for, a particular problem or situation.

Similarly, in relation to deep learning, reflection can provide new insights when connecting theory to practice. Schön (1983) refers to practice as 'the swampy lowlands' because it is uncertain, even 'messy', while theory is the high ground, dealing as it does with, say, prescribed patterns of behaviour. It can therefore be difficult to reconcile the two extremes. Knott and Scragg (2007) explain that reflection can provide a bridge between the two to provide a middle ground. Theory on the page can seem flat and unrelated to real life, but reflection can reveal the connection between the two. For example, students in some disciplines are often asked to carry out a child observation to gain a better understanding of child development theory, but many of them struggle to articulate the links between the child's behaviour and theory in their explanatory accounts. However, by encouraging them to reflect on the child's behaviour, and then on their knowledge of child development theory, for example Erikson, they are able to see the connections and how the outward actions of the child can be explained by the theory.

Legislation can also be included in Schön's 'high ground', dealing as it does with sometimes inflexible eligibility criteria. By reflecting on an individual's circumstances and perspectives, and considering relevant theory, practitioners are able to exercise 'professional artistry' (Knott and Scragg 2007: 105), thereby providing a holistic assessment of the situation which provides more satisfactory outcomes for the service user. Arguably, this is perhaps one of the most important and also the most difficult skills for practitioners to master: holding the 'middle ground' by managing to balance the needs of the service user with what can realistically be provided by ever-shrinking services. The demands required of the practitioner to accomplish this balancing act can bring their own difficulties, not least feelings of stress caused by trying to achieve it, and here yet another aspect of reflection and reflective writing can help.

There is much to support the benefits of reflective writing in helping to relieve pressure and tension created by stressful situations (Adams 1999). Moon (1999b) refers to Cooper's observation that reflective writing such as a journal can be used as an 'emotional dumping ground', functioning as a valve to release tension and stress, while

Bolton (2005: 62) asserts that 'writing has an evidence base for alleviating the symptoms of anxiety and depression', although much more research is needed in this area. The very act of transmitting confusing thoughts and feelings to paper can help to provide relief, because forcing the writer to acknowledge their existence is cathartic, possibly because the act of reflection helps an individual to organise thoughts and rationalise emotions, restoring a feeling of control and perhaps even release.

❖ ACTIVITY 6

What did you observe?	Which child development theory does this equate to?
Child was able to build a tower of five bricks.	
Child was anxious when the mother left the room, even though she had explained she was going to get a drink and would return.	

Similarly, the passage of time can alter our reflections because it lends distance to the event, allowing the reflector to remove themselves from the situation and therefore to become more objective. The reflective writing exercise 'The Park' (Watton et al. 2001) provides an excellent example of this in a series of reflections progressing from the descriptive and ineffective to the deeply reflective and self-aware. A simple example of this in a work context could be to delay replying to an upsetting or even infuriating text or email message until we have considered it from every angle (Knott and Scragg 2007) – see case study in Activity 7.

❖ ACTIVITY 7

Case study

You are a final-year student social worker on placement, working on completing your practice portfolio. You have just received an email from your manager about a foster family you have been working with. A year ago, an emergency placement had been required for two siblings and the Local Authority suggested a certain foster family. You were aware, and had pointed out at the time, that the family was only authorised to take one more child, but because of the emergency nature of the situation, the decision was made to place both siblings with the foster parents. They have been with the family for a year and are thriving. You are now being asked to explain your actions and it has been suggested that the two children will have to be separated and one placed with a family far away. The email has been copied to your lecturer and your practice-based assessor.

1   What are your immediate feelings on reading this email?
2   What else is occupying your thoughts as you read it?
3   What might your manager have been feeling when they wrote it?
4   What is your best course of action?

Delaying the response and reflecting on all the prevailing factors would give you time to consider how to respond appropriately and professionally. (You are perhaps already stressed about your practice portfolio; you are feeling aggrieved for being made accountable for something you raised at the time; perhaps your manager is unaware of your input at the time of the emergency foster placement and so is feeling frustrated at your seeming lack of professionalism. How many more factors can you identify?) Bolton (2005: 46) asserts, 'Reflection in writing facilitates a wider view from a distance, a close acute perspective, and authority over practice' and, throughout this chapter, the value of reflection has been discussed, especially the value of written reflection. Moreover, reflection has a variety of applications. It can contribute to many areas of personal and professional life because it aids learning by helping practitioners to engage with the learning process at a deeper level. Effective use of reflection promotes self-awareness and develops empathy and the emotional intelligence essential for effective practice for any practitioner working with other people: youth worker, social worker, medical worker, health and social care professional. Cowan, Kolb and Gibbs demonstrate how reflection can become a catalyst for change, because it encourages the individual to examine, challenge and alter their ways of thinking and approaching situations, while Bolton and Moon commend its therapeutic use as a means of relieving stress and pressure, both personal and professional and teacher. The distance and objectivity it brings to a situation can even help to defuse awkward and potentially aggressive interactions. Above all, it is the active engagement in the reflection process that writing can bring which makes it a useful skill to master, and an indispensable skill for certain professions, especially when working with society's most vulnerable individuals.

References

Adams, K. (1999) Writing as therapy. *Counselling and Human Development*, 31(5) [online]. Available at: http://search.proquest.com/docview/206834060?accountid=14 693&rfr_id=info%3Axri%2Fsid%3Aprimo (accessed 4 February 2016).

Bolton, G. (2005) *Reflective Practice: Writing and Professional Practice*. London: Sage.

Boud, D. and Walker, D. (1998) Promoting reflection in professional courses: The challenge of context. *Studies in Higher Education*, 23(2), 191–206.

Boud, D., Keogh, R. and Walker, D. (eds) (1985) *Reflection: Turning Experience into Learning*. Abingdon: RoutledgeFalmer.

Cottrell, S. (2003) (2nd edn) *The Study Skills Handbook*. Basingstoke: Palgrave.

Cowan, J. (1998) *On Becoming an Innovative University Teacher: Reflection in Action*. Buckingham: Society for Research into Higher Education and Open University Press.

Dewey, J. (2010 [1910]) *How We Think*. San Diego: The Book Tree.

Elbow, P. (1998) (2nd edn) *Writing with Power: Techniques for Mastering the Writing Process*. Oxford: Oxford University Press.

Francis, H. and Cowan, J. (2008) Fostering an action-reflection dynamic amongst student practitioners. *Journal of European Industrial Training*, 32(5), 336–46. Available at: http://dx.doi.org/10.1108/03090590810877067 (accessed 8 February 2016).

Hargreaves, J. and Page, L. (2013) *Reflective Practice*. Cambridge: Polity Press.

Knott, C. and Scragg, T. (2007) (2nd edn) *Reflective Practice in Social Work*. Exeter: Learning Matters.

Moon, J. (1999a) *Reflection in Learning and Professional Development: Theory and Practice*. London: Kogan Page.

Moon, J. (1999b) *Learning Journals: A handbook for Academics, Students and Professional Development*. London: Kogan Page.

Moon, J. (2004) *A Handbook of Reflective and Experiential Learning: Theory and Practice*. Abingdon: RoutledgeFalmer.

Schön, D. (1983) *The Reflective Practitioner: How Professionals Think in Action*. London: Temple Smith.

Stevenson, A. and Waite, M. (eds) (2011) (12th edn) *Concise Oxford English Dictionary*. Oxford: Oxford University Press.

Watton, P., Collings, J. and Moon, J. (2001) *Reflective Writing: Guidance Notes for Students* [online]. Available at: www.exeter.ac.uk/fch/work-experience/reflective-writing-guidance.pdf (accessed 4 February 2016).

Chapter 11
Contemplating 'career' across disciplines
Reflexive explorations of 'career'

Ricky Gee

Chapter outline

This chapter is a means of provoking the reader's thoughts on the concept of 'career'. It aims to do this in the following way:

- by acknowledging that there are multiple perspectives on 'career', both within the literature and also via individual subjective notions of 'career'
- by considering how career is a political and social project which occurs in contexts that involve others
- by examining important dimensions of career found within the career theory literature
- by considering the notion of duality in such dimensions and how this evokes notions of 'paradox', which is argued to be an important mode of analysis of 'career'
- for students to apply the concepts within the chapter to their own 'career'.

Many contemporary public spaces, such as university buildings, have a tendency to incorporate the use of glass. Such buildings tend to utilise glass as a material for not only windows but also walls, walls where one can view inside rooms which they have yet to enter. For example, when walking through a contemporary, recently refurbished university building one may walk along a corridor with a cascade of glass walls, reminiscent of Bentham's panopticon (see Foucault 1977), where all can be seen and where one is affected by their intrusion of presence. The transparent walls allows an insight into collected communities; for example, in the case of a university building, accountancy, law, sociology, psychology and health and social care pedagogic interactions are all on show. What also becomes apparent is that each community appears similar; however, on closer inspection one can notice certain physical differences. Having taught on the Health and Social Care degree, over a number of years, one can acknowledge the ethnic diversity of the group as well as its gender homogeneity, especially when comparing it to certain other courses. One has to question why this might be the case. How have such demographics been magnetically pulled toward a specific educational destination, especially as such demographics re-occur over many years? Just via these observations one is invited to read 'career', sociologically, politically and philosophically.

To aid such reading this chapter intends to explore some of the important dimensions of 'career' across a number of disciplines. By doing so it invites the reader to contemplate their own experience of 'career', including interactions with others' careers, and how acknowledgement of important dimensions of career might provide different readings than the first that come to mind. The chapter invites you to reflect upon your experiences of being a student, how this strand may be considered as part of 'career', and where the engagement with higher education is likely to have resulted in what sociologists, for example Roberts (1977, 1997, 2009) and Cote (2014), express as a pro-longing of youth − or a return to aspects of 'youth'. Such sociologists would suggest that contemporary society tends to place expectations upon individuals to elongate their educational careers so as to reduce the risk of not engaging with the labour market. There has been a long history of education providing space within the curriculum to aid students' 'career management', for example Law and Watts (1977) for many years have advocated the use of their DOTS system (Decision-making, opportunity-awareness, transition and self-awareness), focusing on the student's ability to 'decide' on their future trajectory and increase their chances of being 'employable'. Since the Browne Report into higher education (HE), which reviewed the remit and purpose of HE and its subsequent rise in tuition fees, employability within the HE curriculum has become an HE policy concern. This chapter explores some of the important conceptual assumptions in the employability agenda within HE. It seeks to deconstruct such conceptions so as to reveal political and ideological positions, therefore arguing that much of the employability agenda in HE provides a neo-liberal and conservative ideological stance that exacerbates inequality, especially when taking into account a student's class, gender and ethnic identity. The chapter concludes by highlighting how exploring such aspects of identity and how they interrelate with opportunity structures provides a more radical reading of an individual's career. It questions whether choice may well be illusionary, both in terms of your own career and the careers of others you come into contact with within the practice of health and social care, and how the study of such a subject area is to take into account such policy considerations.

Have you ever wondered who you are, who you have been and who you are likely to become? It is argued that the asking of such reflexive and temporal questions is a key characteristic of contemporary life (Giddens 1991; Beck 1992). It is relatively easy to ask these questions, yet the answering is much more of a challenge. To answer such questions is likely to evoke the contemplation of 'career'. Yet what exactly does the word 'career' actually mean? How might you conceive such a word and how might your conceptualisation relate to the culture in which you are immersed? It is evident that words play a crucial part in any culture. Words and the concepts that they seek to elucidate provide meaning and expose position (Gellner 1972; Derrida 1992; Ricoeur 1976; Heidegger 1962). One of the striking developments that the author has experienced during his academic journey is how a word utilised in everyday language can provide a perspective that is counter to the meaning of the word within academic discourse. The use of an everyday dictionary provides a useful insight into the layperson's usage of a word, what phenomenologists would call the 'natural attitude', and can provide an analytic lens of the layperson's assumptions about such words and how they relate to the culture in which the words are immersed. The Oxford online dictionary definition of career provides a good starting point, with interesting cultural insights into the concept of career: 'A course of professional life or employment, which affords opportunity for progress or advancement in the world' (Oxford English Dictionary Online, accessed June 2011). This definition, like many online definitions, is concise and to the point. However, such concision can result in a simplification and narrowing of a concept, highlighting bias and at times ethnocentricity. The idea of work is central to the above definition, as work is presented in the guise of employment and a career is only induced if such employment is of a professional nature and encapsulates the philosophy of enlightened thinkers – that of 'progress'. One quickly realises that such notions of career appear exclusive. Someone in a position without employment, or a person in employment that does not 'progress', or those looking after the long-term sick or children or relatives – an important dimension of health and social care – even people of 'leisure', are all deemed career-less. This is a paradigm that excludes people from career and one which makes career vulnerable and in a position to be 'broken' – such as the notion of a 'career break'.

Reflecting upon everyday discourse one can acknowledge the layperson's view of career depicted by the above definition: 'I need to get myself sorted and get a career'; 'I decided to take a career break and look after my children'; 'There is no future in this job, no progression, I need a career'. Yet do such views of career resonate with the lives of many people? What of education and the role of being a student? The role of being a non-paid carer? Are these part of 'career'? There is evidence within the literature – particularly policy literature – to suggest that career may encompass a range of roles, such as being a student; for example, 'An individual's lifelong progression through learning and work' (National Curriculum 2007). However, is such a definition, which widens career to include learning, a means of serving work? Does learning via formal education also assume the notion of 'progress', that one makes a series of ascending steps up a hierarchy from primary school to, potentially, HE? Again, does this resonate with everyone's experience? Do lives progress in such a neat linear fashion? What of those who do not attend formal education – young carers for example – or those whose health may prevent them from accessing formal education? Does this mean that people in such positions are career-less?

Both Donald Super (1994) and Erving Goffman (1961) would challenge the above definitions. Donald Super, a very prominent academic within the field of career development, would suggest that the development, sequence and combination of the roles we play within the life span constitutes an individual's career. Such a perspective therefore brings many roles into play, for example the role of student, parent, citizen as well as the role of worker. Erving Goffman, a prominent sociologist, very much harmonises this view by suggesting that careers can encompass an individual's social strands, that which is significant to the individual that connects aspects of their narrative together, for example housing, caring and leisure careers. Such broad perspectives of career place the dictionary and National Curriculum definitions under stress and lead the reader of such definitions to ponder why career tends to be perceived in such narrow terms. It is also important for the professional worker in the domain of health and social care to explore positional views of career and to ponder why such positions evoke such views.

❖ ACTIVITY 1

PQ

- What are your views on the concept of career?
- Who/what may have influenced your views on this concept?
- If you are to work in the field of health and social care, when might you be required to contemplate career, both your own and others'?

Both Super and Goffman ask us to contemplate career from a broad perspective and also to acknowledge that careers are temporal and are likely to experience transitions, moments and episodes when our careers – to include numerous inter-connecting roles/ strands – significantly adapt. Taking a broad perspective upon career also asks us to contemplate the expectations that society may well place upon us, especially when such expectations are assumed without question. Therefore, within the realm of HE, are there certain expectations in relation to career? A brief historical analysis of career education is required to consider the answering of such a question.

Career education – a brief history

Education policy-makers regard 'career development' work – such as 'career guidance' and 'career education' – as a significant activity to aid people to make short-term 'career decisions' as well as helping to lay 'the foundations for lifelong learning and lifelong career development' (Watts 2003: 4; Office for Standards in Education/Audit Commission 1993; Morris et al. 2000; DfES 2005 cited in Colley et al. 2010). It has long been acknowledged that careers develop over time and therefore policy asserts that to achieve its goals requires further input than a brief one-to-one interaction with a careers adviser (Law and Watts 1977; Law 1996; McCash 2006). Policy therefore perceives that educational curricula can make a useful contribution, via career education (McCash 2008: 2), to supplement career guidance so as to aid such policy objectives.

In the UK in the 1950s, there were policy concerns in relation to 'youth' employment and thus the 'Youth Employment Agency' – which later became the Career

Service – was born to provide young people with 'vocational knowledge' (Heginbotham 1951). At this time compulsory education in school was seen as an arena where career education could develop, in conjunction with career guidance, so as to aid young people's decision making and transitions at the critical interchange between school and the world of work (Law and Watts 1977; Law 1996; Watts 2006; McCash 2006). Career education proliferated during the mid-twentieth century and became common practice and knowledge by the early 1970s across UK schools (Schools Council 1972; Barnes and Andrews 1995), where it was defined as consisting of planned experiences designed to facilitate the development of:

- decision learning – decision-making skills
- opportunity awareness – knowing what work opportunities exist and what their requirements are
- transition learning – including job-search and self-presentation skills
- self-awareness – in terms of interests, abilities, values, etc.

(Watts 2006: 10)

It is argued that this form of career education – commonly known as DOTS – has underpinned much career work within the UK, as well as North America via Hillage and Pollard (1998), where it is still a prominent influence of school as well as HE career curricula (McCash 2006). What becomes apparent is how career education has been incorporated within areas of the curriculum where perceived important transitions are to take place, especially concentrating on the connection between education and the world of work (Heginbotham 1951; Law 1996; Roberts 1977, 1997, 2009; McCash 2006). Such transitions have become extended during the latter stages of the twentieth century, mirroring the elongation of 'youth' due to the post-industrialisation of Western democracies (see Furlong and Cartmel 2007; Beck 1992; Roberts 1997, 2009; Cote 2014). With a large number of young people leaving full-time education in their early twenties, especially with the increased numbers of young people being encouraged to undertake higher education, there has been an increased concern with aiding young people's/young adults'/emergent adults' transition to work within the HE curriculum (Henderson et al. 2007; Furlong and Cartmel 2007; Roberts 1997, 2009). This prominent policy concern for the HE sector appears to have come at the expense of statutory-school-age input, with the previous Coalition Government's removal of the statutory right for career education within school occurring at the same time that an increased emphasis on career within the HE curriculum was being advocated in the influential Browne HE review (Watts 2006; Roberts 2009; McCash 2006; Browne 2010; Andrews 2013). At present, 'career' within the HE curriculum very much becomes operationalised under the guise of employability where it has become a key policy priority due to the major changes facing the HE sector, such as the rise in tuition fees (Browne 2010; CBI 2011; Mercer 2011; Willetts 2011). Such a rise in fees therefore increases the level of financial investment for the majority of undergraduate students. Given this scenario there is a policy assumption that students will become active and rational consumers within a marketised HE sector, looking for a return on this investment via future employment that satisfies financial expectations (Browne 2010; CBI 2011; Mercer 2011; Willetts 2011). This is further exacerbated by the unquestioned underpinning policy principle that HE contributes to the development of a nation's human capital and that employable students will provide a greater national economic yield (NCIHE 1997 in Watts 2006; Browne 2010; Purcell et al. 2012).

Taking the above into account the arena of 'employability' has a tendency to touch upon the concept of career development, with the promise of aiding student contemplation of future employment trajectory (Watts 2006; Yorke and Knight 2006). Anticipating the proliferation of such activity, the Higher Education Academy (HEA) published a series of papers to aid curriculum input in this arena in the early part of the twenty-first century. Tony Watts – a prominent figure within the field of career policy – provides a central contribution within this series (Watts 2006), supplying an overview of important terms and explicitly linking the notion of career development learning – incorporating aspects of DOTS, career management and lifelong learning – to employability. In doing so, Watts (2006) encourages a broad exploration of employability to move from the notion of 'immediate employability' – commonly concerned with student possession of attributes to obtain a 'graduate job' and being 'work ready' – toward 'sustainable employability' – a concern with the ability not only to secure a first job but also to remain employable throughout life. It is within this realm of employability that Watts argues that career development learning can come into play. Watts' argument is that the encouragement of career development learning and the utilisation of career development theory can provide a broader approach to employability – and therefore avoid the conceptual narrowing of a skills approach. Watts is keen to point out that 'much of the now-extensive literature on employability in higher education … pays little attention to the conceptual work on career development or to the work that has been done on career development learning' (2006: 8). What becomes apparent is that although Watts' intentions are laudable his broadening of the employability curriculum stays tightly contained within a rational paradigm that overly embraces the agented notion of career enactment of the student. Much of Watts' argument concentrates upon deployment – the extent to which individuals 'are aware of what they have got and how they choose to use it'. There is little scope within Watts' argument to provide space in the curriculum to contemplate how wider social forces influence the student's career enactment – ideas heavily espoused by Roberts (2009), Young and Valach (2000), Patton and McMahon (1999) and the discipline of the sociology of work (see Fleming 2009). Also, the only mention of political notions of career occur under the confines of future employing organisations, for example students contemplating where there 'may be hidden tensions and power struggles within organisations' or being 'aware of the location of power and influence within organisations' (Watts 2006: 14–15). Watts' attempt to widen the employability curriculum therefore becomes inherently workcentric, apolitical and therefore lacking in criticality.

Within the HEA Employability and Learning series, McCash (2008) provides a view of conceptually widening the employability agenda by the encouragement of career studies. Building upon the arguments of Yorke and Knight (2006), McCash promotes the notion of employability connecting with multiple discourses to include a student's home subject of study, as well as other/further disciplines, so as to promote a transdisciplinary exploration of career. This resonates with one of Watts' (2006) central tenants 'that much of the employability literature has neglected conceptual work on career development' (McCash 2008: 3). McCash's (2006, 2008) promotion of a career studies approach therefore endeavours to break open agented rational work paradigms of career prominent in DOTS. It is via the role of the student as career researcher that McCash promotes the extent of career studies within the curriculum where

> students (and staff) [viewed] as career researchers is potentially liberating for both groups, and also suggests some fruitful connections. The role of career researcher is congruent with the familiar role and function of universities and other educational institutions but wide enough to fit with the developmental needs of the employability movement.
>
> (McCash 2006: 446)

Career studies therefore provides a useful endeavour to open space within the HE curriculum, where career may be explored via a broad perspective, so as to not succumb to the hegemonic paradigm of DOTS.

With the growing trend toward universal higher education provision, and the widening of participation to include previously under-represented groups, student transition into higher education and beyond has increased in importance in recent times (Gale and Parker 2014). Educational and employment policy is therefore becoming increasingly interested in how students, from various backgrounds, engage with education – especially higher education – and destinations beyond. The Futuretrak study is one study (Purcell et al. 2012) which provides a longitudinal view upon undergraduate transition. Its focus is on how students who applied in 2005/06 to go to university, have 'progressed' from the application stage to six months post-graduation. A particular interest is how this cohort compared to previous students as it is acknowledged that this cohort have the additional challenge of transitioning into a labour market experiencing one of the worst recessions within history. The study utilised a large sample of approximately 130,000 participants that it considered covers different categories – such as ethnic groups, subject groups, or types of HE institution – so as to be able to draw conclusions confidently about the impact of different variables on experiences and outcomes. The study is considered to provide important quantitative and qualitative data, which it collected via online surveys. Such a panoramic view provides some useful policy data – for example, that 75 per cent of students feel they have gained skills that employers want. However, given its methodological focus, the study does not provide sufficient detail of how career – which is not operationalised and appears to be underpinned by the assumption that career is equated with work – is lived as an experience that incorporates the numerous roles/strands articulated by Super and Goffman. The Futuretrak project does have a chapter, in its fourth stage of study, that could have the potentiality to open exploration into wider social strands in graduate lives; however, chapter 8 – 'Non-academic HE resources available to students: the impact of participation in extracurricular activities and careers services on access to opportunities' – only concentrates on aspects of extracurricular activities such as being a student representative, as well as support offered by the career service. This chapter does not explore in any depth the interrelations of social strands outside the parameters of work or education, such as caring responsibilities, and also does not take into account how such strands interrelate.

This chapter is therefore advocating for a deeper and broader exploration of career, one that does not become so narrow as to overly concern the notion of employability, where employability may become placed within the realms of 'career development' to include the many strands within people's lives. It advocates that career studies has the potential to aid student exploration of career and will now move toward a contemplation of how a framework of dualities may aid the exploration of career.

❖ ACTIVITY 2

- What roles/strands/themes do you currently enact in your 'career'?
- How do they interrelate? Do they provide any tension?
- What have your experiences of career education been?
- What value, if any, does Watts and Law's DOTS system provide?
- Are there any limitations to such an approach?

Exploring career via the notion of duality

The previous sections have opened up the notion that career tends to be viewed as simply involving a linear progression of work experiences. It has then been argued that there are political and ideological underpinnings to such notions. The chapter is now to demonstrate that if we are to explore career via a broad paradigm, which takes into account numerous roles/strands, it would be useful to have some kind of framework to aid such explorations. The chapter therefore advocates that the notion of duality becomes a useful means to frame such an exploration. This chapter advocates that duality *is a conceptualisation of reality that provides a paradoxical relationship between opposing yet entwining entities.* Everyday examples include day and night, light and dark, male and female. It is evident that to contemplate one entity makes no sense without the other and that the boundaries between the two entities become blurred when placed under scrutiny; dawn and dusk are both and neither day nor night. To conceptualise via a duality is to simplify reality. This can prove to be both enabling (for example, help gain meaning of the complex social world) and constraining (for example, preventing other ways of seeing). As Adorno (1973: 74) warns, 'to perceive resemblances everywhere, making everywhere alike, is a sign of weak eyesight'. It is hoped that this chapter can provide an initial and accessible simplification of key dimensions of 'career' – via dualities – yet with complexity to aid a 'good eyesight'.

The dualities to be explored here – although others could come into play – are self and other, agency and structure, and being and becoming. Such concepts are prevalent in the career development theory literature; however, they are rarely conceived as dualities. The tendency in the literature is to present such concepts as dualisms where they are viewed as separate entities. As a result this creates a hierarchy that places emphasis upon certain concepts over their dual related entity. So, for example, self tends to be valued over other, agency over structure and being over becoming. The chapter will take each of these dualities in order to explore their interrelationship, an interrelationship that avoids hierarchy. It will then move toward concluding remarks in how the reader can utilise such a framework to aid their own career exploration.

Self and other

We live in societies with others, what the influential continental philosopher Heidegger (1962) would describe as 'being-in-the-world-with-others'. Notice how Heidegger insists on hyphenating the words. He does this deliberately to demonstrate how the notions are inseparably linked. Lyotard (1979: 15) provides a similar view, suggesting that a 'self does not amount to much, but no self is an island; each exists in a fabric of relations that is now more complex and mobile than ever before'. What both these philosophers are asserting is that we live in a social world and that a contemplation of self requires a contemplation of other and vice versa.

What does it mean to be a 'self'? A self that can contemplate 'who am I?' Such questions are what Giddens (1991) and Beck (1992) would describe as reflexive questions, where the self contemplates the self. Yet to answer the above questions invariably requires contemplation of the social world and thus others. Let us take a simple example. If someone was to ask me who am I, I would probably provide an answer in the form of a story; for example, that I am, at the time of writing, 41 years old and that I was born in Greater London and that I am now a father of two young boys. Even in this brief answer my story has acknowledged 'other' both in terms of place and other people – reminiscent of how Russian dolls require many to configure a whole.

Our understanding of the self requires an understanding of other in relation to our biography – our story/stories of self. For another example, the prominent academic Noam Chomsky, when asked about his emancipatory politics in the film *Manufacturing Consent*, responds with a story from childhood. He suggests that when he was young he experienced a child being oppressed and bullied by a number of others. Chomsky then laments the fact that he did nothing to help this individual and that he felt terrible about this. As a result Chomsky refused to let such an episode occur again, suggesting that since this occurrence he has always stood by the 'underdog'. What is of importance here is that the interaction with others provoked a change in behaviour for Chomsky. This is obviously not the full story; this event would have related to previous events in Chomsky's life and certain values, shaped by experience, that Chomsky held and holds. The social shaping of our values – deep-rooted aspects of self (Gothard et al. 2001) – are therefore social constructs, likely to be influenced by social interactions with others. Much of self is thus paradoxically other, where aspects of biography – that which constitute and configure our own sense of self, which is constantly under construction (see Giddens 1991) – connect with the stories and biographies of others and vice versa. The 'self' therefore cannot be considered and makes no sense without 'other'.

As already indicated, this is not all one-way traffic. We as a self can also influence the other, the socialiser is socialised (Law 1981). Caputo (2000) asserts that the 'self's' notions of 'other' become entwined with a sense of 'self'. What becomes apparent is 'self's' interplay with 'other', via interaction with 'other', invites an understanding of difference. To contemplate our difference with the other is to venture toward alterity, to acknowledge such alterity – the quality or state of being radically alien to the conscious self or a particular cultural orientation – so as not to shape toward our own wishes, to become unprepared for such alterity. However:

How is one to prepare for the coming of the other? Is not the other, as other, the one for whom one is precisely not prepared? Does not preparation relieve the other of his or her or its alterity so that, if we are prepared, then what comes is not other but the same, just what we are expecting? Would not extending true hospitality toward the other involve a certain unconditionality in which one is prepared for anything, which means that one is not prepared? Is the only adequate preparation for the coming of the other to confess that we cannot be prepared for what is coming?

(Caputo 2000: 41)

Such problematisation evokes paradox, where paradox draws also toward the very notion of reflexivity and that which appears to be a 'natural' predicament for the self, as indicated in Royle's (2003) reading of Derrida's notions of the 'self'. Royle (2003: 54) suggests that:

Hearing oneself speak – that is to say, even if one is keeping silent listening to oneself in the interiority of one's own head, keeping an ear out, so to speak, in order to be able to hear oneself think – hearing oneself speak is perhaps 'the most natural thing in the world', we also know, or think we know, that hearing oneself speak is not 'really' in the world at all: we like to think and feel that it doesn't involve having to 'pass through what is outside the sphere of "owness" in any way'.

Royle is alluding to what Derrida calls 'the regime of normal hallucination' – 'to hear one-self is the most normal and the most impossible experience' (Royle 2003: 54). Under such a lens our sense of autonomy and self-reflexivity becomes problematised. The important point here is that to consider the self as being an isolated entity that 'knows' its essence in relation to what it 'wants' from career – prevalent in managerial and planning strategies to career, such as DOTS – promotes an overt notion of self over other. The self is therefore presented in a fashion that knows and is 'prepared' for alterity by an un-acknowledgement of 'other' within' 'self' – and vice versa – so as to promote a beguiling 'ghost within the machine' (Ryle 1949).

At this stage you may want to consider how others have influenced your self. This can be via local interactions – interactions with the local community such as friends, family and educators – or the wider community – decisions made by politicians, media images, the global markets, material products and consumption trends. The decisions and actions made by powerful groups within an interconnected world can have major consequences on our lives, adapting the social terrain for individuals and groups of individuals to navigate. Via such a lens an individual is to consider how much autonomy one has. This will be a central aspect for the next section.

The important point of learning at this juncture is that dualistic conceptions are useful yet provide a simplistic view which becomes problematised once placed under scrutiny – especially at the borders. With this being the case, the concept of the *self* is fraught with difficulty – mainly due to its paradoxical relationship with other – even though both have great everyday practical use.

❖ **ACTIVITY 3**

Take into account the duality of self and other to answer the following questions:

- How might you describe yourself?
- Does other come into play to answer such a question? If so, how?
- How do notions of yourself influence your contemplation of others?
- How might ideas of yourself influence your future 'career'?

Please take into account Activities 1 and 2 when answering these questions.

Agency and structure

This duality is not only an important parameter in relation to career, it is also important in relation to the social sciences. You might have already come across these words during your studies. The chapter at this point is to provide time to explicitly contemplate this duality – although it is not always presented as a duality.

Many of us will have experiences within life that, at a later date, provoke reflection. 'Why did I do that?' 'What could I have done differently?' Such questions will revisit the scene and are likely to place you back to the perceiving, contemplative, supposedly autonomous I. Once revisiting the scene one can contemplate a different course of action: 'if only I had …'. Such conceptions – 'if only I had …' – encapsulate aspects of 'agency'. Yet such events, as already discussed, do not occur in a vacuum, as all actions occur within a social world. The chances are that a course of action would have been influenced by others, culture and social norms – social phenomena that constrain and enable personal action – that which encapsulates aspects of 'structure'. As indicated in a picture taken of my eldest son constructing a structure at the London Transport Museum, my son required building blocks to enable him to build his structure, yet at the same time he was constrained by the blocks available, particularly when others also came to play and build. 'Agency refers to the active capacity of the actor to pursue voluntarily chosen goals. Structure refers to the conditions of restraint [as well as enablement] that allocate resources and rules for individual actions' (Rojek 2005: 61).

Such concepts pervade everyday life. When we wake up in the morning we may well consider what outfit we are to wear that day (agency), yet such a 'choice' is constrained/enabled and influenced, by one's wardrobe, which in turn is constrained/enabled and influenced by economics, production, trends, social norms, etc. (structure). With extreme agency comes a sense that the world is our oyster, that we have unlimited choice and that we are the sole architects of our future, yet extreme structure may well paint a picture of a mere dingy floating aimlessly within the forces of a deterministic sea. Yet, as with all dualisms, the two entities are inextricably linked. Giddens' (1984) structuration theory is a means of reconciling this supposed divide. Giddens (1984: 19) asserts that:

The actions of all of us are influenced by the structural characteristics of the societies in which we are brought up and live; at the same time, we recreate (and also to some extent alter) those structural characteristics in our actions.

Giddens argues that our everyday actions are influenced by social structures yet actors – people – are not helpless pre-programmed robots, they can contemplate their actions within such structures. He also acknowledges that the structures are social in nature and thus occur due to actors' actions. If actors care not to follow or adhere to the structures then they lose their influence. This is a concept that relates explicitly to work careers. Pallas (1992, quoted in Ecclestone 2007) highlights that when considering our futures we more than likely consider plausible routes. There will be pre-determined routes heavily influenced by social structures – namely 'pathways'. Examples of pathways are college courses and graduate employment schemes. These, however, need to be navigated by the mover and are not extensive. Individuals may be able to pave their own pathways – what are described as 'trajectories' – for example, in terms of work within a pioneering field/role. Once many actors evoke trajectories to pave a pathway they are invariably shaping social structures. An example here might be pioneering employment opportunities. Today there are many employed IT consultants in many work environments, yet there would have been a time when this position did not exist. Yet due to the advent of computers and the prominent use of such technology such roles were brought into being and these in turn advocated the becoming of courses and graduate schemes – pathways – for many to navigate.

Giddens' structuration theory highlights that our agency and actions play their part in the formation, demise and reproduction of social structures. Therefore when contemplating our own transitions through life we need to acknowledge that structures will influence our intentions and enactment. However, we must not forget that we have a say – even though at times minimal – on the advent, reinforcement, reproduction and demise of such structures and our own biography as discussed in the previous section.

When contemplating social structures it would be useful to consider how this interplays with people's identities and social circumstances, where social structures – such as the formal education system – may provide privilege to certain groups in comparison to others. For example, in the 2010 Labour leadership contest each of the five candidates studied at either Oxford or Cambridge:

David Miliband – Philosophy, Politicvs and economics (PPE) at Oxford
Ed Miliband – PPE at Oxford
Ed Balls – PPE at Oxford
Andy Burnham – English at Cambridge
Diane Abbott – History at Cambridge

(Mulholland 2010)

Also, when considering the formal education structure there appears to be a privilege in relation to those who are privately educated in comparison to those who have been educated within state comprehensives, as indicated below:

Students from state schools:
Oxford – 54.3%
Cambridge – 59.3%

RICKY GEE

Durham — 59.2%
Manchester — 78.1%
Manchester Metropolitan — 95.4%

(O'Leary 2012)

What such statistics demonstrate — which may be further researched by exploring the Equality and Human Rights Commission's 'How Fair is Britain?' report (Equality and Human Rights Commission 2010) — is that one's position within the HE sector is heavily influenced by the secondary school that one attends, where there is a large correlation between being privately educated and attending a prestigious pre-1992 university. Not that such disparity does not occur in the labour market, as the quotes from the EHRC report indicate, on the grounds of the interconnections between ethnicity, disability and educational attainment.

● Moreover, Black people and disabled people in their early 20s are twice as likely to be not in employment, education or training (NEET) as White people and non-disabled people.
● Young Muslims are also more likely than Christians to spend periods out of the labour market.
● Overall, a more demanding job market is less forgiving of those **without qualifications**.

❖ ACTIVITY 4

Take into account the duality of agency and structure to answer the following questions:

● How much agency do you have in life?
● How might such ideas of agency be limited or enabled by social structures?
● What social structures do you perceive to influence your 'career' enactment?

Remember to utilise answers in previous tasks to aid you here.

Being and becoming – a tale from ancient Greece

Now almost all the hypotheses that have dominated modern philosophy were first thought of by the Greeks.

(Russell 1961: 57)

What does it mean 'to be'? 'To be a being'? Such questions bring back the notions of self and other. To be is to have an identity, to have some understanding of one's characteristics. Yet this has a temporal dimension requiring a diachronic as well as a synchronic analysis. For example, I am 41 and a proud father of two young boys, yet I have not always been such. If I had the ability to ask my previous self at sixteen, 'What does it mean to be? To be a being?', I am sure I would have answered very differently as I was, in many senses, a different *being*, the major contrasts being that I have now *become* 41 and a father, as opposed to a carefree, naive sixteen-year-old. Paradoxically, such *becoming* has now *become* my current *being*. Therefore 'being' – as a noun – adheres to the present – a name of a person or place evokes a concreteness. On the other hand, becoming evokes a sense of life in a state of flux therefore forever changing – discontinuity, a sense of startlement (Love 2008). Becoming acknowledges the ever-changing nature of life and thus we are never the entirely same person as we were a minute ago. In such a state one constantly has to evaluate 'being' to an infinitesimal degree therefore being is never pinned down. One can argue that such a state is timeless as one cannot acknowledge the abstract memorial marking of time and would be placed in a constant state of startlement (Love 2008).

The relationship between being and becoming has a long history opened and formed by an argument between two pre-Socratic philosophers. Such an argument provides a story of personality, value and material form. Writings on Heraclitus and Parmenides (Russell 1961; Guthrie 1979; Nietzsche 1962) paint a debate argued by different characters. Heraclitus is depicted as a mystic opposed to a man of science and described as loathing rational, logical thought, with many of his assertions being purposely paradoxical – 'We are and at the same time are not'; 'Being and nonbeing is at the same time the same and not the same' (see Nietzsche 1962). With disdain for rationality Heraclitus appeals for intuition, seeing the changing world of experience conditioned by never-ending variations in time and space with all individual objects perceived through time and space as existing relative to other objects. Nature and reality are seen as a continuous action in which there is no permanent existence.

What is clear is that Heraclitean philosophy adheres toward becoming as opposed to being, valuing chaos over order, which is encapsulated by his famous account: 'You use names for things as though they rigidly, persistently endured; yet even the stream into which you step a second time is not the one you stepped into before' (Nietzsche 1962: 52).

The archiving of Parmenides paints a different philosophy from a different character. Parmenides refuted the Heraclitean claim that everything changes by asserting that nothing changes. This argument pushes human conception to its outer limits, yet the argument strangely still seeks equilibrium via a containment of conception. Parmenides arrived at his truths through pure logic by concluding with a doctrine of being. Such logic refuted Heraclitean claims due to them being illogical; something cannot exist without existing, therefore that which 'is' must always be forever present. Asserting such logic is at the expense of the senses, which Parmenides believed to be deceptive.

When considering such a debate in relation to an individual's lifespan/life course, transition encapsulates moments of discontinuities which very often are associated with disorientation and anxiety. Startlement becomes a striking way to emotively engage with aspects of transition – of the initial conceptual sense of how transition affects the self-narrative. Giddens (1991) thus describes fateful moments as turning points in a person's self-narrative. Such moments, he suggests, are threatening to our protective cocoon shielding our ontological security. The fateful moment is thus a moment of startlement where the future is to play out in a different form alien to the continuity of the previous enacted narrative. Yet such moments of ontological despair will adhere toward previous associative notions of the transition to be anticipated. This provides difficulty, especially if the person has little or no notion of what is to come. It places the individual in a similar state of disorientation that Gregor Samsa (in Kafka's (1995) famous *Metamorphosis*) found himself when awaking as an embodied bug yet still had a sense of being human. Gregor's predicament is unfolding at a pace and it is unclear as to how his metamorphosis is to ensue and how he can come to begin to understand such a transformation. Does he rely on notions of being human, or previous conceptions of bugs – yet from the point of view of a human? Therefore it is important to acknowledge that moments of transition are episodes where an individual, or group of individuals, are to contemplate the paradoxical relationship between being and becoming, a never-ending interplay of conception.

Transition as a concept is heavily entwined with the duality of being and becoming. 'Trans' means 'to cross'. Transition thus evokes a sense of movement, a crossing from one state, stage, status and/or environ to another. To do so evokes a contemplation of the displacement of being and becoming highlighted above, where transition is an important subset of career.

❖ ACTIVITY 5

Take into account the duality of being and becoming to aid you here.

- What do the terms being and becoming mean to you?
- How might previous transition within your career have influenced where you are today/in the future?

Duality and paradox

The above three sections have invited the reader to consider important dimensions of career found throughout the career development literature. Taking into account wider social science theory, the chapter has provided a framework of such dimensions via the notion of duality. The importance of viewing via duality – as opposed to a dichotomy – is that it avoids the notion of hierarchy; what the chapter demonstrates is that when we consider a duality – *a conceptualisation of reality that provides a paradoxical relationship between opposing yet entwining entities* – dual entities paradoxically entwine, therefore aspects of other are found within self, being within becoming and structure within agency; one entity does not make sense without the other. This is important when considering many career development theories and models, as there is a tendency to place prominence on one entity over another, i.e. self over other, agency over structure, and being over becoming, what Bowman et al. (2005) would describe as the dissatisfactory 'folk theory' of career – as many argue that such conceptualisations no longer relate to people's 'realities' and are insufficiently nuanced to deal with ambiguity, for example Gelatt (1989), McAdams et al. (2001) and Ruppert (2010). The Activities within these sections have been a means of applying the notion of duality to your own 'career' – whatever you deem, hopefully informed via the literature, your position on 'career' to be. What you will hopefully have experienced is that duality evokes notions of paradox, where self is paradoxically entwined with other, as is the case for agency and structure and being and becoming. The chapter suggests that the acknowledgement of paradox is to be welcomed, a space where the complexity of career may be contemplated, to seek different and radical readings, to potentially challenge normative notions of 'career'.

Concluding remarks

This chapter has provided a tour of important dimensions of career that it asserts will be useful in considering a reflexive exploration of one's career. The intent of the chapter is to challenge the simplistic, agented and apolitical notions of employability that are found in many educational institutions. It argues that employability tends not to take into account how aspects of society can influence a person's career, which also embraces a simplistic notion of career equating work. The chapter therefore opens up the notion of duality and how this can be utilised to consider career so as to be aware that career is a social pursuit involving others-in-the-world, where class, gender and ethnicity interrelate with the opportunity structure and where individuals still have a sense of agency. It has also been acknowledged that careers are lived experiences that involve transitions where one is to question the paradoxical relationship between being and becoming. Such exploration allows for a broader notion and exploration of career, which it is hoped the reader will engage with so as to avoid the narrow managerialist notions of career that are unpopular among the student body (Atkins 1999; Watts 2006; McCash 2006; Knight and Yorke 2003).

References

Adorno, T. W. (1973) *Negative Dialectics*. London: Routledge and Kegan Paul.

Andrews, D. (2013) The new duty on schools to secure careers guidance: Case studies of good practice. *Careers Education and Guidance: Journal of the Association for Careers Education and Guidance*, Spring 2013.

Atkins, M. J. (1999) Oven-ready and self-basting: Taking stock of employability skills. *Teaching in Higher Education*, 4(2), 267–80.

Barnes, A. and Andrews, D. (eds) (1995) *Developing Careers Education and Guidance in the Curriculum*. London: David Fulton.

Beck, U. (1992) *The Risk Society*. London: Sage.

Bowman, H., Hodkinson, P. and Colley, H. (2005) *Employability and Career Progression for Fulltime UK Masters Students. Final Report for the Higher Education Careers Service Unit* (HECSU). Manchester: HECSU.

Browne, J. (2010) *Securing a Sustainable Future for Higher Education: An Independent Review of Higher Education Funding and Student Finance*. www.bis.gov.uk/assets/biscore/corporate/docs/s/10-1208-securing-sustainable-higher-education-browne-report.pdf (accessed 20 May 2011).

Caputo, J. (2000) *More Radical Hermeneutics: On Not Knowing Who We Are*. Bloomington, IN: Indiana University Press.

CBI (2011) *Working Towards Your Future: Making the Most of Your Higher Education Experience*. www.cbi.org.uk/ndbs/press.nsf/0363c1f07c6ca12a8025671c00381cc7/6 0519e9e213d34268025788f003808ef/$FILE/CBI_NUS_Employability%20report_ May%202011.pdf (accessed 20 May 2011).

Colley, H., Lewin, C. and Chadderton, C. (2010) *The Impact of 14–19 Reforms on the Career Guidance Profession in England*. Final Report for the Economic and Social Research Council. Manchester: Manchester Metropolitan University.

Cote, J. (2014) *Youth Studies: Fundamental Issues and Debates*. Basingstoke: Palgrave Macmillan.

Derrida, J. (1992) Force of law: The mystical foundation of authority. Trans. M. Quaintance, in Cornell, D., Rosenfeld, M. and Gray Carlson, D. (eds), *Deconstruction and the Possibility of Justice*. London: Routledge, pp. 3–67.

Ecclestone, K. (2007) Keynote presentation to Researching Transitions in Lifelong Learning conference, University of Sterling, 22–24 June 2007.

Equality and Human Rights Commission (2010) *How Fair is Britain? Equality, Human Rights and Good Relations in 2010*. Manchester: Equality and Human Rights Commission.

Fleming, P. (2009) *Authenticity and the Cultural Politics of Work*. Oxford: Oxford University Press.

Foucault, M. (1977) *Discipline and Punishment*. London: Penguin.

Furlong, A. and Cartmel, F. (2007) *Young People and Social Change: New Perspectives*. Buckingham: Open University Press.

Gale, T. and Parker, S. (2014) Navigating change: A typology of student transition in higher education. *Studies in Higher Education*, 39(5), 734–53.

Gelatt, H. B. (1989) Positive uncertainty: A new decision-making framework for counseling. *Journal of Counseling Psychology*, 36(2), 252–56.

Gellner, E. (1972). *Thought and Change*. London: Weidenfeld and Nicolson.

Giddens, A. (1984) *The Constitution of Society: Outline of the Theory of Structuration*. Cambridge: Polity Press.

Giddens, A. (1991) *Modernity and Self-Identity. Self and Society in the Late Modern Age*. Cambridge: Polity Press.

Goffman, E. (1961) The moral career of the mental patient. In *Asylums*. New York: Anchor.

Gothard, B., Mignot, P., Offer, M. and Ruff, M. (2001) *Careers Guidance in Context*. London: Sage.

Guthrie, W. K. (1979) *A History of Greek Philosophy: The PreSocratic Tradition from Parmenides to Democritus*. Cambridge: Cambridge University Press.

Heginbotham, H. (1951) *The Youth Employment Service*. London: Methuen and Co.

Heidegger, M. (1962) *Being and Time*. Oxford: Blackwell Publishing.

Henderson, S., Holland, J., McGrellis, S., Sharpe, S. and Thomson, R., with Grigoriou, T. (2007) *Inventing Adulthoods: A Biographical Approach to Youth Transitions*. London: Sage.

Hillage, J. and Pollard, E. (1998) *Employability: Developing a Framework for Policy Analysis. Research Report RR85*. London: Department for Education and Employment.

Kafka, F. (1995) *The Metamorphosis*. In *The Penal Colony and Other Stories*. New York and London: Simon & Schuster.

Knight, P. and Yorke, M. (2003) *Assessment, Learning and Employability*. Maidenhead, UK: Open University Press.

Law, B. (1981) Community interaction: A 'mid-range' focus for theories of career development in young adults. *British Journal of Guidance and Counselling*, 9(2), 142.

Law, B. (1996) Careers work in schools. In Watts, A. G., Law, B., Killeen, J., Kidd, J. and Hawthorn, R. (eds), *Rethinking Careers Education and Guidance: Theory, Policy and Practice*. London: Routledge.

Law, B. and Watts, A. G. (1977). *Schools, Careers and Community*. London: Church Information Office.

Love, K. (2008) Being startled: Phenomenology at the edge of meaning. *PhaenEx: revue de théorie et culture existentialistes et phénoménologiques* [*Journal of Existential and Phenomenological Theory and Culture*], 3(2), 149–78.

Lyotard, J.-F. (1979) *The Postmodern Condition: A Report on Knowledge*. Minneapolis, MN: University of Minnesota Press.

McAdams, D. P., Josselson, R. and Lieblich, A. (2001) *Turns in the Road: Narrative Studies of Lives in Transition*. Washington, DC: American Psychological Association.

McCash, P. (2006) We're all career researchers now: Breaking open career education and DOTS. *British Journal of Guidance and Counselling*, 34(4), 429–49.

McCash, P. (2008) *Career Studies Handbook*. York: Higher Education Academy.

Mercer, J. (2011) Education, business and government: A new partnership for the 21st Century. In *Blue Skies: New Thinking about the Future of Higher Education*. http://pearsonblueskies.com/wp-content/uploads/2011/05/36-pp_149-152.pdf (accessed 25 May 2011).

Morris, M., Rudd, P., Nelson, J. and Davies, D. (2000) *The Contribution of Careers Education and Guidance To School Effectiveness in Partnership Schools*. National Foundation for Education Research, DFEE.

Mulholland, H. (2010) Who are the Labour leadership candidates? www.theguardian.com/politics/2010/jun/09/who-are-the-labour-leadership-candidates (accessed 22 December 2015).

National Curriculum (2007) *PSHE: Economic Wellbeing and Financial Capability*. London: QCA.

Nietzsche, F. (1962) *Philosophy in the Tragic Age of the Greeks*. Washington, DC: Regnery Publishing, Inc.

Office for Standards in Education/Audit Commission (1993) *Unfinished Business*. London: OFSTED/Audit Commission.

O'Leary, J. (2012) *The Times University Guide*. London: Harper Collins.

Patton, W. and McMahon, M. (1999) *Career Development and Systems Theory: A New Relationship*. Pacific Grove, CA: Brooks/Cole.

Peim, N. and Flint, K. (2009) Testing times: Questions concerning assessment for school improvement. *Educational Philosophy and Theory*, 41(3), 324–361.

Purcell, K., Elias, P., Atfield, G., Behle, H., Ellison, R., Luchinskaya, D., Snape, J., Conaghan, L. and Tzanakou, C. (2012) *Futuretrak Stage 4: Transitions into Employment, Further Study and Other Outcomes, Full Report*. Warwick: Institute for Employment Research.

Ricoeur, P. (1976) *Interpretation Theory, Discourse and the Surplus of Meaning*. Fortworth, TX: Christian University Press.

Roberts, K. (1977) The social conditions, consequences and limitations of careers guidance. *British Journal of Guidance and Counselling*, 5(1), 19.

Roberts, K. (1997) Prolonged transitions to uncertain destinations: The implications for careers guidance. *British Journal of Guidance and Counselling*, 5(1), 1–9.

Roberts, K. (2009) Opportunity structures then and now. *Journal of Education and Work*, 22(5), 355–68.

Rojek, C. (2005) *Leisure Theory: Principles and Practice*. Basingstoke: Palgrave Macmillan.

Royle, N. (2003) *Jacques Derrida*. London and New York: Routledge.

Ruppert, J.-J. (2010) Life design: here to stay or just a fad? At the 2010 NCDA-IAEVG-SVP International Symposium, Bridging International Perspectives of Career Development, 28–29 June 2010.

Russell, B. (1961) *History of Western Philosophy and Its Connection with Political and Social Circumstances from the Earliest Times to the Present Day*. London: Allen & Unwin.

Ryle, G. (1949) *The Concept of Mind*. London: Hutchinson and Co.

Schools Council (1972) Careers education in the 1970s. Working Paper 40. London: Schools Council.

Super, D. E. (1994) A life span, life space perspective on convergence. In Savickas, M. L. and Lent, R. W. (eds), *Convergence in Career Development Theories: Implications for Science and Practice*. Palo Alto, CA: Consulting Psychologists Press.

Watts, A. (2003) Working connections: OECD observations. Presentation to 'Working Connections: a Pan-Canadian Symposium on Career Development, Lifelong Learning and Workforce Development, Toronto, 16–18 November 2003.

Watts, A. G. (2006) *Career Development Learning and Employability*. York: Higher Education Academy. Also available via www.heacademy.ac.uk/resources/publications/learningandemployability

Willetts, D. (2011) Putting students at the heart of higher education. In *Blue Skies: New Thinking about the Future of Higher Education*. http://pearsonblueskies.com/wp-content/uploads/2011/05/01-pp_017-019.pdf (accessed 25 May 2011).

Yorke, M. and Knight, P. (2006) *Learning and Employability, Series 1: Embedding Employability into the Curriculum*. www.heacademy.ac.uk/assets/York/documents/ourwork/employability/id460_embedding_employability_into_the_curriculum_338.pdf (accessed 20 May 2011).

Young, R. A. and Valach, L. (2000) Reconceptualising career theory and research: An action theoretical perspective. In A. Collin and R. A. Young (eds), *The Future of Career*. Cambridge: Cambridge University Press.

Chapter 12
Personal development planning as reflection

Catherine Goodall

Chapter outline

This chapter introduces:

- personal reflections of professional development planning
- introduction to Knowledge Transfer Partnerships as a model for reflective professional development
- the impact of formal professional development planning on practice.

Introduction

As a case study, this chapter will explore experiences of personal professional development during a 30-month Knowledge Transfer Partnership project between a university and a local authority. The project was situated in the Children's Services department, with a focus on reviewing and improving services for local children and families. The formal process for development required by the project will be examined, and the relevance and degree of applicability of such a model for reflective practice in health and social care professions discussed.

I will describe the role and the professional development process it entailed. In this case, the formal process required by the project was both beneficial and rewarding, but models of professional development are not without critique. The project offered a valuable and unique setting to reflect on my skills and experience, and to improve my professional practice. With a dedicated development budget, it also afforded significant opportunity to plan to enhance my professional capacity.

Critical reflection on skills, knowledge, experience, capacity and professional practice was crucial to this project. The regularly scheduled reviews provided sufficient space and resources to reflect effectively. Alongside taking up formal and informal opportunities for development through training, qualifications and coaching, I was also able to capitalise on the chance to develop and improve general skills and experience, and to increase confidence in my professional capacity.

This chapter has a wide relevance. It describes personal professional development in a project which bridged the worlds of academia and practice. As a unique and small-scale case study, the experiences described are relevant to theory and practice alike. There were unexpected benefits to the formalised personal development planning process dictated by the project. These benefits may be of significance to organisations and individuals far beyond the scope of this small case study. There can be value in professional development planning beyond that which is commonly expected from formal processes. The experiences of this project are linked to wider theory on the impact of critical reflection.

Overall, personal professional development is found to be of great potential benefit to individuals and organisations alike. Organised and formalised models can enhance and support professional development, if designed and implemented appropriately. Challenges for professional development included limitations on costs and resources, ensuring the focus of activities and plans rests on outputs and impact rather than inputs, and ensuring that learning from development activities can be adequately implemented in practice.

Knowledge Transfer Partnerships

The professional development process considered was part of a Knowledge Transfer Partnership project running from January 2014 to July 2016. Knowledge Transfer Partnerships (KTPs) are a unique form of relationship between a university, a business and an associate. KTPs allow businesses to tap into the wealth of knowledge, technology and experience held by universities, to meet strategic business needs. With sustained funding from government through Innovate UK (formerly the Technology Strategy

Board), KTPs have been running for over 40 years. Usually ranging from 6 to 36 months, KTP projects vary greatly in topic, focus, discipline and industry. The majority of KTPs take place with technical and manufacturing companies. The prevalence and impact of KTP projects is significant in the UK economy, and there were over 700 different projects running at the end of 2014 (Technology Strategy Board 2015: 5).

Alongside the clear benefits of sustained relationships between academia and industry, the partnerships are credited with average increases in annual profit for companies of around £1 million, increased employment opportunities, and investment in plant, machinery and research (Technology Strategy Board 2015: 5). University partners benefit from gaining real-world experience and data, by increasing links to industry and by identifying future prospects for collaboration. Many KTP projects lead to academic publications and research outputs, as well as increased visibility for universities in industry.

The partnerships are also extremely beneficial to the associate delivering the project, who occupies a multifaceted role usually involving research, project management, analysis, product or process development and implementation. The associates benefit from supervision at both organisations, coaching from a KTP advisor and a dedicated personal development budget. The projects are also designed to allow associates time and space to complete professional training and development, with around 10 per cent of the project time allocated to this. Associates are also encouraged to produce research outputs, and many study for further academic and professional qualifications, within and beyond the KTP project.

Our project

The period of professional and personal development described here took place during a 30-month KTP project between Nottingham Trent University and Nottinghamshire County Council. The project was situated in the Children's Services department, with a focus on reviewing and improving services for local children and families.

Partnerships of this kind with public sector bodies are rare, and represent different opportunities for the partners involved. From the outset, our project was unlikely to generate substantial income or increased profits, for example. Given the significant reductions in funding and resources faced by local authorities, generation of new jobs or investment in plant or research and development were also not plausible goals.

Our project instead provided a wealth of opportunities to improve local service design, delivery and evaluation. This could lead to significant cost savings and improved outcomes for local children and families. Ensuring that services provided by local authorities are effective and cost-effective is an increasingly vital endeavour, as 'children's services struggle with scarce resources and decisions on how best to allocate these' (Stevens et al. 2010: 145). Indeed, during the course of the project Nottinghamshire County Council, along with many other local authorities in the UK, faced drastic cuts to funding and a shortfall in excess of £60 million (Nottinghamshire County Council, 2016). Such shortfalls require local authorities to make significant cuts and efficiencies to services, which can lead to a negative impact on families' lives and outcomes (Department of Health 2004: 47). It is therefore crucial to ensure that local authorities target services towards families most in need, and use evidence-based methods which have been demonstrated to have a positive impact.

To meet these needs, the project was designed to review and evaluate current service delivery in a range of areas, and to design and implement improvements. One element of the project was to facilitate Participatory Action Research (PAR) with children and young people. PAR seeks to involve participants in research to improve a social problem affecting their lives (Ward and Bailey 2012: 165). Involving children and young people in evaluating and improving services which are designed to meet their needs is essential. Children are assured the right to be heard, and to participate in decisions made about their lives, by the United Nations Conventions on the Rights of the Child (UNCRC 1989).

In line with this, the council follows a locally designed Participation Strategy, which governs the participation of children, young people and their families (Nottinghamshire Children's Trust Board 2014). The KTP project afforded the chance to facilitate in-depth, sustained participation of children and young people in research to improve services. PAR had the potential to inform and improve a wide range of services and their impact on children's lives.

Overall, the KTP project was designed to map, review and improve service design and delivery in the Children's Services department at the county council. The project would take a specific focus on parenting support, the approaches taken to working with children and families, and facilitating Participatory Action Research. The KTP also involved significant professional development opportunities for the associate, as will be described.

Professional development planning

Knowledge Transfer Partnership projects follow a formal and rigid structure. Designed in line with established project management protocols, the projects also include a structured professional development process. Professional development will be discussed, and the relevance of the process dictated by the KTP will be examined in relation to the wider field. In this chapter professional development, personal development and personal professional development will be used interchangeably to refer to the development of skills, knowledge, experience and professional capacity of an individual in relation to a specific professional role in an organisation.

Organisations are social bodies, built from and reliant upon the individuals who work for them (Boddy 2014). To function effectively and efficiently, these individuals need to be able to perform at the optimum level. Commitment, motivation and focus are all crucial for staff to perform at their best and in order for organisations to function effectively. In any role employees may start with differing skills, experience and aptitude, which can affect their ability to perform that role sufficiently. To overcome these differences and ensure that staff are effective, organisations can employ a range of methods. One such method is personal professional development.

There have been innumerate conceptions and iterations of professional development and the impact it can have on individuals and organisations (Clegg and Bradley 2006: 59). At its core, professional development 'encapsulates the idea that professionals are in the process of becoming' (Boud and Hager 2012: 20). Within any one company, discipline or career there may be a range of mechanisms or structures for professional development, and requirements may be specified by statutory or professional bodies, or by the tasks demanded by the role.

Professional development can be observed at two levels, that of the individual and of the organisation (Atkinson 1999). An organisation can take a wholesale approach to professional development, requiring individual employees to acquire specific skills and experience, or stipulating continued training, education or qualifications be undertaken. Alternatively, professional development can be viewed at an individual level, as designed to overcome a perceived skills gap or to build up an individual's experience or performance in particular areas (Kennedy 2005: 239).

As will be discussed, professional development is not always a straightforward endeavour, and may not 'achieve lasting and significant change' for individuals or for organisations (Atkinson 1999: 502). Many factors can influence the degree of success of professional development. One complicating factor is that it is often difficult to define and describe the requisites of a role and its relation to wider organisational needs. Another difficulty can arise where there is a perceived or real mismatch between the needs of the individual professional, and the organisation as a whole. A mismatch requires organisations to display a degree of flexibility, acknowledging that on specific occasions the development of an individual can be of sufficient indirect benefit to the organisation to make it a worthwhile investment (Alvesson and Willmott 2012).

This can be difficult to achieve in large, complex organisations such as universities or local authorities, as in this case. Professional development demands careful planning, investment and resources in order to be effective (Walmsley 2010: 77). An organisation may value investment in its employees in principle, but be unable to sufficiently fund or support individuals to undertake development activities.

My personal development planning

Knowledge Transfer Partnership projects have a long history in the UK, as described. They have been designed and adapted in line with established theory and good practice of project management. KTPs dictate that the associate follow a structured process to review their skills and experience in line with the role specification, and to plan to improve on these throughout the course of the project. Scheduled, regular reviews are a feature of KTP projects, and associates are expected to critically evaluate their progress and professional capacity on a number of occasions.

An established method to facilitate personal development is to produce a Personal Development Plan (PDP). A PDP is used to identify the key skills, knowledge and experience required for a role, to assess the extent to which an individual possesses these, and to set clear goals and targets to address any gaps or areas for development (Kennedy 2005). Both the core skills (such as assertiveness, organisation, problem solving, etc.) and job-specific skills (such as safeguarding or teaching for example) can be evaluated in relation to the defined role (Walmsley 2010: 67).

Development can be achieved through training, coaching, mentoring, private study, professional qualifications, academic qualifications, or any combination of these. A plethora of learning and training opportunities exist in modern health and social care. The degree of relevance, applicability and usefulness of a development opportunity is by no means assured, which in part explains why development activities might not achieve lasting positive impact or change (Atkinson 1999: 502).

This project was situated at an intersection of a number of fields, disciplines and established occupations. The project necessitated skills in project management, research, analysis and practice within the local authority. This unique mix of required skills and experience made professional development planning a difficult and complex process. This was further complicated by the dynamic and changing structure of the role in its initial stages.

Table 12.1 PDP – action plan

Name: Catherine Goodall Date: 2/2/15

High priority development need: Develop skills in drafting strategies and related action plans		
Success criteria: Successfully developing the Family and Parenting Strategy for the department		
Actions	**Start/end date for each action**	**Resources/help needed (including costs, time, etc.)**
Plan workshops with managers	Feb 15	Time for preparation. Possible training/ materials in running workshops
Plan workshops/ engagement with families and parents	Feb 15	Organising workshops, gathering feedback and evidence
Engagement with strategy group for feedback and amendments to initial draft	Mar 15	Time for meeting and amendments
Engagement with group to develop action plan for strategy	Apr 15	Time for planning, meetings and amendments
Anticipated evidence of effective work performance: Developing a new Family and Parenting Strategy		
Date for reviewing progress: 31/3/15		

Table 12.1 is part of an early iteration of planning in the project, and highlights one particular task and the skills and resources I required to complete it. A key difficulty in completing an effective PDP is to be able to identify and clearly articulate both the requirements, or tasks, of a role and the potential development opportunities which will address these needs. This particular example did not require any formal or external training or development, but it did require time and general resources.

Over the course of the project my skills in planning for and completing professional development records were improved. The act of repetition of the planning process enhanced my ability to plan effectively, and as such increased the potential impact on my professional capacity and work.

Professional development budget

As discussed, professional development entails investment of time and resources which can be problematic where organisations face limited funding or scope to invest. KTP projects usually have a dedicated professional development budget for associates, and this project had fairly substantial allocated funds for use over its 30-month duration. Taking on development opportunities requires an evaluation of the costs, time implications, barriers to access, applicability and potential impact. Costs are crucial in situations with controlled and limited budgets, and it was important to select the most beneficial options, whilst attempting to account for potential future development needs. It is common that individuals are required to produce detailed plans which describe the costs and resource requirements of an opportunity alongside the potential impact on their development and work. Table 12.2 is a simplistic example taken from this project. An improved table might also include details of any alternative opportunities, as well as demarcating impact for the individual and the organisation over time. This can be beneficial for organisations to be able to identify where any benefits of professional development may be indirect.

Table 12.2 Resource requirements table for development activities

Date	PD opportunity	Total days	Total costs	Planned initial impact
13 Feb 2014	Safeguarding Children Training	0.5	£0	Minimum standard for safeguarding children met
June 2014	Residential modules for KTP	9	£100	Improved project management skills, networking
2 June 2014	Early Intervention Foundation Evidence Forum, London	1	£70	Increased understanding of work of EIF, the guidebook and networking
4 July 2014	Safeguarding Children Conference, Loughborough	1	£20	Increased understanding of theory of safeguarding and networking
Oct 2014–15	Certificate in Teaching and Learning at NTU	10	£0	Skills developed in designing and delivering teaching in HE, preparation for HEA Associate Fellowship application
6 Feb 2015	PAR Training, Durham	1	£60	Skills developed in facilitating PAR

This dedicated budget provided the project team with sufficient scope and support to identify a range of different development activities to meet the needs of the project and of the broader teams and partners involved. Using the resources available throughout the project I was able to undertake professional qualifications, practice-based training, personal study and training in specific research methods. Financial support and the provision of adequate resources is crucial to ensure that individuals can identify and complete professional development activities. Clear and detailed identification and explication of the benefits of professional development opportunities to both the individual and the organisation can ensure that employers are able to target resources efficiently.

Experiences of the PDP process

Prior to taking on this role, I had no experience of professional development planning. I was unaccustomed to critically reviewing my skills and experience in line with what was required of me by a particular role. Beginning the structured PDP process required by the project was therefore a completely new endeavour, and one which I initially found quite daunting. The PDP for the project was long, complex and, owing to the varied nature of KTPs themselves, covered a very wide range of knowledge, skills and experience.

From the outset this project was characterised by dynamism and responsiveness to emerging needs from both partners. As such, the structure of the project was broad, flexible and changeable, and the role of the associate mirrored this structure. This presented a slight disconnect with the formal PDP process. However, the critical reflection the PDP encouraged was particularly beneficial in this case. Not only did the exercise allow me to identify my strengths and areas for development, but it also allowed us as a team to more clearly define the role, which provided us the opportunity to make stronger links to unexpected areas of the department and to target the project to the areas of greatest need.

Initially I was much more at ease with identifying discrete job-related skills or training opportunities than evaluating more general personal or professional traits or aptitude. In this respect, the PDP was beneficial as it provided a formal and structured process to follow, which was focused on achievable and measurable goals. However, there was a section in the plan entitled 'Long-term aims and aspirations' which I found a continuing challenge. The section required the associate to envisage their life in five to seven years, and to provide a summary overview of their aims and aspirations for that time period. The plan provided the following guidance:

Picture yourself in five to seven years' time and write a short paragraph or list of points that describe what you will be. Refer to the following points in this 'pen picture':

- Job/type of work, including your expectations of salary/income.
- Position (for example, responsibilities for people/finance/other resources).
- Location (where you would like to live/work).
- Employment status (employed/self-employed/family business/co-operative/etc.).
- Personal aims (foreign language, domestic situation etc.).

Whereas I found the process of reviewing my professional skills, experience and capability challenging only at the beginning of the project, I found the aims and aspirations section to be problematic throughout. As I do not wish to follow a standard or established career path, planning more general aspects of my life felt more difficult. A traditional career would be likely to follow a particular trajectory, with expected salaries, requirements for qualifications, and perhaps with stronger ties to a specific region or location. Without this guiding framework, and without personal dependants to influence my decisions, I found it difficult to create a realistic and achievable vision over such a long time period.

Over time repetition of planning for professional development led to a positive realisation, however, as it highlighted that I have a significant degree of autonomy and opportunity with my long-term career plans and personal aspirations. Rather than experiencing anxiety over the lack of focus, I found the process freeing. In the absence of a set course, I was left with the ability to craft my own, to determine my future.

Unanticipated benefits

Unaccustomed as I had been to critical evaluation of my skills and abilities, I benefited significantly from the outset. Whilst focusing on a current lack of skills or experience or on areas of weakness might be problematic for some individuals, I found the process to be enlightening. I gained confidence by being able to clearly articulate my capability and experience. This was bolstered by being able to plan attainable and measurable improvements.

Initially, creating bounded and achievable goals during the project was challenging, and was made more complex by the nature of the project and my lack of experience in this area. Yet I found the process of critical reflection this required in itself to be beneficial and rewarding. By taking stock of my position in relation to what would be required of me during the project, I was able to formulate effective plans to improve my practice and professional capacity. Whilst the formal structure of the PDP may have limitations, in this case I found the process informative and valuable.

Learning from this could hold great importance for organisations, particularly those where funding and investment for formal professional development activities may be limited. Providing space and time for employees to critically evaluate their practice, skills and experience can be extremely valuable in and of itself (Hickson 2011). This type of evaluation demands that an individual identify their professional skills, experience and capabilities and the strengths and weaknesses of their practice.

Yet it is important to acknowledge that critical reflection is not an uncontested concept or practice (Brookfield 2009). As with professional development itself, critical reflection has been considered and debated at length, and there are many models and theoretical frameworks to guide its use in practice. In some organisational cultures, critical reflection is not particularly valued, and individuals may find it difficult to receive sufficient time, space and support for this in their organisations (Fook and Askeland 2007: 526). Critical reflection on weakness and skills gaps has the potential to cause unrest or distress in an individual if they do not feel supported by the organisation, or able to overcome any deficiencies which are identified.

Yet when conducted judiciously in a supportive environment, critical reflection of professional development can be of great benefit to professionals and organisations. In the case described here, critical reflection was valuable to me as an individual, to my professional capabilities, and to the wider project team.

Critique of personal development planning

The PDP process in KTP projects exemplifies a rigid and formalised process of professional development. There has been extensive and wide-ranging critique of organised professional development across a variety of fields and professions. Whilst the idea that professionals can and should continue to develop their skills, knowledge and experience over the course of their careers is generally accepted, the methods to ensure that this occurs are highly contested (Webster-Wright 2009). Professional development appears to be anything but a straightforward notion which can be easily measured or facilitated (Friedman and Phillips 2004).

Part of this critique centres on the notion that professional development can be discrete and manageable, and facilitated externally to the role, which is embodied by development processes such as the KTP's PDP. Boud and Hager have argued that 'most learning takes place not through formalised activities, but through the exigencies of practice with peers and others, drawing on expertise that is accessed in response to need' (Boud and Hager 2012: 20). Professional development structures that require individuals and organisations to identify opportunities which are external to the required role overlook this possibility. By creating distinct professional development opportunities, individuals may be unable to fully capitalise on this organic process within their own roles and teams. Whilst learning and development is possible from opportunities which are removed from everyday practice, a professional might gain significantly more from their day-to-day experiences. This can be particularly problematic where individuals are required or able to attend differing development activities, as mismatches between theory and practice, and between employees, can arise.

Another concern relating to formalised development processes is that they can focus more upon an input, rather than the output. As such, the measure of development is seen as the individual attending or completing an activity, rather than the impact upon their practice. This can be particularly prevalent in standardised or statutory CPD frameworks, where professionals are required to attend a set number of activities or receive a fixed number of hours of training over the time (Friedman and Phillips 2004).

Reflections

This project provided an ideal opportunity to reflect upon and improve my professional practice. Whilst a formal, rigid professional development planning process can have limitations, it was extremely useful and beneficial in this case. Dedicated time to reflect on what was required for the role allowed me to review my skills and experience, and plan effectively to enhance my capability.

A dedicated personal development budget is an increasingly rare resource, particularly in the public sector. The financial support allowed me to take advantage of a range of training and qualifications I would otherwise have been unable to access. Investment in professional development is crucial, and organisations need to be able to find balance in providing for their staff where funding may be limited. The benefits to an individual, their team and the wider organisation can be significant if development activities are well planned and aligned to both the role and broader organisational needs.

Over the course of the project I became accustomed to reflecting on my practice and progress, and to planning for the future. Reflecting and planning in this manner increased the confidence I have in my skills and experience, and increased my ability to identify areas for improvement. Personal and professional development planning need not be a particularly formal or rigid process in order to be of benefit. This case demonstrated that simply allowing time and space to reflect and to plan for the future can have significant value. This is important for organisations with limited capacity to fund professional development opportunities. The acts of critical review and planning can be of benefit, and can aid individuals in developing their professional capacity.

References

Alvesson, M. and Willmott, H. (2012) (2nd edn) *Making Sense of Management: A Critical Introduction*. London: Sage.

Atkinson, S. (1999) Personal development for managers – getting the process right. *Journal of Managerial Psychology*, 14(6), 502–11.

Boddy, D. (2014) (6th edn) *Management: An Introduction*. London: Pearson Education.

Boud, D. and Hager, P. (2012) Re-thinking continuing professional development through changing metaphors and location in professional practices. *Studies in Continuing Education*, 34(1), 17–30.

Brookfield, S. (2009) The concept of critical reflection: Promises and contradictions. *European Journal of Social Work*, 12(3), 293–304.

Clegg, S. and Bradley, S. (2006) Models of Personal Development Planning: Practice and processes. *British Educational Research Journal*, 32(1), 57–76.

Department of Health (2004) *All Our Lives: Social Care in England 2002–2003*. London: Department of Health.

Fook, J. and Askeland, G. (2007) Challenges of critical reflection: 'Nothing ventured, nothing gained'. *Social Work Education*, 26(5), 520–33.

Friedman, A. and Phillips, M. (2004) Continuing Professional Development: Developing a vision. *Journal of Education and Work*, 17(3), 361–76.

Hickson, H. (2011) Critical reflection: Reflecting on learning to be reflective. *Reflective Practice*, 12(6), 829–39.

Kennedy, A. (2005) Models of Continuing Professional Development: A framework for analysis. *Journal of In-Service Education*, 31(12), 236–42.

Nottinghamshire Children's Trust Board (2014) *Nottinghamshire Children, Young People and Families Participation Strategy 2014–2016.*

Nottinghamshire County Council (2016) *Joint Report of the Chairman of The Finance and Property Committee and the Leader of the Council – Report to Full Council 25/02/2016.*

Stevens, M., Roberts, H. and Shiell, A. (2010) Research review: Economic evidence for interventions in children's social care: Revisiting the What Works for Children project. *Children and Family Social Work*, 15, 145–54.

Technology Strategy Board (now Innovate UK) (2015) *Knowledge Transfer Partnerships: Achievements and Outcomes 2013 to 2014.* Swindon: Technology Strategy Board.

UNCRC (1989) *United Nations Convention on the Rights of the Child.* Geneva: United Nations.

Walmsley, B. (2010) *Instant Manager: Managing Yourself.* London: Hodder and Stoughton.

Ward, J. and Bailey, D. (2012) Consent, confidentiality and the ethics of PAR in the context of prison research. In Love, K. (ed.) *Ethics in Social Research, Studies in Qualitative Methodology*, Volume 12. Bingley, West Yorkshire: Emerald Group Publishing Limited, pp. 149–69.

Webster-Wright, A. (2009) Reframing professional development through understanding authentic professional learning. *Review of Educational Research*, 79(2), 702–39.

Chapter 13
Journeys of faith

Personal stories and faith development in church schools

Andy Wolfe

Chapter overview

This chapter will introduce:

- reflection through storying
- reflection in practice
- reflection on belonging and authenticity
- the importance of storytelling.

This chapter is an alternative reflection upon how people can story their own development in a reflective sense. Given a spiritual engagement, the act of narrating experience is seen from a different vantage point in reflection and storying on one's faith journey. In this way narrating the journey provides another way of reflecting that can overcome some of the barriers to reflective practice.

Stories, journeys and context

This chapter is about stories, and their importance in understanding faith development. It explores the way stories are told, the way that they interact and the way that, perhaps more powerfully than any other evidence base, they can help us to understand what is happening as young people and staff alike explore faith in our schools. Stories can encourage and equip, they can confuse and challenge, they can even undermine and wound, but they fundamentally compel us, engage us and, as we read and interact, shape and define us.

Through considering approaches to understanding faith formation, this chapter evaluates the extent to which the narrative language of 'faith journey' equips a school firstly to be more inclusive of all stakeholders, and secondly to imply to all that participation in the community necessitates dynamic engagement in the development of faith. In seeking to understand the importance of personal narrative, the study aims to provide some practical opportunities for schools to explore how to capture that which can be difficult to measure and evidence. It draws particularly on the ONESTORY books in relation to the importance of this personal narrative in capturing a school's ethos or mission statement. These books gather together a collection of sixteen stories from students and staff exploring how their faith has developed as a result of the impact of the Emmanuel School, Nottingham's work and ethos. Alongside the perhaps obvious focus on students' faith development, this book examines the extent to which staff working in a church school are potentially open to developing their own faith journeys, and the key organisational factors that determine this reality. In what conditions is faith most likely to form in students and staff and what implications could this participative approach to faith formation have for the mission of church schools at large?

This is written from a secondary church school perspective where faith development is a central facet of the school's identity, and the language of 'faith journey' is as important to staff and students as academic progression in curriculum subjects. The school's position is clearly defined by its mission statement within a diverse community which it seeks to serve in partnership with the local church. The school's 'ad-mission' policy – namely calling people 'to a mission' – allows for an outward-facing discourse of faith development, which is both open-handed and expectant, providing a range of experiences for students to grow in this area, and accessibly defined by the language of 'faith journey', as opposed to categorising students and staff rigidly by a named faith.

Throughout the chapter, short extracts from the Onestory publications are included by way of illustration of the text, and to encourage the reader to engage with the stories themselves by way of personal exploration of the suggestions being made. In seeking to begin this reflection on the crucial connection between story, journey and faith development in schools, we begin with an extract from the foreword written by the Revd Phil Marsh in the first volume of Onestory, published in 2012:

Ethos. Every school has one.

It is the character of a place, shaped and formed by the underlying values that drive it.

Can you measure it? Can you capture it?

We believe you can, simply through engaging with the real stories of those who inhabit the place, who play their part in the community. Their stories reveal the truth of what lies beneath, and their experience lifts our shared sense of ethos, from aspiration to reality, from words on a prospectus page to the reality of lives moving forward in their own faith journeys.

(Onestory, 2012: 3)

Packing our bags – reflecting the nature of faith development

Although used frequently in church school contexts, 'faith' turns out to be a surprisingly difficult word to pin down in terms of a definition. We might be most comfortable turning to a synonym such as 'belief' or even 'belief in', but ultimately this connection removes the essentially *active* nature of faith – it would be far easier if it became a *verb* 'to faith'. We perhaps need to alter the 'grammar of faith', namely calling the process 'faithing' (Astley 1991: 12), implying movement and narrative. We are concerned with moving from a compartmentalising approach to faith in schools, to a more animated notion of personal journey of faith for the students and staff in our care. Although this chapter is primarily concerned with a range of practical considerations for the facilitation and celebration of faith development in relation to narrative in schools, it is important to see these practical considerations within the context of wider understandings of faith development. In some cases the practical considerations affirm these wider understandings; in other instances they question them.

> My faith journey has been challenging … my friends all believe different things and so it's not quite as simple to know what to think … I still have lots of questions that I don't have the answers to.
>
> (Year 10 student, Onestory, 2014: 14)

Published in 1981, James Fowler's seminal work *Stages of Faith* continues to cast its insightful and persuasive shadow over every subsequent piece of writing in the field. Arguably the most influential contemporary thinker in relation to faith development, Fowler draws helpfully on a range of other scholars, firstly making a key distinction between 'faith' and 'adherence to a religious tradition', urging us not to reduce faith to credal statements and doctrinal foundations. Secondly he uses the linguistic analysis of Wilfrid Cantwell Smith to demonstrate that the words 'faith' and 'belief' are in danger of becoming subject to an overly modernist approach whereby we are primarily concerned with what people believe in. This stands in stark contrast to his more dynamic definition of faith, namely: 'On what, or whom, do you set your heart? … what hope animates you and gives shape to your life, and how do you move into it?', and exemplifying the deliberately empirical and holistic stance of his writing: 'Faith is an orientation of the total person, giving a goal to one's hopes and strivings' (Fowler 1981: 14).[1]

As foundational as Fowler's writing may have become to contemporary understanding of faith formation, he is self-evidently 'standing on the shoulders of giants', drawing incisively on the key developmental research of Piaget, Kohlberg and Erikson (Piaget 1932; Kohlberg 1958; Erikson 1959). The interweaving of these key thinkers reveals many important nuances that separate their arguments to some extent. However, at their core each of these three 'giants' conclude similarly that human development is stage-based, dynamic, and responsive to the stimulus provided by the world in which one is acting.

David Hay's influential work on children's spirituality, *The Spirit of the Child* (Hay with Nye 1998), is important to note here, pointing to the need for church schools to facilitate the conditions for students to conceive of the 'other' and the possibility of God. While this may be accepted more willingly in childhood, the tension evident in adolescence heightens the need for schools to reflect on the day-to-day experience of the student in relation to any exploration of faith. Hay emphasises the 'here and now' (i.e. present experience versus historical study) in 'meaning-making'. This is not simply about the cognitive decisions young people make, but for narrative to make sense it must be rooted in tangible and unique experience. For any school wishing to enact a sense of mission in relation to facilitating faith development, there is a need for clear teaching and instruction, perhaps shaped around the notion of values and distinctiveness. However, more significance is attached to experiential experimentation with faith (for example exploring prayer, bible study or worship), provided within conditions which are relationally safe and emotionally secure. Schools also need to emphasise an acceptance that students' 'meaning-making' will take place in many ways at a variety of speeds. This freedom has been central to Emmanuel's approach, allowing students to explore at their own pace, supported by staff who are fellow travellers on the road. In fact, it has been crucial to emphasise the ability of staff to use the language of 'faith journey' to model to students the journeying about which we are talking. It is no use a teacher or leader encouraging a student to go on a journey they themselves are not prepared to travel. When such an ethos exists, we can begin to see children and teenagers confidently forming lasting frameworks of faith, rooted in personal commitment, that will extend into and characterise early adult life and beyond.

Fowler's staged model extends across the full journey of human life, but we are most concerned with his ideas of *mythic-literal faith* (stage 2 – childhood) and *synthetic-conventional faith* (stage 3 – adolescence). Identifying the first of these crudely with primary-school-age children, there is a clear emphasis on the child's ability to create meaning in an increasingly orderly and linear manner. Fowler stresses the importance of personal narrative and story within this stage – 'The great gift to consciousness that emerges in this stage is the ability to narratize one's experience' (Fowler 1981: 136). This is the age where personal story becomes a central element of faith formation, becoming 'the major way of giving unity and value to experience' (Fowler 1981: 149). He sees meaning as carried by, and 'trapped in', stories, which give coherence to experience. This may illuminate why there has been such an impact from the telling and retelling of stories of faith developing, over against the cognitive instruction in faith development that might sometimes embody an act of worship or tutor activity. Collective worship can miss opportunities to be affective as well as cognitive, most commonly when 'one-way' communication is prioritised over against the facilitation of conversations, debate and reflection together. There is a distinction to be drawn here between primary and secondary practice, where perhaps primary colleagues are more commonly found to be using stories as a way into enabling reflection in a non-didactic manner. In the secondary context of this study, the stories could not have developed without the facilitation and celebration of experience, nor could they have flourished in the absence of concrete teaching and instruction in relation to faith, God and the person of Jesus. However, the dynamism of narrative and the personalisation of meaning-making in this context are rooted very clearly in some elements of the stages of faith as espoused by Fowler's seminal thinking some decades earlier.

In the third stage of faith development, which we crudely align to secondary education, narrative is still critical, but the individual increasingly develops the confidence and need to reflect on the patterns and trends within a range of their stories. Teenagers can draw conclusions that lead to more principled and long-lasting reflections on personal identity. Fowler recognises that they need mirrors, both literally in relation to their changing appearance, and metaphorically in terms of the relationships that they form confirming their own developing sense of self.

> People judge a book by its cover but God sees it so much deeper. Through all the ups and downs, I am so thankful for the input of Christian values at school. I am still at the beginning of my journey and know I am still a work in progress.
>
> (Year 11 student, Onestory, 2014: 21)

Fowler (1981) develops this further, suggesting that teenage conceptions of God need to be to a great extent 'self-validating': 'the adolescent's religious hunger is for a God who knows, accepts, and confirms the self deeply' (Fowler 1981: 153). Fowler sees the primary development of this stage as the formation of socially located 'personal myth' – namely, 'the myth of one's own becoming in identity and faith, incorporating one's past and anticipated future'. The interplay between multiple stories continues to be a significant factor in the development of identity. Thus the model of sharing and celebrating stories provides a strong basis for the facilitation of faith development within the school, again, over and above religious instruction and transfer of knowledge. As he writes elsewhere, 'I am my relationships; I am my roles' (Fowler 1987: 66).

Although it has dominated this discourse for decades, Fowler's linear modelling is of course not above critique and review. There is a growing chorus of voices suggesting that it may be 'a paradigm nearing the end of its useful life' (Heywood 2008: 12). There are a number of broad issues raised by a variety of writers in relation to the overly linear nature of a stage-based model, the lack of engagement with postmodern thinking, and problems raised with the empirical research base and gender bias of the research.[2] The focus of this critique does not find itself explicitly rooted within educational discourse, however, and so a number of reflections on our church school context here will be profitable. Firstly, the movement between Fowler's stages 2 and 3, and its approximate relationship to the transition between primary and secondary schools, may suggest the relative futility of faith development in any school context if it is not connected to the next phase in some way. Perhaps a lack of opportunity to move from primary to secondary church school context (which is, of course, the normal experience for the majority of UK church school students) renders the precious gift given to students in stage 2 somewhat precarious as they move into stage 3. Dioceses, SACREs and multi-academy trusts committed to the notion of faith development for church schools would be advised to consider this potential onward journey for their primary-school leavers. Equally, as Astley rightly emphasises, it can be a mistake to 'rush people through the stages' (Astley 1991: 40). This is not simply because it is unhelpful to do so, but moreover it exacerbates the issues of complicated power relationships between leaders and children which can so frequently cloud genuine personal faith development in children. Furthermore, while an educational obsession with measurable outcomes may lead to a natural attraction to the linear faith development of the kind of model Fowler suggests, we should of course exercise a degree of caution, knowing most people's stories to be more complex, less linear and ultimately all the more interesting for it. This is why a story becomes such a powerful vehicle for exploring what is going on for an individual or a community, and why, in the case of Onestory, the celebration of journeys of faith is a compelling model for reporting such developments in students' lives. Narrative is inherently qualitative and, in this case, ethnological, thus respecting context and experience, neither of which can be easily or meaningfully quantified.

Choosing the destination – belonging and authenticity

Choosing a school is an exciting and daunting step, shaped by a variety of practical realities and emotional responses for students and parents alike. It is not simply a decision about a product, in terms of quality, reliability, recommendation. However much we like to compare schools with an ever-changing set of methodologies and comparison tables, ethos or faith cannot be accurately captured in quantifiable ways. If a school is concerned with faith development as part of its provision, then there are obvious challenges as to how to present this to the outsider looking in. Given that any such developmental journey rests heavily on the authenticity of experience 'as advertised', it is this 'shop window effect' with which we are first concerned, looking to unpick how schools communicate messages about faith, and the extent to which there is an observable congruence between soundbite and reality. Such questions are crucial for the school's prospectus and website in relation to students' potential entry, and equally pressing for the recruitment processes that schools use to attract staff most comfortable with its vision for learning.

Ivy Beckwith's vibrant exploration of faith development in young people, Postmodern Children's Ministry, helpfully contextualises a number of models within a twenty-first-century context, striving to make sense of a postmodern culture and the key issues facing so-called 'millennials' and beyond. There are a number of striking observations, including the core realisation of the rejection of universal meta-narrative. This means that students in our schools do not necessarily come with the same fundamental assumptions about how truth is constructed and negotiated. They give greater priority to the lived-experience of individuals, acknowledging that 'one's beliefs and stories are local' (Beckwith 2004: 23). This clearly gives great challenge to any notion of community-based faith development that is any way aligned with either linear models or religious instruction that focuses on cognitive knowledge transfer. These are children who are comfortable living in the moment, and who frequently 'want to experience something before they learn about it' (Beckwith 2004: 31). Such experiences are never in isolation and therefore the interaction of stories and experiences creates a socially negotiated epistemology[3] within the context of a church school. Therefore the initial presentation of the school should be regularly re-evaluated, considering how the description of the kind of school that we are is impacted by the students' propensity for such meaning-making. (It is, of course, important to stress that this might be in contrast with the thinking of their parents, who, dependent on their age, may exhibit more modernist approaches to this decision.)[4]

> I started to develop in my faith through school ... which really helped me understand things much better, and although one of my parents is still an atheist, the other began to support me a little more in my faith as it began to grow. I would now definitely describe myself as a Christian, but there's no way I could have said that at the start of Year 7!
>
> (Year 9 student, Onestory, V2012: 33)

Beckwith draws upon the thinking of Lawrence Richards in relation to faith development (Richards 1983). While Richards' writing is concerned with a church context, it resonates with a church school context in many ways, including the stress on the need 'to belong'. Belonging cannot simply be in words, or prospectus soundbites, but rather needs to be the lived experience of students on a daily basis, and the extent to which they are involved in the community, forming positive relationships which impact their learning. Second, a sense of 'participation' is highlighted, where activities that characterise faith development need to be focused on students' leadership. This might involve proactively providing opportunities for students to serve, locally or internationally, or be characterised by student-led acts of worship. This is an intentional part of the offering of the school to a local community, because 'children need to experience the stories of faith, not just hear them' (Beckwith 2004: 66).

These two aspects of the church school community are enhanced significantly by the sharing of stories and the language of faith journeys. From the outside, students are empowered to think that their journey is firstly as important as everyone else's, and second, likely to have similarities with the stories that they hear from those that have gone before. The Onestory project is hugely encouraging to those within the school; however, it has an equally tangible impact upon those currently outside the school community, as it illustrates the kind of experience one is likely to have on entering that community. This is not to seek mere repetition of story, but to encourage the notion of personal narrative as meaning-making. This narrative is not the classic 'beginning–middle–end' notion of story-telling, but frequently chaotic, unpredictable, intertwined and without resolution. Nonetheless, this is real. This is how stories go, particularly in the inherently unresolved nature of childhood and teenage years. This approach to narrative has real credibility within a more postmodern approach to faith development, and frequently draws people into the school community in a more compelling and credible manner than the eloquence of the prospectus or open evening speech.

Having established the importance of the initial offer of the school to prospective community members, it is useful to consider what this really means in practical terms for a school setting out its stall. This list is, of course, not exhaustive, but may provide an initial framework for fruitful discussion for school leaders and governors keen to wrestle with this issue.[5]

Ad-missions – all schools have admissions policies, but to what extent are they genuinely reflective of the school's mission as a church school? The word mission itself is important to consider here, and the notion of ad-mission suggesting a 'calling to' the mission of the school. What kind of expectations does your school's ad-mission policy put on those applying for a place, and what notion of faith development is espoused by your paperwork? There are many schools where church participation is a requirement (and in many ways, the beginning of the students' and parents' faith journey perhaps), but how might this form-filling become a dialogue, and a dialogue become a relationship? Also, it is worth considering how the percentage make-up of cohorts may reflect the nature of faith development – schools serving diverse, multi-ethnic, multi-faith contexts may have the opportunity for a richer experience of narrative journey than more deliberately or accidentally homogenous institutions. Either way, it will be difficult to really engage with the questions of what happens to the students when they are part of the school without first engaging with the question of how students enter in relation to their faith development.[6]

> Listening to the stories of others and their experiences with God has really helped and encouraged me in my faith. I think God has a plan for my life but I don't know what it is yet – it's one of those mysteries.
>
> (Year 11 student, Onestory, 2014: 23)

Publicity and soundbites – schools are increasingly sold within a marketplace, with the accompanying need for slogans and straplines. These are frequently compelling and can unite the school around a common purpose – for example, mottos such as 'Together to learn, to grow, to serve', which is used in a wide variety of contexts and with great frequency. Although few will make their decision simply on the basis of this alone, it is crucial to evaluate whether the words that you use really exemplify the values you stand for and, most importantly, if you regard faith development as an important aspect of your work, whether your language reflects this across your prospectuses, websites and other publicity material.

Incarnation – there is not time in this chapter to undertake a broad study of incarnational theology, but in this context we are concerned with what we see, 'embodied' and practised, on the ground. This is contextual theology. Theories of God found to be incarnated in the praxis of the faith school community will be tested in robust conversation with reflections on the experiences of those in the school who see their own faith journeys developing richly. Leaders are certainly comfortable with the wording of ethos statements. However, until Onestory was produced, there was little documentary evidence for internal and external stakeholders that faith development was first a characteristic reality in the school, and secondly a celebrated expectation.

Narrative and word of mouth – what do people in your local community say about your school? No doubt much of this will have to do with the league tables and recent trajectory of results. Equally, there will be the well-rehearsed social prejudice of school admissions where parents ultimately worry whether their child will be safe and well in a context potentially different from their own. Despite these prevailing forces, it is crucial to engage with whether community stakeholders value, notice and report anything to do with faith development of the young people in your care. How is this manifest and, again, how is it celebrated publicly?

Staff recruitment – without effective work in this area, any desire from a governing body to set the direction of the school in relation to faith journeys can prove futile and frustrating for all concerned. Recruitment packs should actively reflect the dynamic approach to faith development (for students *and* staff), and interview processes need to facilitate key personal conversations about faith. Typical questions relating to 'how will you uphold the Christian ethos of the school?' may be better replaced with those that explore candidates' personal faith journey and willingness to further their own personal narrative through their work. It will be difficult to expect adults to lead children on a journey of faith if those adults are not prepared to travel that journey themselves. Equally, where there is a lack of congruence between the school presented to colleagues at the threshold of recruitment and the reality of lived experience, there will be an inevitable tension. Such tension is frustrating and demotivating on both sides, and must be evaluated carefully by school leaders to ensure a consistency of expectation and experience.

Journeys of faith – the importance of telling the story

In order to give some context to these reflections about narrative and journeys of faith, it is important to gain a brief insight into the history, location and identity of the school where the project is growing up. Opened in 2002 in response to a combination of the Dearing Report and local demand for church school provision at secondary level,[7] the school is a medium-sized academy on the banks of a river, serving a diverse range of communities with a broadly comprehensive intake. Its admission policy has led to a rich mix of students and families in terms of their faith, socio-economic and academic backgrounds. The school has a deep partnership with a range of local churches and a foundational commitment to engage in issues of ethos, values and vision at all levels. Throughout the school's development, there has been a consistent focus on defining and revisiting the core values upon which every aspect of the school stands, and this has been captured in a variety of media, including a clear ethos statement and a range of documentation including explorations of teaching from a Christian perspective and policies for behaviour and inclusion which are centred on those Christian values. So far so good, and in many ways this will be entirely congruent with many other church schools in their set-up and orientation.

However, in wrestling with the question of whether the ethos was a genuine reality for students, staff and other stakeholders, the problems of measuring impact empirically became self-evident. What would be measured and what kind of methodology could capture the complexity and reflexivity of faith development in students and staff? In order to address this issue, the Onestory project was conceived with a very simple aim – to capture sixteen stories from the faith journeys of students and staff each year in a book, which would be published to parents, students, staff and a range of local partnerships. All the stories are of course anonymous, but are drawn from across Years 7–13 including also four stories from members of staff, whose faith journeys are equally valued within the school. The methodology involved simple interviews with the students and staff, which were then turned into 300- to 400-word summaries, usually focusing on an interesting or unusual aspect of the faith journey. Some of these stories were then subsequently turned into a display within the school, allowing students, staff and visitors the opportunity to read the narratives, and simultaneously celebrating the notion of faith development in a simple public manner. The project was then repeated in the next academic year, creating Volume 2 of Onestory, and this will continue on into Volume 3. The school is also working on a fascinating development of the project, attempting to capture the stories of students who left the school five years ago, in order to explore whether the experience of being part of a church school community has had a discernible impact on their faith development during the movement into early adulthood. The name of the publication also has some important resonances – firstly it is highlighting the importance of each and every story as equally important and valid – giving priority to each, one story at a time. Secondly, it allows a drawing together and synergy of stories, into one story – namely that of the school at large.

The project is, of course, not without limitation and critique in terms of its aims and methodology. One of the most important questions to ask of the initiative relates to the selection and editing process for the narratives. It is impossible to suggest that the sixteen stories published each year can in any way be taken to represent every other student or teacher in the school – that is certainly not the intention. Equally, the production of the book is subject to the same editorial direction as any other piece of media – decisions are made to highlight particular aspects within the broader meta-narrative of the school's journey. Again, this is definitely not without value judgements, and it is subject to internal and external power relationships which impose a given direction to the ultimate output of the project. However, despite these valid points for reflection, the capturing, sharing and celebrating of narrative has served to highlight the growth of Faith amongst the students and staff in a way that a policy, report or self-evaluation form (SEF) could never achieve. It has underlined themes within the school, encouraged individuals and groups to pursue the development of their own faith, and empowered staff and students with a common and accessible language to facilitate future development. Furthermore it has supported a rethinking of more conventional and modernist views of faith development, and enabled a rereading of stage-based models as enacted in the lives of the students and staff involved.

Terry Pratchett (1991: 19) observes, 'People think that stories are shaped by people. In fact, it's the other way around'. Of course, from a Christian point of view, it is important to emphasise the shaping power of the story of Jesus at this point. The narrative of Jesus, as told in the New Testament, is not merely one that we read, observe and to which we react. The Jesus story is inherently one which shapes, challenges and forms us as we interact with it. In some senses this intertwining of stories is at the very heart of the gospel itself. In the compilation of the Onestory books, there is no direct or deliberate connection between the sixteen stories selected; neither do they explicitly interact with each other within the text. However, in highlighting some simple extracts from the stories, one begins to feel an implicit interaction with the wider school context, and some genuine evidence that faith formation is taking place, rooted in narrative twists and turns, the people indeed being shaped by the stories.

A Year 9 student writes:

> For me being a Christian is about knowing God as a reality in my life instead of believing in a concept. I have so many stories of him helping me, calming me down when I'm angry and even taking away physical pain for my mum when she

broke her foot. One day I know that we'll meet God and see what he's really like in person. For now, I love exploring ideas and thinking things through, and I don't think he minds when we're not sure about him because he wants to help us believe.

(Onestory, 2012: 17)

A teacher writes:

[Thirty] seconds in a corridor literally changed my life. In all the busy-ness and bustle, and the demands of my job, learning my craft, there were people around me who were willing to stop and talk, to stop and pray and to help me too, to stop … There is a difference at Emmanuel – I read it in the prospectus and heard it in the talks. But more importantly, I saw it in the people, the colleagues and the community of which I became a part.

(Onestory, 2012: 12–13)

A sixth-former writes:

It's fair to say things went a bit off the rails. I was only 14 and yet getting into things I really shouldn't have. It seemed easier to go along with it all, going out, drinking, smoking, the lot. In Year 11, it stepped up a gear and I guess I probably let a few people down along the way. I just had a moment where a voice in my head said to me 'you're better than this'. I feel disgusted with myself, but from that moment, my whole mindset changed … There have been a couple of teachers who have been amazing role models for me and have always believed in me and pushed me on. Even in the toughest times, God has held me, and my family, together.

(Onestory, 2012: 28)

Another teacher writes:

If I think back to life 5 years ago, I would never have prayed, or said that faith played a part in my existence at all. However, the regularity and accessibility of this at school has really got this going for me, and I'm now reading the bible regularly and really see myself on a faith journey. Funnily enough, I actually went to a church primary and secondary school, but I don't remember ever having anything like what goes on at Emmanuel. It's great to see that the same sense of faith development that's helped me as an adult is definitely making a real impact on so many young people at an earlier stage in their journey.

(Onestory, 2014: 6–7)

As we have seen in the section of this chapter 'Packing our bags', stage-based models provide stimulating food for thought as to the ways in which people develop their thinking and beliefs. However, the prioritisation and interactivity of story, as a way into understanding what is taking place within a school context, shows that faith development is not at all as causally sequential as such models might suggest. Even in reading these short extracts you will have experienced something very important about personal narrative stories as opposed to other forms of writing – they seem more convincing or compelling than the constructed arguments of the rest of a booklet like this, a kind of dominance of the 'first person' over the 'third person'. Furthermore in reading and rereading such stories, they become dynamic not static, provoking the reader to react and engage with their own story – comparing, evaluating and reshaping accordingly.

Furthermore, our current students do not know a world where life is not negotiated at least in part through the twisting, turning, transient 'multi-logue' of Facebook, Twitter, Instagram, etc. In these worlds, meaning is relentlessly significant yet trivial, permanent yet gone in a moment, utterly individualised yet inherently interactive. It cannot be tracked, predicted or controlled, and yet our students are interpreting this world, frequently seeing it as just as important as their 'real-life' interactions with one another. They are natives to this way of creating meaning and of intertwining narrative, where short epithets summarise life-changing feeling and comment streams uplift and encourage as quickly as they cut down and betray. This is a world where the drama of the story is fast-paced, unpredictable but intensely valuable. It is the world in which our current students are taught about values, narrative and play their own part in creating a community that is constantly changing and adapting to itself and its needs. From this point of view, it is not surprising that a stage-based model of faith development may be on rocky ground and the linear predictability of a faith journey may be challenged. Furthermore, these sociological changes driven by social media mean that almost certainly the students with whom we are working have an inherently different way of making meaning than we can personally appreciate as adults. We can examine it from the outside, and even flirt with it ourselves, but we cannot truly dwell as a native to this cultural norm as they do, not knowing a world where it didn't exist. This generational distance makes it all the more important that as adults we re-examine overly structuralist models of faith development which simply do not resonate in the culture in which children and teenagers are growing up.

Leading faith development in schools – five ideas to explore

Having explored the nature of faith itself and the relevance of traditional models of faith development, we have uncovered some significant questions for any church school to pose itself in the quest to take this element of its identity seriously. Furthermore, the importance of narrative as a vehicle for celebrating and encouraging faith development has shown a need to engage more deeply in the meaning-making processes common to students in our care. Ultimately, this appears to be less about knowledge transfer (in the religious or moral instruction sense that may characterise much of our 'Christian content'), and more about facilitating student-centred narrative journeys where to some extent the adults become fellow travellers as opposed to all-knowing tour guides. In this section, we will endeavour to engage with five simple principles that may assist colleagues at all levels of leadership to meet these challenges in an exciting and creative way. These five ideas are by no means exhaustive, and it is of course the intention of any piece of writing to provoke responses in the reader beyond those suggested in the text. However, they will provide a useful starting point for those keen to engage with this vital area of church school identity.

Wrestle with the theology of faith development for your school

If church schools are to engage with the prospect that their students are on some kind of faith journey, then the debating and formulating of a school's position on faith development will be an important undertaking. Elements of the narrative approach explored in this ethnographic study may be directly transferable into any context; however, it is important that schools and governing bodies spend time and energy working together to understand the extent to which they wish to embrace the idea of faith development within their context. This is not a one-off exercise enabling the completion of a policy or prospectus, but needs to be an on-going dialogue responsive to student and staff thinking. For some leaders, this will feel like a simple activity, whereas for others the language used and the sense of personal faith commitment may necessitate the enlistment of partners (beginning with the local church) to assist and contribute. In addition it will be important to evaluate the impact of leadership of faith-related activity within the school, including the models of chaplaincy[8] employed. It may also be important to consider how the majority shareholders in the school (i.e. the students) are empowered to engage in these kinds of questions, and what genuine leadership opportunities might emerge for students to lead each other in this. In any case, the most effective approaches will be those that are most widely shared and co-constructed as opposed to the imposition of policy and procedures.

Evaluate your provision in relation to faith development versus religious instruction – are we communicating moral messages or facilitating students' exploration of faith?

Church schools organise coherent programmes for acts of worship and other tutor-based activities. Many of these centre on particular themes and content, giving structure and purpose, and in some respects reflecting well-produced medium-term planning and schemes of work familiar to all teachers. This creditable model allows students to visit and revisit themes in different ways as they grow through the school. However, like many church contexts, there may be a tendency for such activities to be quite didactic, and frequently facilitated by an 'expert' imparting knowledge to the many. However common this practice may be, it is poor educational practice and arguably holds back spiritual development.[9] It is thus profitable to reflect on whether these activities allow students to explore faith actively as opposed to being communicated to. Although there are, of course, practical challenges to this, the more active students can become, either during these acts of worship, or in reflecting upon them afterwards, the more likely they are to engage genuinely in 'owning' their own journey of faith. This might involve, for example, opportunities for students to share their own stories within acts of worship, respond practically in prayer activities or for staff to permit discussion points and dialogue. There may also be value in reflecting on the frequently shifting emphasis in lesson observation frameworks on teaching versus learning. What kind of outcomes might we see if our programmes are centred on facilitating students' faith development as opposed to the acquisition of knowledge? Although any such outcomes will be difficult to pin down empirically, consideration of the extent to which we encourage and empower students to explore for themselves, enabling the voice of the child, will be a rich area of reflection.

See the faith journey as an expected element of the wider educational growth of all

All schools rightly spend a lot of time analysing their students' progress across a range of academic skills, both in lessons, between assessment points, and of course in their final outcomes in relation to targets. Academic progress is not something that is merely hoped for, it is an expectation for all. Although challenging to find quantitative measurements of faith development, it is reasonable to expect that students who are operating within a vibrant and empowering church school community should be impacted by this in some way. Of course, the outworking of this may be seen immediately, or may not be evidenced until much later in life. However, for any school taking its church school identity seriously, this aspect of students' development should be an expected, rather than merely hoped for, element. This involves evaluating the impact of certain activities, and will encompass regular student voice activities to engage with growing narratives and journeys. Once a coherent theology is arrived at together, and the conditions for faith development are in place, then schools should be confident to expect the quality of their provision to have an impact.

Use narrative as a way of capturing, celebrating and encouraging

Narrative is of course not the only way of capturing what is going on in the development of your students, but on account of its simplicity and authenticity it does have huge advantages for schools looking to understand the way their students are developing. The celebration of narrative also has a silent pay-off for other students and staff, implying to each member of the school community that their own narrative could be valued in just the same way, and therefore there is a valid expectation that a narrative journey will be taking place. In the Onestory project, the booklets were printed and distributed widely, but were also part of a display in school and available on the school website, which of course helped to shape the impact further. In addition, there is a strong case for such a project being used as effective evidence for any external visits, including both Ofsted and SIAMS inspections, where the personal narratives act as unique case studies of student and staff growth in this area.

Model the approach by highlighting staff journeys of faith

Although the Onestory publications are for obvious reasons anonymous, it is fairly easy to tell which stories come from staff and which come from students. The staff narratives generally focus on the time during which colleagues have been working at the school, but also give some wider context to their journey beforehand. This bold and honest expression of faith development of staff certainly helps model what is hoped for in the lives of students, but equally importantly gives focus to the reality of staff developing in this way, actively co-learning and growing. The highlighting of staff journeys of faith gives further weight to the argument to revisit Fowler and stage-based models as these journeys rarely fit in with a linear sense of faith development. Anecdotally, students, parents and other stakeholders in the school also value reading this kind of story, because it speaks of a community where the school's ethos and values are having an equally transformative impact on staff. The interviewing and editing of staff narrative requires perhaps a greater depth of humility and trust, but in understanding the publication's purpose, colleagues have been happy to be involved.

Telling your own story – leaders' personal journeys of faith

There is a well-known leadership adage which tells aspirant leaders never to ask others to do something that they wouldn't be prepared to do themselves. It is a message about role-modelling and incarnational leadership which is designed to get people on side and motivate them about their own part of an organisational culture. This final section explores the importance of school leaders and governors being prepared to engage in this kind of faith journey themselves, modelling the exploration of faith and interaction of story from the top. The premise for this potentially provocative reflection is simple – is it realistic to consider that a dynamic approach to faith development can become a reality in a church school without leadership that models this approach?

As adults, we may have a keener desire than children to categorise people into static faith stage boxes – we may have a tendency to think for example that it is helpful to designate people as Christians or not, or to use slightly confusing descriptions like 'she's not a Christian herself, but she's very sympathetic I think', or 'he doesn't believe in God himself, but can really appreciate the values like love, charity and forgiveness'. We may stray into the mythical notion that 'professional Christians' such as clergy who work with us in schools are fixed in their faith, lacking questions and with watertight and immovable answers to everything, like a faithful product salesman. All of these positions can be confusing and quite unnerving for colleagues at all levels. However church school leaders categorise themselves, far more important is a willingness to engage in faith journey as a metaphor for growth and development. This needs real thinking about, not least because without a sensible and realistic reshaping of linear stage-based models of faith development, such a metaphor can feel threatening and one-directional. It is not about imposing a simplistic model of evangelism intent on conversion of non-believers, but rather establishing safe and encouraging conditions in which leaders can explore faith and ask questions, using personal narrative as an accessible way in to such conversations.

There is a need to develop better training and development for leaders of church schools to help with the articulation of faith development; equally the establishment of clearer and safer relationships between churches and schools (particularly their leaders) may provide the relational bedrock for stories to be exchanged and mature conversations about faith to grow up. For those recruiting leaders in church schools, a reconsideration of the kinds of questions asked at interview may highlight the dynamism of candidates' engagement in a journey of faith as against static categorisation and church attendance statistics. Governing bodies may need to engage in deep thinking and wrestling over a school's identity, but beginning from personal faith development as against succinct policy statements. Whatever the practical considerations, it is fairly clear that unless leaders are prepared to engage themselves in such thinking, debate, conversation and exchange of personal narrative, it will be very difficult to expect other staff or students to engage in a similar way.

Why not consider beginning by writing your own story, or if it is easier, tell your story to someone else who could pick out the main points and write with you? It could be a great activity to do with a group of senior leaders or governors, and perhaps one to return to at some designated interval – annually for example. Explore how talking about faith may become easier through telling your own stories as opposed to simply transferring knowledge of other people's stories. There are also many practical ideas that could come from this for acts of worship, tutor programmes and other lessons at every age and stage.

The Onestory books might provide a helpful model which schools could adopt or try out fairly easily. They certainly offer a useful way for schools to explore what is actually going on amongst the members of their community, and go some way to providing some evidence of faith development within the school context. The accessible format of a booklet is achievable in-house, or using a design company to assist with the production. Equally a web-based presentation could be just as effective, and would have the further benefit of being able to interact with the stories through commenting online, for example. While the project has been developed in a secondary context, there are no obvious barriers to its transfer into primary or university situations. It would indeed be fascinating to explore the nuances of the thinking for different age groups.

However one chooses to engage practically with the notion of faith journey and personal narrative, it is clear that it can provide a rich and dynamic language with which to explore one's own faith and to talk with others about their faith development. In the context of a church school, the idea of talking about journey and story is accessible and attractive, and for students living in a social-media-driven age, one cannot avoid the importance of the interaction between narratives. Such prevalent cultural forces necessitate a rethinking critique of more established stage-based models of faith development, and provide a fertile ground for exploring faith with young people, and the adults with whom we serve.

Author Neil Gaiman writes the following in his collection of short stories entitled *Fragile Things: Short Fictions and Wonders* (2006: 1):

> Stories, like people and butterflies and songbirds' eggs and human hearts and dreams, are also fragile things, made up of nothing stronger or more lasting than twenty-six letters and a handful of punctuation marks. Or they are words on the air, composed of sounds and ideas – abstract, invisible, gone once they've been spoken – and what could be more frail than that? But some stories, small, simple ones about setting out on adventures or people doing wonders, tales of miracles and monsters, have outlasted all the people who told them, and some of them have outlasted the lands in which they were created.

The heart of the Jesus story, which most closely touches our own, both personally and corporately, is the paschal event of his death and resurrection, as one cosmos-changing paradigm shift. Such is the power of self-sacrifice for the good of others, which stands as a challenge to all our other stories, but also beckons us, winsomely, into the story – so that we might take the risk of also choosing for it to become ours. It is thus this interaction of narrative, between each other, and ultimately our individual interaction with the bigger Jesus story that energises the development of faith. Church schools provide dynamic and fertile ground for this to take place for students and staff alike.

In conclusion, we offer a final quotation, taken from the Revd Phil Marsh's foreword to Volume 2 of Onestory:

God works. Which is why there are more stories to tell.

... as we read the stories of others, we may ourselves become aware of the ways in which God has been and is undoubtedly at work within our own lives. As we share the journey of faith of others, perhaps we see something of our own reflected in theirs.

Our stories both told and untold, of God at work in human lives, are all part of One Story. Our prayer is that these stories would delight and encourage you, and that in sharing them, they may serve to shed light afresh on each of our own journeys.

(Onestory, Volume 2: 3)

Notes

1   This is an important distinction, which, in philosophical terms, is between a rationalist and empiricist approach. Much theological writing was at one stage heavily rationalist, and this was, indeed, in line with a modernist approach. Postmodernity is more potentially holistic, valuing experience as much as reason, and Fowler was writing when postmodernity was just starting to gain credibility in popular thought.
2   The growing chorus of dissenting voices is drawn from a variety of disciplines, and is most succinctly drawn together by Professor David Heywood in his highly critical paper, 'Faith development theory: A case for paradigm Change' (Heywood 2008). This paper mixes together the nuanced thinking of Astley (1991) and Streib (2001, 2004), and is further built upon by psychologist Dr Adrian Coyle in his 2011 paper, 'Critical responses to faith development theory: A useful agenda for change?'
3   Epistemology is one of the core areas of philosophy, and is concerned with the nature, sources and limits of knowledge. In this context, the notion of its social negotiation concerns the way that knowledge, understanding and meaning-making can be seen to be constructed socially between people rather than by individuals in isolation.
4   A range of information is provided for parents in relation to the school's ethos, mission and purpose through the school's website, Parent Handbooks, etc., and indeed a Parent Partnership group meets regularly to discuss school matters. In the course of this, there are opportunities to discuss the nuances of faith development and the rationale behind approaches to prayer, worship, chaplaincy work and ONESTORY.
5   Colleagues working in the primary and secondary sectors will have a variety of practical differences in the outworking of these practicalities, but most of the principles are applicable in both areas.
6   It is important to admit a growing need for coherence of expectation between church schools in this way – to illustrate crudely from business, in the UK there are 18 IKEAs, 43 John Lewises, 338 Waitroses, 808 Starbuckses, 1200 Sainsbury's stores, 4900 Co-op food stores, all of which give a fairly reliable and uniform approach to each business' values and entry points. What questions of coherence are present for the 4700 church schools in the UK and how might these be best articulated in relation to faith development and narrative?
7   For a deep and insightful reflection on the founding and initial growth of the school, see Howard Worsley's informative and perceptive reflections in Helen Johnson's *Reflecting on Faith Schools* (2006).
8   The chaplaincy team is led by a core strategic group made up of around eight staff (including the local vicar and senior staff). This group meets weekly and oversees the work of a wider team of around 25 staff made up from across the staff team, and partnering with other local and city church groups to undertake a wide range of enrichment activities, acts of worship and tutor programme resources.

9   See for instance Ian Terry's recent publication Living the Lord's Prayer (2014) for a compelling example of an alternative practice which leads to a richer and deeper experience for students involved as they explore the prayer dialogically.

References

Astley, J. (1991) *How Faith Grows*. London: Church House Publishing.

Beckwith, I. (2004) *Postmodern Children's Ministry*. Grand Rapids, MI: Zondervan.

Coyle, A. (2011) Critical responses to faith development theory: A useful agenda for change?, *Archive for the Psychology of Religion*, 33(3), 281–98.

Erikson, E. (1959) *Identity and the Life Cycle*. New York: International Universities Press.

Fowler, J. (1981) *Stages of Faith*. San Francisco: Harper and Row.

Fowler, J. (1987) *Faith Development and Pastoral Care*. Philadelphia: Fortress Press.

Gaiman, N. (2006) *Fragile Things: Short Fictions and Wonders*. New York: William Morrow.

Hay, D with Nye, R. (1998) *The Spirit of the Child*. London: Jessica Kingsley.

Heywood, D. (2008) Faith development theory: A case for paradigm change. *Journal of Beliefs and Values*, 29(3), 263–72.

Johnson, H. (ed.) (2006) *Reflecting on Faith Schools*. London: Routledge.

Kohlberg, L. (1958) *The Development of Modes of Thinking and Choices in Years 10 to 16*. PhD dissertation, University of Chicago.

Onestory. (2012) *Journeys of Faith at The Nottingham Emmanuel School*. Nottingham: The Nottingham Emmanuel School, Volume 2. Available from www.emmanuel. nottingham.sch.uk/files/uploads/2015/06/One-Story-Volume-1.pdf (accessed 10 april 2017).

Onestory. (2014) *Journeys of Faith at The Nottingham Emmanuel School*. Nottingham: The Nottingham Emmanuel School, Volume 1. Available from www.emmanuel. nottingham.sch.uk/files/uploads/2015/06/One-Story-Volume-2.pdf (accessed 10 april 2017).

Piaget, J. (1932) *The Moral Judgment of the Child*. Glencoe, IL: The Free Press.

Pratchett, T. (1991) *Witches Abroad*. London: Corgi.

Richards, L. (1983) *Theology of Children's Ministry*. Grand Rapids, MI: Zondervan.

Streib, H. (2001) Faith development theory revisited: The religious styles perspective. *International Journal for the Psychology of Religion*, 11(3), 143–58.

Streib, H. (2004) Extending our vision of developmental growth and engaging in empirical scrutiny: Proposals for the future of faith development theory. *Religious Education*, 99, 427–34.

Terry, I. (2014) *Living the Lord's Prayer* (eD23). Cambridge: Grove Books.

Chapter 14
A personal learning journey

Vicky Palmer

Chapter outline

This chapter will:

- introduce a reflective and personal account of a reflective journey on a professional doctorate
- explore the contribution of 'journaling' to reflective practice
- introduce critical moments.

We have sinned and been sinned against, we have acted as law-breakers. As police, as prosecutors, as defenders ... we strive to control ourselves or others from still other people's attempts to control us. We are all continuously torn between lust and loyalties, confronted with dilemmas; often ending up with regrets for our failures ... The problem is access to ourselves. Access and respect for what we find.

(Christie 1997: 14)[1]

Reflection, in all its various guises, is not easy. Some students and health and social care practitioners take to it more quickly with practice, and others have to work exceptionally hard to understand it, recognise its worth and then incorporate it into their daily practices. I fell into the latter category, having struggled with the basic concepts as a social work student in the 1980s and then finding little to no time for it in my years of practice in the caring professions. It was not until embarking on the professional doctorate course as an academic that I found the space to devote time to its comprehension and practical application. It was certainly worth the wait. Without self-reflection, it is difficult to improve upon what we think we know and how we may do things better. A lack of critical reflection means that moving forward with our personal and professional goals becomes inherently more problematic. Had I not employed a deep level of reflection through the use of a detailed reflective journal during my course, I would never have reached the stage of completion.

This chapter documents my reflective journey through the various stages of the professional doctorate course and may assist the reader to see the similarities of their own progression through either undergraduate or postgraduate studies and beyond, into the world of practice in the caring professions.

Professional doctorate placing

The professional doctorate sits at the top end of academic qualifications and is the equivalent of a PhD in terms of length, complexity and the award conferred. It is generally viewed to be a course that sits on a continuum, with professional researcher at one extremity and researching professional at the other (Bourner et al. 2001; Wellington and Sikes 2006), acting as a bridge between academia and professional practice and acknowledging the multifarious ranges of student experiences (Flint and Barnard 2009). One becomes a doctor of practice rather than a doctor of philosophy. It is suggested that 'practice-based research [is] an area situated between academia-led theoretical pursuits ... and research informed practice, and consisting of a multitude of models of research explicitly conducted in, with, and/or for practice' (Furlong and Oancea 2005: 9).

For me, the professional doctorate represented an extension and consolidation of the complex interplay between teaching proficiency in the field of youth justice and practice acumen required to work with children and young people in the youth justice system who have mental health issues. It was the orientation towards and emphasis upon praxis,[2] in terms of changing working practices, of this form of higher-level learning award that held the edge over the more traditional PhD with its focus on academic praxis. In essence, I needed to acquire the skills required to become an effective researcher, one who could use the results from research to improve upon current practice in Youth Offending Teams and related disciplines.

A good starting point for learning the art of reflection is to understand and acknowledge our personal goals for pursuing our various courses and subsequent areas of professional practice. If these goals are not interrogated, we can potentially leave ourselves open to the pitfall of studying or working in a flawed or biased manner. That is, for example, selecting those theories or methods of working that suit our particular mind-set and discounting others which may in fact be more appropriate (Maxwell 1996). For the practitioner is neither all-knowing nor impartial and there will remain differing interpretations for practitioners concerning mentally disordered offenders and how to address their specific problems in the youth justice system. This is clearly related to the notion of reflexivity; that is the manner that the practitioner's individual identity has impacted upon how and what we learn (Rogowski 2002). As Smith (2009: 25) appreciates,

> it is rarely possible – or perhaps even desirable – to attempt to place oneself outside the subject matter ... it may be more appropriate for the researcher to make explicit her own perspective and beliefs rather than attempt to bracket them out of the investigative process.

It would therefore seem pertinent for me to interrogate my personal goals and drivers.

Identity: Critical moments of biography

We are informed by Wellington and colleagues (2005: 19) that 'human beings are storying beings' and that the lens through which we view our world is grounded in our lived experiences. Consequently, our interpretation of all that we see and feel is filtered through these prior, influential perceptions (Giddens 1991; Moon 2006). It is useful then for the reader to be permitted entry to some autobiographical influences to the product of my professional doctorate thesis, *Mental Disorder, Learning Disability and Autism: A Research-Led Design of a Mental Health Module*. But as Bourdieu (2004: 109) informs us, 'one's social past is particularly burdensome when it comes to doing social science – whatever the past and that identity may be'. He cautions us to avoid over-narcissistic reflexivity if it leads to no practical effect. If I was to meet Bourdieu's criterion, I was tethered to what D'Cruz et al. (2006: 75) have defined as 'first variation reflexivity' – looking at my individual response to my situation in terms of self-development and the choices I have made concerning the trajectory of my life within its own unique biography.

I grew up in a north Nottinghamshire mining village which had an extraordinarily striking landscape, set in the floor of a verdant woodland valley, on a tributary of a small river within the ancient boundary of Sherwood Forest. In my childhood, it possessed secret springs feeding an Art Deco lido, preternatural woodland and stickleback streams – an eternal playground. In this place, a teenaged mainframe knitter met a young draughtsman, whose lives became inextricably linked by virtue of a shotgun wedding. The knitter would progress to designer and then teacher, the draughtsman would resort to blissful dipsomania, and the 'shotgun' product was passed between the two. I would live between pit village and street-life, one foot in the working class, the other in its more interesting underbelly. When not engaged in homework, I spent my days amongst a rich array of societal misfits, bound together by their contempt for state-sanctioned slavery in the form of paid work and a penchant for nicknames from which nobody was exempt. My father and his posse were my lifeline and training ground until running for the hills of Sheffield to attend my only university 'clearing' option, a BA in Business Studies at its then 'polytechnic'.

My identity is rooted in these two people and places, ingrained 'across different ... intersecting and antagonistic discourses, practices and positions' (DuGay et al. 2000: 17). The knitter, my mother, was an apostate concerning politics or religion, but was driven by an elect puritan work ethic, rigidly underpinned by frugality. The dipsomaniac, my father, by contrast was pagan, contemptuous of 'the law' and so unconcerned by any requirement to work that he gave it up, aged 35. Unlike Foucault (1980), my father believed in his knowledge of the power and control of nature, the enthusiasm and contentment that should be central to the human condition and lived only off the land, supplemented by state benefits and an abounding supply of alcohol. He challenged conventional capitalist society and teased my own place within it. My mother's proverbial principle was, 'see no evil, hear no evil, speak no evil'[3] and my father's, 'kila-mon-jiro'.[4] Although both are now 'missing', their presence remains in the haunting of my identity (Bhabha 2000). As Benwell and Stokoe (2006: 3) enlighten us, 'although people may present themselves differently in different contexts, underneath that presentation lurks a private, pre-discursive and stable identity'.

Mizaru, Kikazaru, Iwazaru and 'Kilamonjiro'

When a workaholic mother is preoccupied with a Western societal interpretation of the three wise monkeys' apophthegm and an intemperate father is distracted by intoxication and petty larceny, any meaningful notions of child development or protection are lost. Thus, the seeds were sown for a yearning to 'know' the causality of the marginal, eccentric and occasionally nefarious nature of the human condition, driven by the curiosity and naivety of youth, yet confined by the boundaries of a traditional, moral, grammar school education and a BA in Business Studies which served no useful purpose whatsoever.

Following graduation, my father's own vocation assisted me to secure full-time employment as a 'project manager' at a hostel for homeless ex-offenders. This was not work, this was simply time spent within my father's coterie, albeit in a different location, and I was in a position where the residents' discourse made complete sense to me (Hall 1997). This post formed the foundation of my MA application to university to study and train as a social worker and probation officer.

Studying the discipline of mental health at MA level was revelatory. It involved learning about concepts and constructs of human nature that were as intriguing as they were perplexing. Students were taught various contemplations of mental health from the 1800s, such as French psychiatrist Pinel's (1806) depiction of psychopathic characteristics. This was followed by English psychiatrist Prichard's (1835: 135) interpretation of 'moral insanity', portrayed as,

> a madness consisting of a morbid perversion of the natural feelings, affections, inclinations, temper, habits, moral dispositions and natural impulses without any remarkable disorder or defect of the intellect or knowing or reasoning facilities, and particularly without any insane illusion or hallucination.

Our framework of knowledge was consolidated through required, compulsory reading of autobiographies such as Sylvia Plath's haunting (1963) narrative, *The Bell Jar*, and Primo Levi's (1960) translated Holocaust memoirs, *If This is a Man*. Aspects of the module felt unsavoury and voyeuristic, such as contemplating the psyche and motives of serial killer and necrophiliac, Dennis Nilson. Yet the teaching was striking, having been delivered by a passionate and charismatic lecturer who assisted students to shine a light upon 'madness' by 'interrogating the being of madness itself, its secret content, its silent, self-enclosed truth' (Foucault 1972: 1).

Following graduation in 1989 until 2005, I worked alongside adult and young offenders as a probation officer. This was my calling, as it was my colleagues'. It was with heavy hearts that we witnessed, day by day, the probation profession being challenged at the highest level. The introduction of tedious, unintelligent paperwork infiltrated our working day, such as the introduction of the original *OASys* offender assessment proforma (HM Prison Service 2003). Bewildered and sceptical clients were ushered out of the office so that we could write about their risk, escalate its deadliness and note down their inappropriate language. All of this was to meet ill-thought-out deadlines and political mediation that satisfied the auditors. It was as if I subconsciously evaluated these new approaches to 'enhancing' knowledge concerning offenders, recognised the text of the new procedures as hollow and meaningless and took action (Flint 2008). I watched my colleagues leave one by one, and then in 1998, I myself jumped ship to continue working as a probation officer, but within youth justice.

Idealising a new landscape and then homogenising its features

The youth justice profession bristled with optimism following its radical overhaul by the passing of the Crime and Disorder Act 1998, the flagship legislation of the New Labour government. Experiencing first-hand the amalgamation of five previously disparate agencies,[5] I was caught up with the vitality, excitement and 'arrays of activity' (Schatzki 2001: 10) of this new eclectic mix. There was a family atmosphere and we all adored miscreant children who possessed the ability to make us laugh, recoil, and become frustrated or angry in equal measures. We cultivated a cultural, dry and dark sense of humour. But once the gloss of novelty had tarnished, what I witnessed gradually reduced to something akin to 'an image in a funhouse mirror, the broad contours were similar, but the content and form were misshapen and contorted beyond all recognition' (Shaw 2006: 289). Professionalism became usurped by expediency and form-filling, practitioners were expected to pull 'solutions out of a can' (Hester 2010: 86) and the cold winds of corporate capitalism tightened their icy grip with the introduction of the *Asset* core profile and its multitude of supplementary assessment documents (Youth Justice Board 2003). Professional experience and expertise came under attack and the youth justice social worker's occupational identity was shaken to the core (Souhami 2003). The profession had become subject to zombification (Pitts 2001).

Having entered the profession of youth justice with a passion for working with difference, upholding children's rights and steadying their passage through life's injustices, I left as a result of the imposition of a particular form of the many faces of managerialism; one that was related to New Public Managerialism (Newman 2000;

Kirkpatrick et al. 2005). The centralisation of the service ensured that managers were co-opted to take measures of instrumental rationality within service delivery. The social work value base became increasingly eroded to make way for a heuristical[6] approach, one which placed more value on cost effectiveness (Fisher 1998). Yet as Fisher and Lovell (2009) note, as financial performance improves, social performance worsens. My own stake within the Youth Offending Service became more untenable as managerialism and IT-based case work expanded. With increasingly more time spent at my computer and less time spent working alongside young offenders, I made the decision to leave my original profession of choice. I commenced working as a senior lecturer in youth justice in 2005.

Professional doctorate embarkation

Reinvigorating my passion – my identity – for working with young offenders through teaching others how to 'do it', I noted from the sidelines that the youth justice profession was moving ever further away from its original value base. The creeping poison ivy of managerialism and its outward manifestations of technological enframing (Heidegger 1962) had become overgrown and nobody listened to its more erudite detractors (vide Pitts 2003; Armstrong 2004; Muncie 2004; Smith 2005; Hester 2008). Wishing to explore the extent of the veracity of their claims, a change of position was required, a laterality: a deviation of identity. As Egan (2001: 101) says, 'identity is a contested space; at different times our many affiliations, attributes and experiences – labels – jockey for prominence'. I felt that if there were any means by which I could make a difference at a systems level, I would need to consolidate, structure and articulate my experience and personal ideas by embarking on the professional doctorate course (Lester 2004). This seemed potentially the only way in which I could question contemporary assumptions about the governing variables of youth justice in order to create more informed new insights by changing the 'field of constancy' (Argyris and Schön 1974: 19). What I had not anticipated was the challenge of liberating myself from the grids of my 'own symbolic or social order in order to reconstruct the underlying formations of other such configurations' (Kögler et al. 1992: 4).

As with any course of study in higher education, nothing can prepare you for the professional doctorate experience. Wellington et al. (2005) counsel that it is not something to take up on a whim and that passion is required to undertake it. Mathieson and Binder (2009) sagely advise that it is more about grim determination than academic excellence, a thought embodied by Marshall and Green (2004: 8): 'there is a certain desperation in the successful PhD student, a blinkered obsession with it'. Nothing can prime you either for the reactions of others, epitomised by an email response from a close friend:

> what confuses me is why you are doing a doctorate plus all of the other stuff! … trying to hold down a full-time job, bring up kids including a toddler and then try and pass more exams! Crikey, what are you trying to prove and to whom?
> (Ballantyne, cited in Flint et al. 2009: 8)

At that stage, I simply did not know the answer.

Document one: Learning a new language

The professional doctorate requires students to submit a total of six separate theses or 'documents', all of differing lengths and each testing discrete skills of research and academic writing. On a bleak November day, I packed my new notepad, jumped in my car and arrived for the first two doctoral taught days relating to document one (Palmer 2009a). Looking around the room I saw a mish-mash of people. Who were they and what were their backgrounds? Were they Stephen Fry-clever? What were they doing there? What was I doing there? Would they make me do role-play?

> they didn't. Oh no. They just got right down to business and bamboozled me with a plethora of particularly strange words. I secretly thought they had made some of them up for effect. 'Hermeneutically' – a neutered female cat? 'Phenomenology' – Ufology? 'Ontology' – the performance of autopsies? 'Semiotics' – half-wits? 'Epistemology' – readings given by priests? 'Ethnography' – racism? I was shocked. Very shocked.
>
> (Journal entry, 14.11.08)

The challenge of learning this new language seemed immense, retaining comprehension of the words appeared impossible, and the development of my own 'word bank' seemed the only solution. Upon reflection, my own naivety appeared to expose the sovereign powers of language as a means of exclusion. It was clear that in order to move from a state of exception to one of inclusion, I needed to be inculcated into a grander form of narrative 'practice', a new 'site where understanding is structured and intelligibility ... articulated' (Schatzki 1996: 12). I needed to learn new words and, more importantly, what they meant.

Commencing the process of learning involved reading some 21 handouts provided to get our cohort started and, 'I had never been so bored in all my born days. Topics chewed to oblivion, bloody great lists of authors and dates and mind-boggling long words – how do they get away with it?' (Journal entry, 15.12.08). Drafting the original research proposal, as with the drafting of undergraduate dissertation titles, necessitated an apprenticeship of some magnitude, requiring the assistance of a supervisor's skills, one who possessed,

> the wisdom of Solomon; a positively Delphic prescience in their pronouncements of what will matter; the communicative skills of Martin Luther King; the analytical clarity of Ada Lovelace and a breadth and depth of knowledge that could only come from omniscience.
>
> (Marshall and Green 2004: 27)

It was these qualities that enabled one of my supervisors to stifle his laughter, nod and take notes, when presented with my initial research title, 'How Have Youth Justice Qualifications Enhanced the Lives of Practitioners and to What Extent Have They Improved Outcomes for Young Offenders?' This first supervisory session was thought-provoking, but from the detailed notes and reflections taken during this session, I was later able to crystallise the proposal to the more conceptualised, 'A Critical Examination of the Professionalisation of the Youth Justice Workforce'. I may have moved from *erleben*[7] to *erfahren*;[8] from the technological and simplistic question to that which lies beyond calculation (Vernon 2008).

The first critical moment arose following submission of the first draft for this document. A critical moment may be classified as an aspect of learning that is required for a novel and specific meaning to occur in the student's awareness (Wood 2006). The 'moment' came in the form of supervisory feedback which stated, 'implicitly you have positioned yourself as an emerging theorist who is indeed capable of superior insights compared to those of agents in practice'. This hit me hard. It appeared to reflect back an arrogance to my nature. It made me question my identity, morals, character and the heart of who I am and I did not like what I saw. I had fallen into the trap of Kögler et al.'s (1992: 3) 'theory–agency relationship', according myself a privileged position 'over and above the situated agent'. My writing was living proof of it. I needed to begin to neutralise my stance and take the lead from the practitioner voice, rather than speak on their behalf.

To summarise my learning from document one (Palmer 2009a), it is clear that it formed the beginnings of a reconfiguration of my identity. I had begun the process of change from the pre-doctoral 'self as knowing' to one where ideas were beginning to 'disperse and reconfigure' (Forbes 2008: 450).

Document two: Epistemology and identity

> I am Vicky. I am a mother, a partner, a friend, a lecturer, a doctoral student, a day-dreamer and hard-worker. I am a passionate allotment gardener. I am a registered social worker and remain employable as a probation officer and YOS worker.
>
> (Journal entry, 12.05.09)

Though this was a crude attempt to consider my identity, it still demonstrates the fragmentation that lies within who we actually are at any time and the contradictory voices that jostle for position within our being (Johns 2004; Fisher and Lovell 2009). In document two (Palmer 2009b), we were required to locate ourselves within current debates concerning professional research, utilising our own values and assumptions while assessing our own development regarding critical reading (Flint and Barnard 2009). Writing a critical literature review could be deemed relatively straightforward, but positioning oneself within it was the real test of intellect. Without the benefit of contextualised prior understanding, I believe that such a task may only initially be part-met. Gibbs and Flint (2012: 3) provide some clarity here:

> within our transcendental and temporarily structured world, past epochs ever play out and press in on us in moving towards the future; our understanding of identity will be evidentially an interpretation of the accumulated experience, and choices then in the future.

My past, structured professional life may enable me to partly locate my beliefs and professional identity within the literature, but my deeper, epistemological, existential, philosophical and ontological beliefs may only begin to emerge during and throughout the doctoral programme. It is only the accumulated experience of reading, thinking and writing that has enabled me to begin to grasp and articulate this reflexive awareness. As Ryle (1968: 3) usefully articulates, 'there can be no question of my being able to locate and correct mistakes in my multiplication sum before being able to multiply'. For myself, I didn't manage to fully achieve any location of self within current debates until document five (Palmer 2014). This is because the doctorate, as with many undergraduate courses, challenged my entire belief system.

In document two (Palmer 2009b), focusing and refining my learning felt impossible. My supervisor's suggested amendments to my initial draft seemed unachievable at the time, and were placed to one side never to be worked upon. Concerning the fundamentals of welfare and justice, he said,

> not sure about the possible conflation here of discourses of welfare and social justice – there is too much to do to nuance the differences. Discourses of justice have a long and complex philosophical heritage. Discourses of 'welfare' have also their own distinct history. Perhaps need to problematize the relationship of policy initiatives designed to ensure the welfare of particular groups of people and its complex inter-relationship with conceptions (plural) of social justice.
>
> (Feedback, 13.11.09)

Without ever revisiting this piece of advice owing to its perceived complexity, I found that in the rereading of it for document six, I inexplicably achieved its aim. Either the advice remained in my subconscious psyche, or I felt my way naturally via the reflexive doctoral process. Although, at this stage, I was aspiring to meet the competencies required by the Researcher Development Framework (RDF) (Vitae 2010), I had still not acquired the knowledge, confidence, intellectual abilities or insight that is crucial for the higher levels of development. Through the critical literature review, I had developed the RDF component requirement of argument construction, but had yet to develop techniques of intellectual risk in the form of deconstructing the nuances of pre-given social constructs such as the notions of welfare and justice.

Documents three and four: an apprenticeship in the rigours and processes of research

Just as I thought I was beginning to grasp and play with the rudiments of doctoral discourse, the teaching moved up a gear and we were required to 'understand the nature of positivist, realist and qualitative epistemologies (including non-empirical varieties)' (Flint and Barnard 2009: 27). It is difficult to articulate the terror that this new layer of complexity generated in me. It involved learning more new words alongside their meaning and application. It implied reading the philosophers from source and I attempted Heidegger for the second time around. Unfortunately, I did not make a note of the text that had been perplexing me, but my journal entry of 22.10.09 revealed the following:

> I had to read the passage over and over again to in any way get what he was banging on about. Yet I felt pleased with myself once I'd got it and it did make a lot of sense. He does seem to operate in a vacuum/bubble though – away from the hurly-burly, life's a bitch of everyday life.

It was not until three further years into the doctoral process that I realised that most people struggle with Heidegger's writing; his technical vocabulary being famously complex to comprehend (Buckingham et al. 2011). My observations above seemingly miss the point of Heidegger's work, which was to remove us from the inauthentic existence of the 'hurly-burly' to enable us to reach a deeper understanding of our own existence. He would see this as a means of opening readers to questioning, to language, to thinking and to projected understandings. This was just one further example of a critical moment to my learning, and that was the gradual recognition of the bases of others' perspectives and alternative stances (Wood 2006). It was from these many instances of confusion and misunderstanding that my reflexive awareness developed. As D'Cruz et al. (2006: 78) expound, reflexivity is a continuum of looking 'outward to the social and cultural artefacts and forms of thought which saturate our practices and inward to challenge the processes by which we make sense of the world'.

Making sense of the primary research also held its unexpected challenges, not least because of the emotive content of many of the returned questionnaires for document three (Palmer 2011).

> [S]ome have simply reduced me to tears and I'm dreading reading them again. There have been episodes of practitioners working through the death of their young people whom they had clearly formed close bonds with. Suicides have also featured. One girl went to see her mother with her YOT worker after her mother had set fire to herself in her prison cell. Some are working with young people who have committed offences so horrific, you really have to stand back and praise their skill and dedication.
>
> (Journal entry, 17.04.10)

Though I did not realise it at the time, the critical moment here came with the realisation that I had finally cut the umbilical cord away from my original profession. There were no tears shed during the course of my career and I had worked with scenarios more harrowing than this. I was finally viewing the profession as an outsider. My identity had seemingly shape-shifted and I did not see it coming. Alternatively, it may be the case that where feelings concerning difficult cases needed to be supressed within the purely professional role, undertaking the research process provided space for releasing these emotions within the more secure boundaries of the professional doctorate. Hence both identities had 'merged into one another rather than facing each other as if from separate corners of the ring' (Alcoff 2003: 7). Finally, it has been suggested that the recognition of emotion is pivotal to the reflective process (Boud et al. 1985; Moon 2007).

The learning achieved through gradually finding my way through documents three (Palmer 2011) and four (Palmer 2012) was in acquiring the tools in terms of language with which to frame my research. These tools were not ready to hand and had to be learnt through immersion in the research literature. I still felt that I needed to make the transition between conscious incompetence to conscious competence (Hersey and Blanchard 1977; Guthrie 2007). I seemed to be at the stage described by Pointon (2014: 11) where I was gaining confidence with the language of research, yet at the same time did not feel sufficiently competent 'to enter through those portals where its usage is common parlance'.

Document five: Critical reflection and reflexivity

My continued naivety and confusion concerning theoretical, philosophical, epistemological and ontological positioning (let alone what they meant) continued in earnest right through the crafting of document five (Palmer 2014). I had been reproached for being 'cavalier' in my methodological and epistemological positioning by one supervisor, and in retrospect, this was a kindly understatement since my irreverence was essentially masking my sheer ignorance. A journal entry dated 18.07.12 epitomised my desperation: 'It may be helpful to locate someone in a PhD publication that is coming from a similar perspective to my own. I wish I knew what mine was!' Yet in the same journal entry, directly below this comment, appeared a more enlightened statement, 'progress in youth justice is not linear, it's often ad hoc and circular but I do believe that mental health "knowledge" has been abandoned for many reasons'. In this rudimentary statement, I had unknowingly summed up my position. Acknowledging the circular nature of youth justice practice is a subconscious reflection of an epistemology which rejects the objectivity of social facts, and has similarities with my chosen research framework. Clearly, youth justice practice tangibly exists, and the 'abandonment' of the teaching of mental health 'knowledge' to its practitioners accords with Heideggerian philosophy in terms of phemonena being 'buried over' (1962: 60). From that journal entry to reaching the point of crystallisation took a further period of eighteen months of independent reading and individual and group tuition. Yet even the positional identity-framing articulated for document five (Palmer 2014) may in the future be subject to change, since what holds relevance and application now may be subject to fluctuations over time, depending upon what we are attempting to produce an account of (Benwell and Stokoe 2006).

For the final thesis, I was dreading asking previous research participants for assistance for a third time. I felt sure that few, if any, would respond to my electronic questionnaire and felt guilty asking them to undertake more work on my behalf. Prior to sending the final surveys, in anticipation of a potential poor response and in trepidation of the third marathon of data analysis, my journal entry read:

> I need to maintain dogged determination and persistency, but the doctorate pushes everyone to the limit and it really is like persevering uphill through treacle – thick, black molasses. I still only see a pinpoint of light at the end of the tunnel – but it's something.
>
> (Journal entry, 07.01.13)

On a positive note, this certainly accorded with some aspects of Domain B, the personal qualities required by the RDF which include perseverance, responsibility, enthusiasm and self-reflection (Vitae 2010). In one final leap of faith, the surveys were sent and the results articulated in document five (Palmer 2014) – the longest, most gruelling document of them all and the main one that is interrogated during the final oral examination, the *viva voce*.

Completing document five (Palmer 2014) led me to consider not only whether my own orientations and opinions had impacted on the manner in which I engaged in the field of research, but also whether the process was influenced by the perceptions that participants had of me. This seemed particularly pertinent since I had taught every single participant previously, meaning that they could attribute to me some form of expertise or even identify me as an academic source of power (Smith 2008, Palmer 2009). It may have been that my respondents had deferred to the views they were aware that I held. However, this perhaps could be balanced by the findings having greater depth because the respondents shared similar backgrounds in their learning. Whatever the influence of the two-way process, document five (Palmer 2014) finally made real the multitude of limitations inherent within each of my three empirical studies, and all research has its limitations.

Conclusion: Learning through reflection

The professional doctorate journal of reflection is without doubt the gel that holds together all six documents. It provides catharsis and perspective (Moon 2006), empowerment (Cooper 1991), space for cognitive dissonance and possible resolution (Festinger 1957), and space to learn about self. Johns (Palmer 2004) informs us that reflection may be generated by feelings of frustration, anger, sadness, resentment or even guilt. This helps to contextualise a singular journal entry on 22.08.12:

> this doctorate. Too many blind alleys, way too many mistakes. The frustration, the exasperation, the uncertainty, the pure hard slog, the loneliness; pure isolation. The subject, the hand grenades thrown in the way, the burning criticism … the madness it induces.

Clearly, I had yet to make Johns' (2004) connection. But with this cluster of critical emotions and incidents firmly in the past, there had been evolution through reflection-on-action (Schön 1983). In retrospect, blind alleys, mistakes and frustration appeared both inevitable and essential, promoting skills of crisis management and supervisor–supervisee negotiation. The loneliness and isolation need not have been negative factors, but perhaps are an indication of a reduction in reliance upon my supervisors and a gradual assumption of greater independence (Sambrook et al. 2008).

Concerning the transformation of knowledge, it was clear that until the latter stages of the professional doctorate I had fallen prey to an acceptance of the existing literature, and hence to the assumptions and ideological components of the established approach (Maxwell 1996). Rather than using the literature, I had initially allowed it to use me (Becker 1986). Yet for document five (Palmer 2014), the best literature was that which led me to set aside 'legitimate knowledge', as well as my own experience and speculative thinking. As Somerville and Keeling (2004: 42) reflect,

> [W]e all have personal 'maps' of our world. These develop across our lifetime and our early experience plays a vital role in their development … Personal experience determines how much of our environment we actually 'see'.

I was initially constrained by a traditional, moral, grammar-school-for-girls education which involved accepting knowledge as 'given'. As an undergraduate, I viewed knowledge as an absolute and at postgraduate level knowledge became more context-bound and subjective. However, at doctoral level, the idea of knowledge became one of making 'best approximations' depending upon the most compelling interpretations (Lester 2004). Trevillion (2008: 448) informs us that 'social work research in the UK generally focuses on ways of improving service outcome to particular client groups'. My study attempted to promote improvements in outcomes for young offenders affected by mental disorder, learning disability and autism should they transgress the law. Trevillion (2008) also points out that, 'with some honourable exceptions, it has not for some years sought to extend or develop the core knowledge base or central underpinnings of the social work tradition'. Though clearly not a given, it is hoped that the work undertaken for the professional doctorate of social practice might assist in knowledge development in the, often obscure, practice area of mental 'ill' health; ultimately giving expression to the complexity of movements in this area towards social, political and moral justice.

Notes

1   Here, the veteran Norwegian criminologist, Nils Christie, discusses barriers to insight in the context of our ability to understand others. If this is to be achieved, we must understand ourselves. Though taught as a crucial component of social work, probation and juvenile justice practitioner courses in the psychoanalytical environment of the 1950s and 1960s, it has been lost to their contemporary focus on 'effective practice', organisational procedures and work-based competencies (Smith 2006). Fortunately, reflexive awareness has not yet been lost to the professional doctorate process.
2   One of the central conceptions of change is the notion of praxis, that is, 'reflecting upon the world and changing it within the same process' (Banton et al. 1985: x).
3   Originally a Japanese pictorial maxim attributed to the three wise monkeys – Mizaru, Kikazaru and Iwazaru – it originally meant being of good mind, action and speech. In contemporary Western society, however, it has come to have a darker significance, that of dealing with impropriety by turning a blind eye.
4   Kilimanjaro is a dormant volcanic mountain in Tanzania. Its distortional word-play by my father translates to 'let's blow my giro'; kila (kill) mon (my) jiro (giro). Street alcoholics would synchronise the timings of their cash benefit collections. A group of seven 'associates' would never have a day without money for their chosen liquid of torpor.
5   These agencies were the Social Services Department, the Probation Service, Education, Police and Health.
6   'Heuristics ... is used to explain how public officials make resource allocation decisions if they are working in traditional public services, and how they set about introducing market mechanisms into the systems used for delivering public services if they are working within the context of new public management' (Fisher 1998: 10).
7   Vernon (2008) uses this term to embody technological, lived experience; that which denotes a naive comprehension of where we are.
8   As an alternative, Vernon (2008) categorises erfahren as a more primordial experience, one concerning where we want to be.

References

Alcoff, L. (2003) Introduction: Identities – Modern and Postmodern. In Alcoff, L. and Mendieta, E. (eds), *Identities: Race, Class, Gender and Nationalities*. Oxford: Blackwell Publishing.

Argyris, C. and Schön, D. (1974) *Theory in Practice: Increasing Professional Effectiveness.* London: Jossey Bass Ltd.

Armstrong, D. (2004) A risky business? Research, policy, governmentality and youth offending. *Youth Justice*, 4: 100–113.

Ballantyne, F. (2009) What are you trying to prove and to whom? In Flint, K., Barnard, A., Ching, J. and Flint, C. (eds), *Producing Space for New Forms of Social Research: An Exploration of Henri Lefebvre's Thesis.* Nottingham: Nottingham Trent University.

Banton, R., Clifford, P., Frosh, S., Lousada, J. and Rosenthall, J. (1985) *The Politics of Mental Health.* Basingstoke: Macmillan.

Becker, H. (1986) (2nd edn) *Writing for Social Scientists: How to Start and Finish Your Thesis, Book or Article.* London: University of Chicago Press.

Benwell, B. and Stokoe, E. (2006) *Discourse and Identity.* Edinburgh: Edinburgh University Press.

Bhabha, H. (2000) Interrogating identity: The post-colonial prerogative. In DuGay, P., Evans, J. and Redman, P. (eds), *Identity: A Reader.* London: Sage.

Boud, D., Keogh, R. and Walker, D. (1985) *Reflection: Turning Experience into Learning.* London: Kogan Page.

Bourdieu, P. (2004) *Science of Science and Reflexivity.* Cambridge: Polity Press.

Bourner, T., Bowden, R. and Laing, S. (2001) Professional doctorates in England. *Studies in Higher Education*, 26: 65–85.

Buckingham, W., Burnham, D., Hill, C., King, P., Marenbon, J. and Weeks, M. (2011) *The Philosophy Book.* London: Dorling Kindersley.

Christie, N. (1997) Four blocks against insight: Notes on the oversocialisation of criminologists. *Theoretical Criminology*, 1(1): 13–23.

Cooper, J. (1991) Telling our own stories. In Whitehead, C. and Noddings, N. (eds), *Stories Lives Tell: Narrative and Dialogue in Education.* New York: Teacher's College Press.

D'Cruz, H., Gillingham, P. and Merlendez, S. (2006) Reflexivity, its meanings and relevance for social work: A critical review of the literature. *British Journal of Social Work*, 37: 73–90.

DuGay, P., Evans, J. and Redman, P. (eds) (2000) *Identity: A Reader.* London: Sage.

Egan, K. (2001) *Why Education is so Difficult and Contentious* [Online]. Available at: www.tcrecord.org/AuthorDisplay.asp?aid=4974 (accessed 07.11.13).

Festinger, L. (1957) *A Theory of Cognitive Dissonance.* Stanford, CA: Stanford University Press.

Fisher, C. (1998) *Resource Allocation in the Public Sector: Values, Priorities and Markets in the Management of Public Services.* London: Routledge.

Fisher, C. and Lovell, A. (2009) (3rd edn) *Business Ethics and Values: Individual, Corporate and International Perspectives.* Harlow: Pearson Education.

Flint, K. (2008) *Towards an Exploration of Research Acts Produced in the Name of the Professional Doctorate: Exploring the Interplay of Ethics, Methodology, Epistemology, Reflection, Reflexivity and Identity in Doctoral Level Research.* Nottingham: Nottingham Trent University.

Flint, K. and Barnard, A. (2009) *Professional Doctorate Programme Incorporating the Awards of Doctor of Education, EdD; Doctor of Legal Practice, DLegal Prac; and, Doctor of Social Practice, DSocPrac: Producing Knowledge, Developing Practice.* Nottingham: Nottingham Trent University.

Flint, K., Barnard, A., Ching, J. and Flint, C. (2009) *Producing Space for New Forms of Social Research: An Exploration of Henri Lefebvre's Thesis.* Nottingham: Nottingham Trent University.

Forbes, J. (2008) Reflexivity in professional doctoral research. *Reflective Practice*, 9(4): 449–60.

Foucault, M. (1972) *The Archaeology of Knowledge* [Routledge Online]. Available at: www.marxists.org/reference/subject/philosophy/works/fr/foucault.htm (accessed 05.07.12).

Foucault, M. (1980) *Power/Knowledge: Selected Interviews and Other Writings 1972–1977.* New York: Pantheon.

Furlong, J. and Oancea, A. (2005) *Accessing Quality in Applied and Practice-Based Educational Research.* Oxford: University of Oxford, Department of Educational Studies.

Gibbs, P. and Flint, K. (2012) The phenomenology of practice: The agency of 'We', 'I' or 'Deferred'. Paper presented to *Educational Philosophy and Theory.*

Giddens, A. (1991) *Modernity and Self-Identity: Self and Society in the Late Modern Age.* Cambridge: Polity Press.

Guthrie, C. (2007) On learning the research craft: Memoirs of a journeyman researcher. *Journal of Research Practice*, 3(1): 1–10.

Hall, S. (ed.) (1997) *Representations: Cultural Representations and Signifying Practices.* London: Sage.

Heidegger, M. (1962) *Being and Time.* Southampton: The Camelot Press.

Hersey, P. and Blanchard, K. (1977) (3rd edn) *Management of Organisational Behaviour: Utilizing Human Resources.* New Jersey: Prentice Hall.

Hester, R. (2008) Power knowledge and children's rights in the teaching of youth justice practice. *Inter-University Centre Journal of Social Work*, 17, Fall 2008 [Online]. Available at: www.bemidjistate.edu/academics/publications/social_work_journals/issue17 (accessed 12.04.09).

Hester, R. (2010) Globalization, power and knowledge in youth justice. In Taylor, W., Earle, R. and Hester, R. (eds) *Youth Justice Handbook: Theory, Policy and Practice.* Cullompton: Willan.

HM Prison Service (2003) *Offender Assessment and Sentence Management – OASys.* London: HM Prison Service.

Johns, C. (2004) *Becoming a Reflective Practitioner.* Oxford: Blackwell Publishing.

Kirkpatrick, I., Ackroyd, S. and Walker, R. (2005) *The New Managerialism and Public Service Professions.* Basingstoke: Palgrave Macmillan.

Kögler, M., Herbert, M. and Hendrickson, P. (1992) *The Power of Dialogue: Critical Hermeneutics after Gadamer and Foucault.* Cambridge, MA: MIT Press.

Lester, S. (2004) Conceptualising the practitioner doctorate. *Studies in Higher Education*, 29(5): 1–3.

Levi, P. (1960) *If This is a Man* (trans. Wolf, S.). London: Abacus.

Marshall, S. and Green, N. (2004) *Your PhD Companion: A Handy Mix of Practical Tips, Sound Advice and Helpful Commentary to See You Through Your PhD.* Oxford: How To Books.

Mathieson, J. and Binder, M. (2009) *How to Survive Your Doctorate: What Others Don't Tell You.* Maidenhead: Open University Press.

Maxwell, J. (1996) *Qualitative Research Design: An Interactive Approach.* London: Sage.

Moon, J. (2006) (2nd edn) *Learning Journals: A Handbook for Reflective Practice and Professional Development.* Oxford: Routledge.

Moon, J. (2007) Reflective Learning Workshop. Centre for Excellence in Media Practice, Bournemouth University.

Muncie, J. (2004) (2nd edn) *Youth and Crime.* London: Sage.

Newman, J. (2000) Beyond the new public management? Modernizing public services. In Clarke, J., Gewirtz, S. and Mclaughlin, E. (eds) (2000) *New Managerialism, New Welfare.* London: Sage.

Palmer, V. (2009a) *Document One: A Critical Examination of the Relationship between Higher Education and the Professionalisation of the Youth Justice Workforce.* Unpublished thesis, Nottingham Trent University.

Palmer, V. (2009b) *Document Two: Epistemology and Identity – Critical Review of the Literature and Development of Contextual Framework.* Unpublished thesis, Nottingham Trent University.

Palmer, V. (2011) *Document Three: Designing Research 1: Using Methodology within a Specified Area of Professional Activity.* Unpublished thesis, Nottingham Trent University.

Palmer, V. (2012) *Document Four: Designing Research 2: Using a Contrasting Methodology and Methods within a Specified Area of Professional Activity: Then Fear Drives out all Wisdom from my Mind.* Unpublished thesis, Nottingham Trent University.

Palmer, V. (2014) *Document Five: A Critical Approach towards the Professionalisation of the Youth Justice Workforce: A Research-Led Design of a New Module – 'Mental Disorder, Learning Disability and Autism'.* Unpublished thesis, Nottingham Trent University.

Pinel, P. (1806) *A Treatise on Insanity.* New York: Hafner.

Pitts, J. (2001) Korrectional karaoke: New Labour and the zombification of Youth Justice. *Youth Justice,* 1(2): 3–16.

Pitts, J. (2003) *The New Politics of Youth Crime: Discipline or Solidarity?* Lyme Regis: Russell House Publishing.

Plath, S. (1963) *The Bell Jar.* London: Faber and Faber.

Pointon, A. (2014) *Reflections on the Process of Becoming a Doctor of Education.* Unpublished thesis, Nottingham Trent University.

Prichard, J. (1835) *Treatise on Insanity.* London: Gilbert and Piper.

Rogowski, S. (2002) *Young Offenders: A Case Study of Offending and the Youth Justice System and How this Relates to Policy and Practice Developments over the Post-War Period.* PhD thesis, Manchester Metropolitan University, Department of Applied Social Sciences.

Ryle, G. (1968) *The Thinking of Thoughts: What is 'Le Penseur' Doing?* [Online]. Available at: http://lucy.ukc.ac.uk/CSACS117/Papers/ryle-1.html (accessed 02.08.12).

Sambrook, S., Stewart, J. and Roberts, C. (2008) Doctoral supervision: A view from above, below and middle. *Journal of Further and Higher Education,* 82(1): 71–84.

Schatzki, T. (1996) *Social Practices: A Wittgensteinian Approach to Human Activity and the Social.* Cambridge: Cambridge University Press.

Schatzki, T. (ed.) (2001) *The Practice Turn in Contemporary Theory.* London: Routledge.

Schön, D. (1983) *The Reflective Practitioner.* Aldershot: Ashgate.

Shaw, S. (2006) *The Genesis and Development of a Youth Offending Team: Youth Justice in a Town in South-East England 2000–2003.* PhD thesis, London School of Economics.

Smith, D. (2006) Making sense of psychoanalysis in criminological theory and probation practice. *Probation Journal,* 53(4): 361–76.

Smith, R. (2005) Welfare versus justice – again! *Youth Justice* 5: 2–16.

Smith, R. (2008) *Social Work and Power.* Basingstoke: Palgrave.

Smith, R. (2009) *Doing Social Work Research.* Maidenhead: Open University Press.

Somerville, D. and Keeling, J. (2004) A practical approach to promote reflective practice within nursing. *Nursing Times,* 100(12): 42.

Souhami, A. (2003) *Transforming Youth Justice: A Local Study of Occupational Identity and Membership*. PhD thesis, Keele University.

Trevillion, S. (2008) Research, theory and practice: Eternal triangle or uneasy bedfellows? *Social Work Education*, 27(4): 440–50.

Vernon, J. (2008) Erfahren and erleben: Metaphysical experience and its overcoming in Heideggar's *Beitrage*. *Canadian Journal of Continental Philosophy*, 12(1): 108–25.

Vitae (2010) *Introducing the Researcher Development Framework*. London: Careers Research and Advisory Centre.

Wellington, J. and Sikes, P. (2006) A doctorate in a tight compartment: Why do students choose a professional doctorate and what impact does it have on their personal and professional lives? *Studies in Higher Education*, 31(6): 723–34.

Wellington, J., Bathmaker, A.-N., Hunt, C., McCulloch, G. and Sikes, P. (2005) *Succeeding with Your Doctorate*. London: Sage.

Wood, K. (2006) Changing as a person: The experience of learning to research in the social sciences. *Higher Education, Research and Development*, 25(1): 53–66.

Youth Justice Board (2003) *Guidance Note 1, Asset: The Youth Justice Board's Assessment Profile*. London: Youth Justice Board.

Chapter 15
'Tain from the mirror

Towards an education for reflection in the helping professions

Kevin Flint, Vicky Palmer and Adam Barnard

Chapter outline

This chapter introduces:

- the language of reflection
- deconstruction of reflective language
- reflective practice to come.

Introduction

One of the many challenges that connect those variously involved in the helping professions is a seemingly almost insatiable drive for the improvement of practice. In this matter one is always open to learning from others and from the multiplicity of signs of the 'Other' pointing to possible ideas, theories, narratives and so on at play in any identity. For example, the identity 'author' carries with it the play of numerous different other identities, including woman, professional, artist, challenging, erudite, scholarly, feminist, etc. Collectively these and other possible identities at play in any one identity are categorised in short as the 'Other'. In working with researchers and practitioners from a range of different practices over the past eight years, there is apparent a manifest collective awareness of the transformations made in advancing understandings of what is given in the everyday practices involving 'clients', 'individuals', 'patients', 'participants', 'service users', 'offenders' in a sublime range of different contexts.[1] As human beings, of course, we are always interested in exploring the possibilities of a multiplicity of different identities made possible in what are re-presented as any such 'contexts'. Indeed, it has become customary within the practices of reflection based upon what has been re-presented, too, as rigorous truth claims to knowledge, to employ a seemingly ever-growing range of forms of reflective practice in order to make the connection between ideas, theories, philosophies and so on, and any possible transformations in the multi-layered, rich and complex everyday aspects of social care, nursing, health and social care, psychology, research (Johns 2010; Bulman and Schutz 2008; Knott and Scragg 2013; Maclean 2010; Redmond 2006; Rolfe et al. 2010; Webber 2010).

It is striking, too, in examining the literature on reflective practice in the helping professions, that while most practitioners hold onto the familiar Newtonian optic – where the entity, light, in Newton's express terms 'corpuscles of light' – travelling in straight lines is considered to be reflected in plain mirrors in accord with the 'law of reflection'. A law, indeed, that in its metaphor constitutes a division between the actual object and virtual image of reflection. Not surprisingly perhaps, a number of researchers have variously struggled with the efficacy of this optical metaphor as a basis for understanding what happens in practice.[2]

Indeed, in contemporary physics the radically contrasting *language* of quantum electrodynamics, QED, not only provides another possible understanding of just *how reflection is constituted* at the mirror's surface, it also creates a rich source of new ideas and suggestions for further research within this specialised field. In so doing the metallic tain surface hidden at the back of the mirror comes to have a pivotal significance that has been largely ignored within the application of the Newtonian metaphor of reflection. In the exploration of reflection in the helping professions which follows, the tain is used to symbolise a way of understanding the complex relationship between what is done in everyday practice, and the constitution of the very practice of the *language of reflection* itself, that until now has remained largely dissimulated in such work.

In QED light is no longer viewed as a single entity, but may now be understood in terms of mathematical *languages* describing both electromagnetic waves and particles (light quanta), whose separate and distinctive properties only become manifest depending upon the form of observations made. The *language* of QED then provides other possible understandings of the basis upon which reflection occurs at the tain surface. While the slowing down of light can be explained by refraction as a phenomenon of waves, reflection at the hidden surface of the tain (i.e. polished tin, aluminium, silver etc.) may be understood on one hand as a particulate phenomenon arising from the interplay of particles, i.e. light quanta and metal atoms in the tain surface, and on the other it may also be understood in terms of waves – involving the constructive interference of light waves incident on the surface with electrons from the tain atoms that may also be understood as behaving like waves in their atomic orbitals, or distinct quantised energy levels within each atom.

One should note in passing that the mathematical language of QED does not provide any understanding of just how and on what basis quantisation is constituted in this atomic world. There are parallels here, too, with the modelling of the behaviour of the collective human body according to bioecological theories of human development, to which we will return in the concluding half of this chapter.

Manifestly, then, it is the change of *language* that makes such transformations possible in physics, and it is language that in some way constitutes the basis for understandings of reflection in any professional practice. There are obvious qualitative differences, for example, between the languages of social practice, psychology, nursing, social work and so on, each with its own particular technical terms, historical emphases, specialist discourses and idioms. But just how we understand the *language of reflection* and how the languages of the helping professions work to constitute the basis for reflection is the subject of this concluding chapter.

For some readers, perhaps, the possible challenge of learning about the structure of language may seem far too abstracted from everyday professional practice to be of any practical use. The now very rarely used verb, *tain*, signifying shorthand for the action, in this case 'to obtain', and a number of its other obvious compounds, might at first only reinforce such a position. But, we are using it to symbolise that which remains generally hidden from view: namely the question of just *what constitutes the basis for reflection*.

The suggestions for this hidden language constituting reflection arise not from any arbitrary theory imposed from the outside. Nor are we are suggesting here some kind of analogy with quantum theory. At issue is what can be revealed from a deconstructive reading of discourses of research concerned with reflective practice in the helping professions. In addition to new suggestions for research we hope that the language constituting reflection that is revealed in this chapter will also provide a productive new focus for professional practice in ways that open space for greater understandings of the multifarious everyday practices of human beings.

More controversially, perhaps, what follows suggests that unlike the customs of reflection and reflective practice in the helping professions, and forms of professional activity, this deconstructive reading of the language of reflection at least opens the possibility of coded space and a home in language that no longer serves to alienate human beings.

Concerned with the economy of *what is given* in reflection, the opening half of this chapter seeks to focus upon the issue of the language constituting reflection, while the concluding half seeks a focus upon the questions raised in the complex relationship between those identified as professionals and other human beings. Ordinarily, of course, it is no accident that we employ a range of identities other than human being in our everyday world of practice. Such identities accord with the economy of what is given by reason; its very grammar drawing together subject with object has become so familiar it is easy to forget that 'human being' in its many possibilities sometimes seeks to exceed any such economy. It is no accident, then, that the grammars of everyday practices, including our languages, are continually open to transformation. In terms of our everyday professional practices within the helping professions, it would seem that very few, until now, have given consideration to just how we handle working with human beings in our practices. Is it not the case that the very possibilities sometimes open to us as human beings are ordinarily just viewed as exceptions to everyday rules and protocols?

The very fact that *as human beings* we live our lives continually in a 'state of exception' (Agamben 2005) in our languages has really not been addressed within customs of reflection and reflective practice currently employed in the helping professions, or, indeed, in other forms of professional practice. Moreover, the identity, 'individual', falls considerably short of being an effective synonym for human being; the former, as an isolated discrete and completely dead representation of a completely isolated unit, will always be open to calculation as the subject and object of any economy of practice. The latter vital figure in life, in always already 'being-with' others and the Other at play in any identity, in living in its ever-unfolding temporal world, sometimes opens space for exceeding any such economy. In so doing the possibilities opened by human beings certainly remain beyond the calculus of any statistically based formulation.

Here, we are drawing from leading-edge work in the field of developmental science concerned with the bioecological modelling of human behaviour by Urie Bronfenbrenner. A deconstructive reading of one chapter from his final book, *Making Human Beings Human* (2005), not only opens further questions concerned with human beings and the sovereign powers of being as presence, it raises, too, the question of the powers driving us to exceed any economy of what is given in practice. It also provides another rationale for the new language introduced as a way of understanding how reflection is constituted in practice involved for human beings.

In this way, as professionals with interests in understanding possibilities opened within a wide range of different practices found in the helping professions, we are concerned with the challenge of opening new space for debate on the language of, and so the rethinking of, the structures reiterated in such practices. In moving in this way, our seemingly insatiable desire in the name of the improvement in the helping professions to exceed what is given, may be understood in terms of moves towards social justice.

Consequently in writing this chapter, and in this emerging spirit of moves to exceed economies of what is given in practice, the inclusion of the *tain* symbolises a mission to radicalise the debate concerning the very practice of reflection used in the helping professions, including the very practice of research itself, and to begin to open new frontiers for such practices.

Discursive practices disseminated within the literature on the helping professions use the term 'reflection' and its seemingly ever-growing associated terminology, 'reflective practice', 'reflection-in-action', 'reflection-on-action', 'critical reflection', and even 'reflection-on-reflection', and so on, almost as if the question of reflection itself is somehow beyond questioning. 'Reflection', it seems, carries with it a mystical authority invested in a belief that returns us all, perhaps, to the time as neonates when we first began to understand and to project the possibility of 'the Other' as different from ourselves in some way by looking into a mirror. It is no surprise, then, to find that in their focus upon 'reflection', Donald Schön's (1983) along with Chris Argyris' (1982) writings in the 1980s and 1990s, on questions of learning within a range of organisational settings, is still able to re-tain its standing as the most cited locus of authority on matters of reflection in any professional practice. Given the field of education, too, is always cultivating transformations of culture (Flint 2013) within any professional practice, one is hardly shocked to find that the much-cited work of David Boud and his colleagues (1985), who were concerned with the relationship between experience and reflection, similarly touched a nerve in the public psyche.

But in the spirit of having uncovered the hidden tain of the mirror, and with realisation that it has a pivotal function in the language of QED in providing an understanding of the basis upon which reflection is constituted, it seemed obvious to open questioning concerned with the language constituting reflection in the helping professions and more generally in all forms of professional practice. With this consideration came the understanding of the possibility that rather than in the hegemony of much current professional practice, where we unconsciously and assiduously as human beings hold onto our neonatal experience of reflection as pertaining to some essential quality hidden within our very soul, in the spirit of pragmatism in which the works of Schön, Argyris, Boud and others are located, is it not time to open space for questioning the very practice of language itself, given that its economy as a language constitutes express understandings of 'reflection'?

The language of reflection as a practice

Language, after all, is a practice with which we all become familiar in our everyday repetition and reiteration of words and phrases that we variously employ in making sense of our 'professional' worlds. Languages that we variously learn through our inductive 'training' and 'development' within specialist divisions of the helping professions may be understood in semiotic terms, as the patterned repetitions and reiterations of signs and chains of signs, where in metaphysical terms at least, each of these signs are considered to point to something else. Consequently everyday customs involving the patterned and patterning repetitions and reiterations of signs are always open to transformation, revision, redefinition, idiomatic re-emphasis and so on.

Quite straightforwardly, for example, even without any appeal to semiotics and deconstruction that follows, one can imagine that various individuals, each possessed with their own distinctive theoretical lenses on just how to understand the world of practice, may come to view the very event of reflection in quite different ways. Just how this works in practice has yet to be modelled and examined in research. Working with reflective practice in the helping professions, in education and other professional practices, Kevin Flint, Adam Barnard, Vicky Palmer and others (Flint et al., in preparation) at Nottingham Trent are already working towards the critical examination of such models of reflection drawn from any one of a number of notable theories and philosophies given expression by Michel Foucault, Martin Heidegger, Pierre Bourdieu, Paulo Freire, John Dewey and so on.

Indeed, even closer to the everyday world of practice, don't we each reiterate everyday our own unique identities that ordinarily are given expression in the stories we variously tell about our experiences? The question remains as to just how reflection among helping professionals is to be understood in this particular context.

Reflection is not something that can be summoned at will. Nor is it either a form of practice that can follow straight after an event in a linear fashion. We cannot hope to adequately reflect at the end of a working day by methodically writing in our reflective journals, trying to respond to the standard questions generally accepted to invoke reflection, i.e. that which is *given*. Questions such as, 'how did that make you feel?' and 'what could you have done differently?' become meaningless when the fluid interplay between thought and feelings cause us to 'to and fro', to rise and fall as waves of reflection, some having more significance than others. Yesterday's trough of anxious reflection may be the precursor to tomorrow's crest of exhilarative new insight, but not because the two incidents are necessarily related – as cause and effect – but rather in spite of it owing to the absorption of a random critical moment perhaps two years previously. In the social world, in fact, reflection is often accompanied by diffraction. Counter-intuitively a single space in this world can sometimes be the source of circular waves of energy that come to affect people. There are times when reflection opens space for stillness, allowing for release, calm contemplation and for letting things be in their disorderliness and uncertainty. Perhaps one of the leading and most controversial philosophers of the twentieth century, Martin Heidegger, spoke of an 'ethic of *Gellasenheit*': letting things *be* in their own ground. There are others when reflective practice garners action such as a complete change in practice or merely a tweak.

We do not reflect in a vacuum and there are multifarious obstacles that sabotage our ability to reflect, including the ever-diminishing resource of time, the ubiquitous interjection of corporate bureaucracy and the unbridled imposition of ever-changing responsibilities. Reflection, it would seem, has moved from the realms of necessity in the social care professions to those of indulgence.

Concerning professional identity, Vicky Palmer recalls her earlier experience as a probation officer, an officer of the court. Upon leaving the profession to take up a teaching position at the university, she struggled to accept the identity of 'academic'. Commencing a professional doctorate brought her some respite from this tension, as there was comfort in a number of new identities that the programme opened up for participants. For Palmer the language of research as a new mirror for experience opened space for the possibility of continually reiterating and exploring a new identity as a 'researching practitioner':

> There was never absolute resolution, with my identity continually fluctuating, and then seemingly assimilating, only to revert back to alternating again. Immersion in academic writing was merely a thick veneer, discretely concealing the probation officer through the medium of a pen. Following completion of the professional doctorate process and receiving the title of Dr of Social Sciences, I virtually immediately re-transitioned to 'probation officer mindset' – I still think and feel like a probation officer. I internally assess, appraise my colleagues and students as one would assess clients or service users. Probation practice and social justice lies at the heart of all that I think and do; this position is immovable and cannot be shaken. I defended my doctoral thesis in the viva voce as one would a vulnerable young defendant before a crown court judge – with practicality, empathy, rationality, yet mindful of the rules of the court and protective of its future readership.
>
> In returning to my thesis and deconstructing the reading of my professional doctorate, there is internal conflict within the work. I rarely merged the

identities of probation officer and academic and clearly kept both 'in separate corners of the ring' (Alcoff, 2003: 7). There are connotations, denotations and changing contexts in the writing. Differing perspectives and ideologies clash. It would not be conceivable to operate as a probation practitioner using the neutrality of language that at the time I felt had been so necessary in writing a doctoral thesis. Hence there are contradictions and dichotomies around professional identity, which never fully resolve themselves. Although the textual signs may indicate that my identity is entrenched in academia, the persona behind the mirror is unyieldingly 'practitioner'. It is not about hierarchy, rank or positionality, I simply found myself having to 'not be myself' in the writing, the style and form being dictated by the language of the academy. That stable identity and pre-discursive self never fully permits me to present myself as an authentic academic.

(Benwell and Stokoe 2006: 3)

The language of reflection in this case may be understood, then, as moves towards understandings of spatial differences, signified by others and by the Other in any identity. In terms of the law-like language of reflection, is there not some sense of moving towards justice in this possible revision and reconstitution of such a law-like structure in our practice? Indeed, it is such spatial differences there in our languages that make possible this deconstructive reading. In the name of moves towards social justice, then, we just need to give ourselves time for deconstruction, where there is more to be revealed about the constitution of 'reflection'. Clearly while the foregoing philosophical and theoretical discourses may be appealing, by themselves they do not address the question of the basis for the constitution of the language of reflection.

In the everyday practices of the helping professions, and in any associated practices of research, however, it has also become a customary and generally unquestioned assumption, within the hegemonies shaping such practices, that some sense may be made of innumerable patterns of everyday work by drawing from a variety of 'meaning-makers'. 'Reason', 'the voice', 'assessment', even 'writing' itself, have now all become regarded as meaning-makers. Somehow, and tacitly, such meaning-makers are assumed within economies of what is given in practice to sustain a direct connection with the 'is', being as presence, finding expression in every verb and nominalisation in our lexicon.

There is another radical possibility, too, suggested earlier by our brief consideration given to understanding the constitution of reflection. What is almost always elided in the hegemonic grammars of everyday practice in nearly all professional practices, including forms of qualitative, social and educational research, is the presupposition structuring such meaning-makers used in our practices; namely, concerning truth itself. We hold onto the guardrails of our metaphysical representations of truth claims as if our very lives depended upon them. Indeed, this observation alone suggests another fruitful line of research into practices in the helping professions and other professional spheres; namely, studies directed towards understanding more about the mystical authority we variously invest as human beings in particular beliefs about aspects of our world of practice.

Many researchers and professionals around the world, for example, still hold on with great tenacity and resolve to a set of beliefs about the way rigorous and formal adherence to methods of science creates what they regard as objective scientific knowledge about the social and educational world. The study of knowledge, its justification, its claims to truth, its production, is called epistemology. This still dominant, mechanistic epistemology, called positivism, or variants of it, permeates and shapes knowledge production in most Western cultures (Kincheloe 2008). As a mirror on the world this positivist epistemology purports to reflect the objective truths about the world in which we all live.

As might be expected there have been some challenges to this position. Over the past 100 years or more, a diverse group of researchers have become wedded to a radically contrasting set of theories concerned with the production of knowledge. They call themselves 'critical theorists'. In place of positivists' single mirror, the languages of critical theory/critical thinking constitute a multiplicity of mirrors on this complex world.

In part the mystical authority invested in one of these epistemologies, or others, is that they each seek to constitute in their own different languages a focus for us upon the objects formed in those reflective discourses. Let us not forget that as human beings we are always different from such objects formed in the mirror. Is there not a matter of justice at stake here, that we take account of the possibilities open to human beings? Moreover, as with the earlier transformation in the language of physics, there are other languages of reflection and with them other ways of understanding moves towards truth in our social world that will emerge from this deconstruction.

But, as readers can we not already hear a ghost knocking at the door of much everyday experience? It proclaims loudly:

> Why bother with such 'meaning-makers' – whatever that means – let's just get on with what's important. Our priority is to care for others. We haven't got time for such considerations.

The language of reflection as a historical and cultural practice

Sure, we have not got time for consideration of the constitution of reflection if we intuitively in various ways understand time as an empty sequence of now ... now ... now ... that has to be filled up every day. As Walter Benjamin once suggested, the very form of such clock-time that presses into us in this modern world seems to constrain, delimit and to contain us in some way within economies of what are given in practice. In the hegemonic cultures of everyday practice in the helping professions, as in other professional practices, are we not in our own different ways so jammed into what is demanded of us in our practices that we do not entertain the possibility that time itself is an invention which may also be understood in other ways, including for example, in terms of the projection of a possibility, and of history?

> Ghost of experience: 'I'm just exasperated that we've got so many priorities that have to be addressed as soon as possible, what is the point of this deconstruction?'

Our ghost certainly has a point. But, given the pressures in every dimension of practice in the helping professions, is there no possibility, not of clock time, but constituted in historical time, in examining more from this deconstruction of reflection and its impact upon us as human beings?

Taking seriously Schön's 'reflection-on practice', and in the spirit of deconstruction drawing from Derrida's oeuvre, have we yet in the helping professions taken historical time to examine critically what Derrida calls the 'catastrophe of memory' that leaves us only with the cinders of past experience? Derrida, just like those working in the police, raises questions not just about the efficacy of memory, but also his notion of catastrophe points to the complication and the impossibility of ever separating with any certainty constative statements of fact concerning past experience from performative injunctions inscribed in earlier promises to undertake particular actions. Here we return to parallels with the language of QED used to explain light phenomena involving particles/waves. Again, the issue of the possible catastrophe of memory suggests another fruitful area of research that has yet to be addressed in reflective practice.

There is also another significant issue at stake already in this deconstruction of reflection. There remains the question of whether it is possible for the deconstruction to open space beyond the mystical authority currently invested in the ontological grounding of what is done in the practice of reflection, and any theological exegesis variously delimiting the highest possibilities projected from such practice. Certainly a response to such questions remains to be addressed, as they were never posed by any of our main protagonists concerned with reflective practice from the 1980s.

More concretely it is possible to grasp what is at stake in the practice of the reiteration of signs from Schön's (1987) work, Educating the Reflective Practitioner, which he saw as correcting and giving a new focus for some of his earlier exploration. Here his practice of writing already involves deferment of signs from the pragmatist philosopher and educator, John Dewey (2009 [1934]). Albeit unconsciously, too, Schön's text defers the sign 'thinking', in this case 'like a doctor' (Schön 1987: 34), from the writings of any one of three possible philosophers, René Descartes, Immanuel Kant, Edmund Husserl. Similarly, too, in Boud and his colleagues' (1985) chapter, 'Promoting reflection in learning', cultivated by that transcendental 'meaning maker' reason (unconsciously drawn from Kant's writings), the sign 'thinking' becomes reiterated in terms of 'intellectual and affective activities in which individuals engage to explore their experiences in order to lead to new understandings and appreciations' (Boud et al. 1985: 19). There is no suggestion, too, that our protagonists identified here constitute the only show available as grounds for the training and education of professionals in all forms of professional practice, including the helping professions.

Indeed, John Dewey, David Kolb, Kurt Lewin, Paulo Freire, Max van Manen, Barbara Carter, Jack Mezirow, Jürgen Habermas and others, have all been cited as authority figures in the field of the helping professions. Like our earlier main protagonists, their discursive practices have been deferred from signs iterated in the practices of Descartes, Kant, Plato, Aristotle, Parmenides, Heidegger and others. Ordinarily, of course, and in radical contrast to such deferment of signs, in the hegemonic customs of everyday practice such authority figures are represented as the original source of 'ideas'. As the voice of such claims they are implicitly and falsely considered to give expression to the being of what are represented as original ideas. It is ironic therefore that it turns out that 'idea' is itself a sign deferred from Plato's discourse.

Unconsciously or not, there is no question here of the intentionality of our main protagonists or, indeed, these many authors, in eliding such deferments of signs, nor that their discursive practices preclude possible agency in other spheres of activity.

Unfortunately, neither of our main protagonists, Schön and Argyris along with Boud and his colleagues, it would seem, have taken seriously the possible reiteration of signs from Husserl's and others' works. Indeed, each of them delimited their deferral of signs to Dewey's writings about learning and experience. In contrast, in his readings of Descartes and Kant, Husserl had considered his discourse to be the culmination of a whole tradition that has been traced back to what Derrida felicitously identifies as 'Plato's Pharmacy'. Much modern Western thinking and language can be traced back to Plato's school of thinking. Indeed, in making further sense of such connections Husserl's phenomenology of consciousness proved pivotal. Using an approach in effect not dissimilar to archaeologists, his philosophical study of phenomena, entities, events in the world where all of their dressings, layers of materials, coverings and other accoutrements are first removed, enables people to 'see' aspects of the everyday world in their own naked reality. This particular approach also headlines an understanding of the pivotal role of signs, of language, in helping us as human beings to make sense of our worlds. It created the basis for the so-called 'language turn' in the social sciences.

The language of reflection in the disseminative drift of signs

In attempting to stand outside of the disseminative drift of signs from 'Plato's Pharmacy', that is, Roland Barthes' *Empire of Signs* that continues to grow with many historical cultures both inside and outside Europe, Martin Heidegger's texts at least open space for understandings of the barriers, disarticulations and dislocations between specialist modern forms of practice. One issue raised earlier is the mystical authority invested in the *language* of claims to truth as correctness; Heidegger's discourse, in radical contrast, opens understandings of truth in terms of the harbouring and making secure entities in the world (Stambaugh 1992). We will return to this possibility a little later in concerning ourselves with justice in reflective practice.

Another associated issue for 'reflection-on practice' that ordinarily makes it difficult to stand outside the disseminative drift is that of the anthropology of specialisation; Foucault (1984) saw this in terms of the discursive practices of 'regimes of truth'. Here, in the context of the helping professions, such a regime may be identified 'as … system[s] of ordered procedures for the production, regulation, distribution, circulation and operation of statements' (Foucault 1984: 132). In this way 'truth' is understood as a 'regime' constituting the basis for the governance of the helping professions, being 'link[ed]' with systems of power that produce and sustain it, and to effects of power, which it induces and which extend it' (Foucault 1984: 132, emphasis added).

Reflection constituted in the differences and deferrals of signs

Unlike the concerns expressed in this chapter with reflection that place an emphasis upon the *language of practice* itself, i.e. the express way people talk about their everyday work, it is already becoming clear that reflection may be understood provisionally as constituted by differences and deferrals of signs, including their associated signifiers and signified possible understandings, in which individuals are decentred. For example, if a social worker spoke of working with a client, then her discourse would be centred upon the actions of herself and her client. In decentring one moves the reflective mirror to the language in which we live our lives, so that language rather than human beings becomes the pivotal concern, so providing a basis for understanding the possibilities open to us. But, ordinarily, of course, our main protagonists, along with regimes of practice in the helping professions and associated regimes of educational practice, simply and conveniently hold onto the individual at the centre of such practices. Such emphasis certainly remains expedient for economists' statistically informed calculus for the isolated 'individual'. In this way language, our essential home in this world, becomes the province of other specialised regimes of truth claims concerned with semiotics, linguistics and so on that, ironically, rarely see the light of day in the helping professions.

The language of the regime operative within the helping professions also largely excludes consideration being given to Heidegger's critical reading of specialisation. This is unfortunate because his writings sought to uncover other forces 'viz-a-tergo' (Gadamer 2004), operating from behind, as it were, in historical terms, that variously structure and so delimit understandings of what is possible in the helping professions. His texts point to the metaphysical and ontological grounding of such practices – largely opening consideration of 'ideas', 'what' is done in practice along with its 'reasoning', its 'content', and even our 'subjective' express 'consciousness' of it. Ironically, on the other hand, in this dominant secular world, in metaphysical terms Heidegger's texts also reveal what he calls their 'theological' structuring that always already delimits the highest beings attainable within such practices: expressions of 'that' 'paradigmatic idea', its 'subject', 'form', 'organisation', are all constitutive of a theological structuring of practice.

Despite the sociologist Max Weber's observations made more than a century ago, to the effect that little consideration has been given to the spirit of theology in capitalist societies, it still remains the case that in the helping professions and more generally in the social world, little consideration has been given to researching the theological structuring of its practices.

Moreover, in 'reflecting-on' the practice of language it is important to keep in mind, too, that as long as we hold onto presuppositions concerned with the metaphysical determination of truth claims to knowledge, herein lies another dimension of the mystical authority invested in our beliefs. The belief in such a presupposition structuring the practices of the helping professions, given expression in its verbs and nominalisations, means that professional practice is driven by the naming force and gathering powers of being as presence. Counter-intuitively, perhaps, especially for those schooled in the languages of empiricism, Cartesianism and so on, it is such ontotheological structuring of the metaphysical representations of being as presence in every aspect of our professional practices that is driving us as human beings every day. Ironically, it drives us by constituting only one way for revealing the world of the helping professions in accord with all such metaphysical exigencies, i.e. metaphysical assumptions connecting each sign with a particular thing or event. We will return to this point shortly in consideration of Bronfenbrenner's theories of human development.

In the metaphysical determination of signs, of course, a given sign purports to point towards a particular entity, event, phenomenon, etc. Like the identities inscribed within the discursive practices of policy-makers, and their dominant express concern for 'transparency', there is rarely any consideration given to others and indeed 'the Other' at play in any such identities. As we suggested earlier, the identity 'woman', for example, may be variously inscribed by the identities of others, including 'mother', 'daughter', 'sister', other siblings and so on, along with the symbolic Other, taken from roles, characters, etc., including 'professional, leader, politician, writer, happiness, sobriety'. Recall, too, the ghost of policy-makers' egregious dissimulation of the practice of language with their snapshots of various figures that are 'required' in practice: 'It's vital, they say, that everything we do in practice is "transparent", open to "audit", "objective", "evidence-based", "effective" in doing the right things and "efficient" in doing things right'.

Whether or not, as suggested here, policy-makers view themselves as distinguished in some way, towering above their flock of sheep, as the Latin *ēgregius* suggests, is just another elision of what really matters. Unconsciously, at least, our ghost here gives some clues as to the structuring of the *economy of what is given in practice*. It places emphasis upon ethical reflective practice that is 'conditioned' in relation to what is 'possible' and 'calculable' in the practices of the helping professions.

Indeed, such an ethic really amounts to a reiteration of Aristotle's text in the *Niomachean Ethics* (NE). The text of the NE distinguishes 'deliberation' as a type of inquiry constituted by rational 'calculation'; 'comprehension' as 'the application of a belief' which is itself 'conditioned' by its being comprehended in a 'proposition', a policy, a theory, etc.; and, in this deconstructive reading, 'understanding' is considered as a projection of possibilities.

Moreover there is always a close relationship between economy and spirit expressed by those hidden ghosts in our practices. Economy, from the Ancient Greek, *oikos* – household – and *nomos* – law – names the laws inscribed in that which is *given* in practice and how it is managed; spirit being the animating principle in human beings, which *gives* life to our practice. Keep in mind, too, that the space–time between any such economy of signs and the vital actions of that body we call 'human being', is constituted in some way in our professional languages.

In the spirit of Aristotle's words deferred from the NE, alongside words of managers deferred from the helping professions, 'consideration' of this brief 'reflection-on' the very practice of language begins to reveal some of its sovereign powers used in the helping professions. In so doing we sought to present the 'outcomes' of this deconstruction of the *language* of reflection, which are never complete, in terms of a numbered list presented as follows:

1   The language of reflection, like any language, is constituted with a threefold structuring that opens space for the inclusion/exclusion of particular entities, people, events and so on, along with its capacity to hold matters in a state of exception, not least the matter of human being. Herein lies its sovereign power as a *language*. In this way the articulation of any identity carries with it the sovereign power to include, exclude and make exceptions, consonant with the structure of its law. With its focus upon the economy of the individual within the discursive practices of the helping professions, ironically, the language of 'reflection-on' the practices of human beings has largely been re-*tained* as a matter of giving idiomatic expression to exceptions.

2   Our deconstruction has revealed how the language of reflection used in the helping professions is constituted in terms of the interplay of differences between signs, signifiers and what is signified and largely contained within dominant forms of the ontotheological structuring of practice. In so doing it has also begun to uncover for consideration other languages of semiotics and of deconstruction and an associated framework that could be employed in developing from practices in the helping professions, including research, other understandings of such practices. Not least, such language already opens space for concerns regarding the theological structuring of such practices, and the mystical authority invested in particular beliefs.

3   In foregrounding the repetition and reiteration of signs, constituted in the *delimited* and *delimiting* language of reflection, we have shown how much practice is mediated by concerns about what is happening in the present. Such expressions of concern about the present not only fill up every moment in the empty sequence of now … now … now constituting our modern invention of clock-time. In so doing, the regimes of governmentality and of government for the helping professions, both *retain* and *sustain* the naming force and gathering powers of being as presence in economies of what is given in the customary reiterations of the customary language of reflection.

    3.1   Placing an emphasis upon re-presentations of truth claims about practice within its delimited economies, remains in line with Freud's so-called 'death drive' − his particular way of giving expression to the unconscious drive arising from the fact that we will all return to being inorganic matter. Paradoxically, in holding onto presuppositions about the language of truth claims in practice, such regimes of reflection largely elide the possibility of justice to come for human beings held within such law-like structures. Indeed, rather than addressing the issue of our lives being decentred and in the throw of the 'disseminative drift of signs', imagine that Plato's school of thinking worked just like a pharmacy that cultivated new and special words rather than medicines, and Plato's ideas, his special words, have come to be repeated and reiterated in different ways by generations and generations of people. If you know what to look for you can find Plato's ideas and words being repeated in our everyday workplaces around the world. This is the disseminative drift from Plato's Pharmacy. In placing the 'individual' at the centre of professional practice, within this disseminative drift of signs, what is created is an ever-growing fog from the polysemy of re-presentations of meanings constituted in practice. In the fog of this current polysemic space we variously continue to work daily in constituting and thereby mourning a whole range of dead 'objects', 'subjects', 'individuals', 'selves', and other *re-presentations* created every day in line with the drives of Thanatos, and given expression in Freud's 'death drive'. In Ancient Greek mythology Thanatos was the god of non-violent death. His was a gentle touch, like that of his brother, Hypnos [sleep], from which we now derive a number of words: hypnotic, hypnosis, hypnotise, hypnotherapy, etc.

    3.2   Moreover, in largely eliding all but the most instrumental forms of philosophical discourse used to shore up current regimes of governmentality employed in the helping professions, little consideration has been given to what Friedrich Nietzsche identified as the 'eternal return' of the same 'will to power' in any representations of practice. As suggested earlier, Nietzsche realised that every day in our practices we each repeat and reiterate signs, phrases, words and other symbols in our writing and speaking etc. What he is alerting us to is the fact that in our repetitions of reflective practices we have become concerned almost exclusively with the objects formed in the mirror. As objects they can be connected to any economy and constitute the basis for power and control. Tacitly what Nietzsche was also alerting us to is the question of the possibilities open to ourselves as human beings. With all this focus on the objects formed in the mirror of reflection on the world of practice, as human beings have we not come to accept that our behaviours are sometimes unpredictable, surprising, exceptional, idiosyncratic and so on?

Given the explosive increase in the sovereign powers of the language of information over the last twenty years or so, within its very own eponymous age-mediating practices within the reflection of helping professions, in historical terms is it not time for newly constituted languages that might open the possibility of space for life-affirming moves towards justice? In this decentred world that privileges language and the repetitions of signs, justice may be understood as moves towards creating languages and practices that constitute an openness to new understandings as possibilities in the world. Such moves are created through the deconstruction of existing languages.

Indeed, the very question of moves towards justice also raises the issue of the complex relationship of those identified as professionals with other human beings. The case example of such a relationship that follows is taken from the writings of, perhaps, the leading 'bioecologist' of the twentieth century, Urie Bronfenbrenner. Deconstructing and so uncovering new aspects of his professional language that are already hidden there in his discursive practice, reveals something quite remarkable about representations of both 'reflection' and its associated 'reflective practice' in the helping professions. It brings us back to the very question of 'improvement' and its relationship with ourselves as human beings, which is driving so much practice in the professions.

Reflective practice to come

At first glance this may seem a strange sub-heading. We have used it to signal albeit unconscious moves towards justice taken in Bronfenbrenner's writings that are simply and unconditionally impossible and incalculable. Hence, rather than the seemingly more familiar metaphysical representation of 'reflective practice' in the present, the injunction 'to come' is there to signal a possible movement no longer delimited or restricted in any way by the sovereign powers of such metaphysical language.

Urie Bronfenbrenner lived most of his life in America, following his family's move to Pittsburg from Russia when he was six years old. His father had been a neuropathologist who had worked at a hospital for the developmentally disabled called Letchworth Village. Bronfenbrenner is generally now regarded as one of the leading developmental psychologists of the twentieth century. In the UK, for example, his work was instrumental in shaping the 'Head Start' programme.[3]

In his 'Foreword' to Bronfenbrenner's last book, Making Human Beings Human, which brings together a series of leading papers by the author, Richard M. Lerner's (2005) text identifies a number of 'cutting-edge' ideas attributable to Bronfenbrenner's work in developmental psychology. Particularly noteworthy is 'the theoretical focus on temporally [historically] embedded person-context relational processes; the embracing of dynamic change across the ecological system; and [the] relational, change-sensitive methods predicated on the idea that individuals influence the people and institutions of their ecology as much as they are influenced by them' (Lerner 2005: ix). Here ecology constitutes the study [logia] of the house [oikos] in which particular species live.

Morally, in Lerner's terms, what had charged Bronfenbrenner's writings and research had been a concern with the 'plasticity' and thereby the 'potential for systematic change associated with the engagement of the active individual with his or her active context'. At issue, then, in Bronfenbrenner's research had been albeit tacit reflective concerns with the possibility that 'developmental science' may in some ways 'improve the course and contexts of human life' (Lerner 2005: ix).

Before uncovering any more from Lerner's prefatory remarks, let us just pause for one moment, as readers, to reflect again with Hegel's discourse on that earlier point about reflection in the form of its traditional metaphor borrowed from Newton and Freud. Like all philosophical discourse, in Hegel's practice he sought to constitute a whole for reflection, which ordinarily remains divided; opening a gap between being and thinking. But, despite Hegel's best efforts in this direction by way of his dialectic, the identity, 'whole', unconditionally it turns out from Derrida's incisive deconstruction, like any of our identities, to be impossible and incalculable. It points to a heterogeneous ethic consonant with the unconditional and unrestricted space for cultivating possibilities open to human beings that always already remain incalculable and impossible to define. This is the decisive ethic for any improvement involving the practice of human beings.

Let us now uncover more about just how Bronfenbrenner's discourse handles such moves towards the ecological development of human behaviour. Certainly from Lerner's (2005) preface concerning Bronfenbrenner's approach to his professional work, the latter's seemingly indomitable spirit is consonant with the aspirations of many working to improve practice in the helping professions. In evaluating Bronfenbrenner's contribution, Lerner points not only to 'the persuasive articulation and refinement' of 'singularly creative, theoretically elegant, empirically rigorous' theory at the cutting edge of developmental science, but is also careful to note Bronfenbrenner's 'humane and democratic scholarly contributions' extending over 'more than 60 years'. Here, too, the spirit of Bronfenbrenner's practice, along with its associated ethic and moral principles, accords with the aspirations and ethos driving much practice in the helping professions that has been more than evident in every chapter of this very book.

In beginning to understand a little more about the constitution of reflection in practice, then, let us now look more closely at the space and time between the moral agency of this obviously purposeful human being, and in this case aspects of his particular practice of the reiteration of signs in his particular language. In Article 10: 'Ecological Systems Theory' (EST), which distinguished his identity as a cutting-edge 'developmental scientist', his writing begins with an open admission of the 'inherent conflict of interest' he experienced in being both 'critic and creator' (Bronfenbrenner 2005: 106) of his own work.

One might consider the moral agency of this particular human being as a professional scientist in terms of the *style* of his practice of writing, revealed in his reiteration of signs. His particular and customary *style* (Spinoza et al. 2007) of practice is revealed in the representation of 'theory' that is coordinated from the opening lines of his article with questioning; it articulates what matters for his agency as a scientist, namely critical and informed dialogue about EST through his writing with other 'readers' (Bronfenbrenner 2005: 107). Indeed, in its style, his express humanity is apparent in his 'phras[ing]' that continually returns to possible sources of 'clarifi[cation]', 'revision', 're-definition', 'consideration' and so on concerning 'possible answers' to his questions (Bronfenbrenner 2005: 151), along the 'limitations' of, and any possible 'retrospection' upon, his theory along with his re-formulation of 'behaviour as a function of person and environment' and 'development as a function of person and environment' (Bronfenbrenner 2005: 106–73). His style of writing, too, is not without its own sense of 'irony' (Bronfenbrenner 2005: 108) in acknowledging that his criticisms, at some points, apply to his own 'development' of theory.

But, in a similar manner to professionals working in the helping professions, the *language* of Bronfenbrenner's customary practices, as a scientist, a writer, and a communicator, in its express terms of training, education, specialisation, focus for concerns upon evidence, on what is done under particular conditions, together with any measurable outcomes, and so on, rarely encourages consideration being given to *languages* of such practices themselves. But it is the sovereign powers of languages governing our professional practices that have largely excluded matters involving:

- as we have mentioned before, the repetition and reiteration of signs, phrases, sentences;
- the matter of the ontotheological structuring, which is pivotal (the ontology or being of what is done in practice creates its ground or basis for action, while its theology, such as its organisation or its form, constitutes the upper limit of what is possible in practice). It is such ontotheological structuring of the naming force and gathering powers of being as presence that is driving such practice – not us, we are being driven along by it; along with,
- the matter of the possibility of exceeding the economy of what is given in any metaphysical determination of signs; and, not least,
- the matter of the constitution of reflection connecting the agency of human beings with the practice of language.

It is, perhaps, doubly ironic that all such exclusions have significant bearing upon how we might understand the possibilities open to that body – individual and collective – we variously identify as human being, which Bronfenbrenner's language in the title of his book is purporting to be 'making ... human'. Ironically, a body, indeed, that in its being, is sustained in a state of exception in this very book, largely unconsciously dissimulated within his professional, methodological and epistemological languages drawn in this case from science, mathematics, logic and bioecology.

Reflective practice to come: reiterations and repetitions of signs

Language, our essential home in this world, is always already on the move. We all live in this endlessly moving drift of the dissemination of signs. In such drift of signs there are only differences, as Ferdinand Saussure revealed more than 50 years ago. Bronfenbrenner's discourse makes numerous references to 'consideration', as a move to reveal constellations of possibilities, which is unconsciously deferred from Aristotle's NE. The latter's writings can be traced back to Plato, Parmenides and others. There are no origins in language, only differences.

But the collective and mystical fixation upon truth claims to knowledge in practice, constituting its own sublime locus of power, has almost invariably blocked us from seeing things in our practices in other ways, including, for example, in moves towards what appears to be justice when confronted with the delimiting economies of what is given in extant law-like structures in professional practices. Indeed, almost every page of Article 10 involves the appearance of such moves through Bronfenbrenner's on-going partial deconstruction of his own discursive practice. But the possibilities opened by such moves are continually closed down. For example, after introducing what is represented in the text of Article 10 as 'the cornerstone of the theoretical structure', it subsequently returns: 'obliged to acknowledge a first infirmity [in this cornerstone] of equal magnitude' (Bronfenbrenner 2005: 107). The text then continues to elaborate additional revisions and reconceptualisations of the law-like structures inscribed in the principles of 'Ecological Systems Theory'.

But, while this movement towards a more sophisticated modelling of the ecology of human behaviour might be understood in political philosophy in terms of justice, in terms of the closer match between representation and practice, in remaining largely within a homogeneously structured economy of what is given in practice – in terms of the conditional, calculable, possible dimensions of such practice – the economy of the text of Article 10 always falls short of moves towards justice in the full sense accorded to the possible unrestricted unfolding of historical movements of human beings in a heterogeneous economy.

Justice to come is not precluded by such modelling in EST. Ordinarily, however, in the fog of obfuscation conflating any possible distinction between the text and human agency, and the continual movement to close down any possibilities outside the homogeneous economy of language constituting the language of Bronfenbrenner's reflective practice, any movement towards justice in the text remains largely blocked.

Reflective practice to come: the movement of being as presence

In this particular text an understanding of human being is projected in terms of the 'properties of a person' (Bronfenbrenner 2005: 120); an entity located within the metaphysical economy of what is given in EST. As in its gift to almost every professional discourse in the helping professions on the matter of human beings, there is no possibility of distinction to be made between beings, entities or things and 'traces' of being. The latter, moreover, which is ordinarily elided, constitutes the basis upon which beings are understood. In fact, though being as presence is not thematised in the text of Article 10, it is there in every hypothesis, principle, proposition, theory, critical dialogue … indeed, it is there in all of its verbal affirmations and nominalisations, constituting the actions and organisation, content and form of this very text. Moreover, in its 'protension' and 'retention' of the words constituting Article 10, being as presence delimits and shapes, in this case Urie Bronfenbrenner's writing, in accord with the metaphysical and ontotheological structuring of his very practice.

The 'upon which' in the projections of understandings of beings, too, which is not considered explicitly in this text, which shapes, delimits and determines such projections, just like the lens in an electronic projector, is constituted by the principle of 'assessment', along with its express twelve scientific 'principles', including the principle of 'reason' identified in Article 10. Counter-intuitively, perhaps, when understood in terms of the language constituting this style of practice, 'being as presence', coupled with the empty now … now … now of clock-time, constitutes the seemingly insatiable drive for the improvement of practice in the helping professions.

It is no surprise, therefore, that such modelling identified in Article 10 is viewed in terms of 'development'. All of the naming forces, viz-a-tergo, gathered together by being as presence in any application of the EST model, will necessarily delimit and shape the 'development' of human beings in their practice. But the multiplicity of unrestricted possibilities open to beings is simply constituted as a 'standing reserve' of energy, which paradoxically is driving the whole system. Until now such possibilities have been largely unconsciously sustained in a state of exception outside by homogeneous economies of practice; the latter, the product, as we have seen, of the mystical authority held by science and the pursuit of supposedly rigorous truth claims to knowledge. Moreover, this standing reserve is continually available for use in the system. Ironically there is no basis for justice to come in this system of modelling.

Justice to come: exceeding the metaphysical economy of the gift

There are points in the text of 'Article 10' where the gift of the delimiting and homogeneous economy of what is given in practice is exceeded. But, again these are not thematised or even considered as such. As we uncovered earlier, all of the signs gathered together as a presence in this article are always already constituted from deferred and spatially separated signs within the disseminative drift of the 'empire of signs' mediating the world of the helping professions. And, unconditionally as identities each of those signs carries with it an incalculable interplay of 'others' and the 'Other', which makes impossible the fulfillment of any identity in practice. For example, in Article 10 reference is made to 'context', which as the text itself illustrates, unconditionally remains impossible to define completely; it lies beyond any possible calculation.

Here we should keep in mind that Bronfenbrenner's theoretical work had constituted a significant transformation in the context of his developmental science, enabling it to move from earlier descriptive science concerned with cataloguing changes to his later work in engaging with what Bronfenbrenner called 'real' experimentation. But, unconsciously and unconditionally as a human being, his very practice of writing, theorising, experimenting and so on, itself presupposes what at the moment remains impossible and incalculable dimensions. His very own practice as a developmental scientist, therefore, presupposed, albeit unconsciously, not only a heterogeneous ethic, but also, again unconsciously, his very own reflective practice was constituted in the law of absolute hospitality; unconditionally it remained continually open to what is currently considered impossible and incalculable.

Paradoxically, his language of developmental theory, however, blinds itself to the possibility of the heterogeneous ethic, to the possibility of the absolute law of justice and to the possibility of his own living in a state of exception. Yet in his reflective practice in living in a state of exception, his very practice finds its sense of moves towards justice in remaining unconditionally and continually open to its impossible and incalculable dimensions. Nevertheless, the logic and the sovereign powers of the language constituted in his writings concerned with ecopsychological development never open space to make visible the manifest other vital and heterogeneous dimensions constituted in a state of exception by such powers. Ordinarily many such possibilities are simply excluded by the homogeneous economy of the language in which his theories are constituted.

Consequently and ironically, there is a sense of moves towards justice in his reflective practice constituting models for the development of Ecological Systems Theory. But, in being in receipt of such language, the behaviours and environment of all recipients of such modelling is already constituted by the naming force and gathering powers of being as presence at work in the model. In this way, their very possibilities of being are conditioned and delimited by what is projected as possible and calculable within the model. And, in living in a state of exception, their express sense of being in accord with the heterogeneous ethic is always made available for use within the model development system.

As it stands, therefore, such EST modelling simply constitutes a system for driving human beings in accord with the sovereign powers of the language of its emergent models. And we return to a sublimely powerful and completely reiterated version of Foucault's regime. In this case it is a regime constituted by and driven by the powers of being as presence.

Justice to come: the matter of the constitution of reflection

Provisionally at this point it has become apparent from the deconstruction that in the social and educational world of the helping professions, the language of reflection is constituted in the play of differences and deferrals of signs. Such deconstruction is constituted in the law of absolute unrestricted hospitality to both homogeneous and heterogeneous ethics of practice. In pursuing the question of the constitution of the language of reflection we have uncovered the order constituted as law-like structures in our languages. Alongside such laws we have also begun to understand the possibilities opened by moves towards social justice in such practice. The latter moves are always constituted by deconstruction, itself, as we noted earlier, always mad about justice.

What has become apparent in pursuing the deconstruction of Bronfenbrenner's writings is that albeit unconscious absolute hospitality constituting his own practice of writing is simply never extended to all possible constituents of such modelling. It has also become apparent that the constitution of reflection in practice may be understood in terms of the language, economies, ethics of laws and aligned moves towards justice. Unconditionally, the latter, in moves towards making whole the division between being and thinking in any reflective practice for professionals, practitioners and their clients, are always already impossible and incalculable. Herein lies the law of absolute hospitality. Thus, although this comprises a provisional understanding of the language constituting reflection, there remains much to uncover about just how such understandings of reflection and reflective practice using this new language might work in a range of different practices in the helping professions.

In reflection-on the dominant form of reflective practice in the helping professions, therefore, given the dominant homogeneous economy in which such practice is located, there remains much to be done in opening space for unrestricted education in both the heterogeneous economy, the laws inscribed in the language of practice, any moves towards justice and its very own law of absolute hospitality. In the latter case we have not even begun to open questioning concerned with democratic practice demanded of any such possible moves towards justice. Nor has any consideration been given to the complex effects of the policing of any of the laws inscribed in the governmentality of the helping professions.

Notes

1   The International Association of Practice Doctorates (IAPD) continues to hold a series of conferences concerned with understanding practices involving a wide range of professional activities.
2   While a number of contemporary readings of Schön, Dewey and others on reflective practice have contributed to a realisation of some of its limitations, until now no one has raised the question about the possibility of different languages constituting reflection in practice; see Wigg, R. S. (2009) *Enhancing Reflective Practice among Clinical Psychologists and Trainees*, University of Warwick, http://webcat.warwick.ac.uk/record=b2334215~S15
3   www.acf.hhs.gov/programs/ohs

References

Agamben, G. (2005) *State of Exception* (trans. K. Attrell). Chicago: University of Chicago Press.
Alcoff, L. (2003) Introduction: Identities – modern and postmodern. In Alcoff, L. and Mendieta, E. (eds), *Identities: Race, Class, Gender and Nationalities.* Oxford: Blackwell Publishing.
Argyris, C. (1982) *Reasoning, Learning and Action: Individual and Organisational.* San Francisco, CA: Jossey Bass.
Benwell, B. and Stokoe, E. (2006) *Discourse and Identity.* Edinburgh: Edinburgh University Press.
Boud, D., Keogh, R. and Walker, D. (1985) *Reflection: Turning Experience into Learning.* London: Routledge.
Bronfenbrenner, U. (ed.) (2005) *Making Human Beings Human: Bioecological Perspectives on Human Development.* Thousand Oakes, CA: Sage Publications.

Bulman, C. and Schutz, S. (eds) (2008) *Reflective Practice in Nursing*. Oxford: Blackwell.

Dewey, J. (2009 [1934]) *Art as Experience*. New York: Perigee Books.

Flint, K. J. (2013) What's play got to do with the information age? In Ryall, E., Russell, W. and Maclean, M. (eds), *The Philosophy of Play*. London: Routledge, pp. 152–63.

Flint, K. J., Barnard, A. and Palmer, V. (in preparation) Pedagogy of reflection: Constituting spacing for practices of education without violence. Paper to be submitted to the *International Journal of Pedagogy*.

Foucault, M. (1984) Truth and power. In Faubion, J. D. (ed.), *Michel Foucault: Power – Essential Works of Foucault, 1954–1984*, Volume 3 (trans. R. Hurley and others). New York: New York Press.

Gadamer, H.-G. (2004) *Truth and Method* (trans. J. Weinsheimer and D. G. Marshall). London and New York: Continuum International Publishing.

Johns, C. (ed.) (2010) (2nd edn) *Guided Reflection: A Narrative Approach to Advancing Professional Practice*. Chichester: Wiley-Blackwell.

Kincheloe, J. L. (2008) *Knowledge and Critical Pedagogy: An Introduction*. Dordrecht: Springer.

Knott, C. and Scragg, T. (eds) (2013) (3rd edn) *Reflective Practice in Social Work*. London: Sage.

Lerner, R. M. (2005) Foreword: Urie Bronfenbrenner: Career contributions of the consummate developmental scientist. In Bronfenbrenner, U. (ed.), *Making Human Beings Human: Bioecological Perspectives on Human Development*. Thousand Oaks, CA: Sage Publications.

Maclean, S. (2010) *The Social Work Pocket Guide to Reflective Practice*. Litchfield: Kirwin Maclean Associates.

Redmond, B. (2006) *Reflection in Action: Developing Reflective Practice in Health and Social Services*. Aldershot: Ashgate.

Rolfe, G., Jasper, M. and Freshwater, D. (2010) (2nd edn) *Critical Reflection In Practice: Generating Knowledge for Care*. London: Palgrave.

Schön, D. A. (1983) *The Reflective Practitioner*. New York: Basic Books.

Schön, D. A. (1987) *Educating the Reflective Practitioner: Towards a New Design for Teaching and Learning in the Professions*. San Francisco: John Wiley.

Spinoza, C., Flores, F. and Dreyfus, H.L. (2007) *Disclosing New Worlds: Entrepreneurship, Democratic Action and the Cultivation of Solidarity*. Cambridge, MA: MIT Press.

Stambaugh, J. (1992) *The Finitude of Being*. New York: State University of New York Press.

Webber, M. (2010) *Reflective Practice in Mental Health: Advanced Psychosocial Practice with Children, Adolescents and Adults*. London and Philadelphia: Jessica Kingsley.

Conclusion

This has been a journey, a learning and professional journey through the terrain of professionalism and developing professional practice in health and social care. As a keen, committed and sharp-eyed reader, you will have navigated the chapters according to your needs and found much of value to inform, influence and invigorate your professional journey. It is as much about the journey as it is about arrivals and departures, so although it is hoped this book is a critical friend to accompany your travels and adventures, the story is far from over.

There are many ways to cut a cake and navigating through the book resembles the professional practice journey. Each chapter can be read alone but is also in dialogue with the other chapters and forms a 'game of two halves', with the first half of the book being part of thinking and the second half of the book being about doing.

Each chapter, just as with literature reviews, can be read in three dimensions. The first dimension is the 'landscape' or 'terrain' of the issues that are being examined. This usually forms an x axis, although it is not a simple linear line or dimension but a sculpted, shaped and contoured dimension. For example, Chapter 1 on definitions and history works with the peaks and troughs, highs and lows, fields and dales of professionalism and what is means to be a professional.

The second dimension is the y axis, or the reaching upwards to overarching philosophical concerns but also reaching downwards to singular points of reflection. For example, Chapter 2 provides a visual presentation of ideas that form an overarching school or tradition of philosophical thought but also provides the singular philosophical contribution of each thinker. As such, each chapter works in a vertical dimension.

The third and final dimension of each chapter is the z axis, or temporal or time or chronological dimension. Ideas unfold in time and have a history, present and future. Each chapter attends to the history of ideas and the future projection of where this might lead.

As you develop your individual professional journey and develop your professional practice a similar process of highs and lows, overarching and singular encounters, and times of history and future projections will add to your experience and journey.

Chapter 1: The current context and climate of professionals

Drawing on an extensive and eclectic range of sources to give a multi-layered perspective on what 'professionals' and 'professions' are, this chapter introduced reflection and its history to open debate and discussion on developing reflective practice.

The contours and landscape of professions, the overarching aspiration and singular points of professions, and the history and future of professions add to the contribution this chapter makes to informing the development of professional practice.

Chapter 2: Philosophy for professionals

This chapter used a different register to introduce the value of theory and philosophy to reflective practice. Using individually created portraits it presented a 'picture' and thumbnail sketch of each philosopher, their impact, contribution, key concepts and key works, and includes criticism. An invitation to further reading also accompanied each entry. This is a catalytic stimulus to theoretical engagement. The landscape of philosophical ideas is provided, the traditions that each 'picture' informs and the history and possible futures precipitate professional development. This is an area that demands further development.

Chapter 3: Values and ethics for professionals

This chapter reviewed the challenge of values and ethics for professionals and the need to develop a reflective approach to ethical decision making in practice. This approach is informed by the landscape and 'swampy lowlands' of values and ethics, the overarching singularities of values and ethics, and the history and future of ethical decision making.

Chapter 4: Professional identity

This chapter reviewed the contributions of understandings of self and identity and the way in which personal and professional identities contribute to professional practice. The concept of professional identity in areas such as social work education is a relatively neglected topic. The difficulty in formation, maintenance and review of a stable identity in problematic circumstances is enhanced by reflective exercises. The change of identity across a career and the forming of an identity as a central element in the promotion of social justice were considered, along with the psycho-social constructions of identity.

The landscape of identity, the overarching and singular themes, and the history and future of identity were also considered.

Chapter 5: Working in organisational systems

Howard's chapter explored the nature of organisational systems, with examples from social work's adult and child care practice, to reflect upon current workplace culture and values. This discussion is relevant for health care practitioners within the 'force field' of public services. The chapter enables the reader to reflect on their own current or future organisational and professional role in their working systems. Using practical reflective activities throughout the chapter, Howard illustrates how practitioners can promote service-user-focused values and social justice within their own (or other) organisations, even with new public management and managerialism.

The challenge for reflective practitioners of professional judgement and creative thinking from rule-based managerialism mitigates against critical reflection on practice. Processes that prevent rather than enable direct work with service users are counterproductive to all those involved in practice.

The 'reflective pluralist' framework for organisational leadership and management is an antidote to managerialism as it recognises the emotions in practice and seeks to construct knowledge and support which deals with the reality of practice and working in an organisation. The integration of service users' capacity and capability to manage upwards in distributed leadership to achieve authentic leadership and effective supervision, to critically engage with practice issues, also contributes to authentic leadership. The learning organisation as a relationship-based, value-led practice promotes social justice and empowerment to challenge a shame-and-blame culture for individual workers. Developing an active social learning culture, a community of practice and appreciative inquiry are key building blocks in an effective learning organisation.

Chapter 6: Critical practice: 'Touching something lightly many times'

In this chapter, Linda Kemp was 'touching something lightly many times' and she provided some thoughts on language and reparation in relation to mental health and social justice. Discussing language as a medium of dwelling and the expression of experience through language, the relationship between professional and service users in health and social care was considered in relation to mental health. The measurement used by professionals was critiqued from a service-user perspective and the use of the 'Unrecovery Star'. Using Foucault, the fixity of discourse and its limiting effects of 'discursive formations' were opened up for ongoing investigation and the possibilities of a creative life. The reparative work of art affords integration, reintegration, based on a social model where rather than an individual isolated from the social culture in which they live, they (re)integrate within the cultural terms of that society. The continual and dynamic becoming offers the possibilities of overcoming an economy of distorted desires. Linda offered a reflective account of an unbearable lightness of unbeing, as an antidote to turning people into things. Individualisation becomes the possible dark side of therapeutic interventions.

Chapter 7: Globalised practice

This chapter reviewed the current state of play of globalised health and social care. Tracking different definitional approaches to globalisation, the contours of this process were mapped and the challenges for health and social care from this process were discussed. It was suggested that increasing homogeneity for communities, the winners and losers of globalisation, and the need of professionals to have a global awareness were other elements of reflective practice. The dangers of reflective practice being pushed into technologically mediated and unreflective practice could make a McDonaldised reflective practitioner. Being aware in the world, understanding the landscape, the overarching themes and singularities of experience, and being historically informed and future orientated are essential parts of developing professional practice.

Chapter 8: Reflections on conditionality

Towers' chapter is a reflective account of the issues of conditionality in social policy teaching. Using enactment, the issue of rights, entitlement and the morality of decision making in relation to welfare were discussed. The condition of category and conditions of circumstance reveal diverse moral compasses in trainee professionals. The chapter reviewed the historical emergence of entitlement and the 'golden age' of social justice, solidarity and universalism. The rise of conditional welfare and a creeping conditionality in entitlement is part of reciprocity linked to citizenship. Reflecting on how the situations of service users bring together new knowledge and new insights on how social justice is linked to fairness, rights and responsibilities, and reflecting on the context, circumstances, measures and outcomes, allows the reflective practitioner to make informed judgements on practice in social policy.

Chapter 9: Professional supervision

Supervision plays a key role in professional education and practice and underpins the development of professional identity. Supervision is viewed as a reflective process, distinct from mentoring and coaching. The challenge of supervision as a process and positive force for social justice, or as a subtle way of controlling individuals, was discussed.

Chapter 10: Reflective writing for professional practice

In this chapter, Trafford provided a reflective account of writing. She addressed the pre-reflection and anxiety of starting to write and the value of a learning journal to experiment with different styles of writing. She provided a spiral for the process of writing and reflection for, in and on action. Using case studies and activities the process of reflection in continuous professional development and in developing self-awareness was addressed. The skills development of 'deep learning' and 'cognitive housekeeping' provide ways to practise in swampy lowlands and reduce stress through writing. The 'emotional dumping ground' of speaking to stress and anxiety is an essential tool for professional practice. Written reflection facilitates deeper learning, self-awareness, empathy and emotional intelligence, works as a catalyst for change and is therapeutic.

Chapter 11: Contemplating 'career' across disciplines

Gee provided a reflective tour of the important dimensions of career. He challenged simplistic notions of employability for a more holistic and reflective exploration of career that recognises and attends to the intersections of structuring dynamics in society. The lived experience between being and becoming challenges the current managerialism of career.

Chapter 12: Personal development planning as reflection

Goodall's chapter provided an insight into tried and tested methods for reflection through personal development planning in an actually existing project. Although providing a reflective 'moment' where a professional takes stock of the situation and is invited to reflect on performance, the act of reflection and the recording of reflection is determined more by performance management than an authentic form of reflection. The chapter includes reflective exercises as an example of the support for PDP offered.

Chapter 13: Journeys of faith

Turning to different strategies for reflection, this chapter examined 'faithing' of a faith journey of different movements and narratives in schools. The dynamism of narrative, the personalisation of meaning and the value of mirrors are all important in faith journeys. Personal myth-making provides an interesting alternative to the more regimented personal development planning of the previous chapter. The linear model of reflection is not without criticism and the chapter focused on the contribution of the rejection of metanarratives. The chapter then reflected upon those issues relevant to schools through admissions, publicity, incarnation theology, narrative and recruitment. The chapter offered an empirical methodological discussion and the editorial decision on narratives, to propose a reflective engagement with faith. As such, it contributed to the reflective lens and armoury for reflective practitioners to compare, evaluate and reshape their own stories. The chapter ended with a call for five moments of faith-based reflection.

Chapter 14: A personal learning journey

Beginning with 'critical moments of biography', Palmer's chapter was a personal reflection on her professional doctorate journey. She charted the journey from professional doctorate embarkation, learning a new language, epistemology and identity, an apprenticeship in the rigours and processes of research, to critical reflection and reflexivity. Significantly, learning through reflection is core to the doctoral process and the becoming a researching professional and this chapter gave 'voice' to that process.

Chapter 15: 'Tain from the mirror

In the final chapter, a challenge formed to the existing ordering of reflective practice in health and social care and helping professions. The identity of those in these professions was discussed through the lens of reflection in the mirror and the language of reflection. This provided an appropriate concluding discussion and a fertile springboard for future and further development by radicalising the debate about the practice of reflection. The opening of space for justice to come concluded the reflective conversation.

What this book has been is an invitation to readers to engage in reflective practice on the journey from being to becoming professional. There have been many high points on the way and a range of challenges for reflective practitioners to engage with. The activities in the chapters have provided milestones to explore reflection from a range of vantage points to inform best practice in health and social care. The three dimensions of landscapes, highs and lows, histories and futures, inform each chapter but offer the invitation to read across, though, within, above, below, forward and back, to make a full experience of being a professional.

The different narratives in the book come from different perspectives and approaches and are written at different levels with different styles. The eclecticism and multiplicity of voices is one of the strengths of these collected narratives. For the reader, this presents different degrees of challenge and engagement that allows you to pick your own path through professionalism and reflection. It is hoped that the ultimate goal of becoming professional, motivated by social justice, is one of the achievable events from the journey.

Index

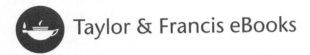

Taylor & Francis eBooks

Helping you to choose the right eBooks for your Library

Add Routledge titles to your library's digital collection today. Taylor and Francis ebooks contains over 50,000 titles in the Humanities, Social Sciences, Behavioural Sciences, Built Environment and Law.

Choose from a range of subject packages or create your own!

Benefits for you

» Free MARC records
» COUNTER-compliant usage statistics
» Flexible purchase and pricing options
» All titles DRM-free.

Benefits for your user

» Off-site, anytime access via Athens or referring URL
» Print or copy pages or chapters
» Full content search
» Bookmark, highlight and annotate text
» Access to thousands of pages of quality research at the click of a button.

REQUEST YOUR **FREE** INSTITUTIONAL TRIAL TODAY

Free Trials Available
We offer free trials to qualifying academic, corporate and government customers.

eCollections – Choose from over 30 subject eCollections, including:

Archaeology	Language Learning
Architecture	Law
Asian Studies	Literature
Business & Management	Media & Communication
Classical Studies	Middle East Studies
Construction	Music
Creative & Media Arts	Philosophy
Criminology & Criminal Justice	Planning
Economics	Politics
Education	Psychology & Mental Health
Energy	Religion
Engineering	Security
English Language & Linguistics	Social Work
Environment & Sustainability	Sociology
Geography	Sport
Health Studies	Theatre & Performance
History	Tourism, Hospitality & Events

For more information, pricing enquiries or to order a free trial, please contact your local sales team:
www.tandfebooks.com/page/sales
